Urological Oncology

Edited by

Jonathan Waxman
Department of Clinical Oncology, Royal Postgraduate Medical
School, Hammersmith Hospital, London

and

Gordon Williams
Department of Surgery, Royal Postgraduate Medical School,
Hammersmith Hospital, London

Edward Arnold
A division of Hodder & Stoughton
LONDON   MELBOURNE   AUCKLAND

© 1992 Jonathan Waxman and Gordon Williams

First published in Great Britain 1992

British Library Cataloguing in Publication Data

Waxman, Jonathan
  Urological oncology.
  I. Title   II. Williams, Gordon
  616.99

ISBN 0-340-54926-2

Whilst the advice and information in this book is believed to be true and accurate at the date of going to press, neither the author nor the publisher can accept any legal responsibility or liability for any errors or omissions that may be made. In particular (but without limiting the generality of the preceding disclaimer) every effort has been made to check drug dosages; however, it is still possible that errors have been missed. Furthermore, dosage schedules are constantly being revised and new side effects recognised. For these reasons the reader is strongly urged to consult the drug companies' printed instructions before administering any of the drugs recommended in this book.

Typeset in 10/12 pt Century Old Style by Rowland Phototypesetting Ltd, Bury St Edmunds, Suffolk. Printed and bound in Great Britain for Edward Arnold, a division of Hodder and Stoughton Limited, Mill Road, Dunton Green, Sevenoaks, Kent TN13 2YA by Butler and Tanner Ltd, Frome, Somerset

Introduction

The last fifteen years have seen an extraordinary change in the management of urological malignancy.

This revolution in urological cancer has come from the extension of modern techniques of oncology to urology. As a result of this fusion of the two sciences, urological oncology practice has altered. Thus, patients with prostatic cancer are now offered medical orchiectomy, patients with advanced bladder cancer may be cured by combination chemotherapy and previously incurable patients with testicular carcinoma now survive. Along with these changes in the treatment of urological cancer there have been advances in basic science. The development of the techniques of molecular oncology has led to an analysis of the importance of oncogenes in urological tumours. It is hoped that the next decade will bring molecular oncology into the clinic so that treatment tailored to control the malignant genome will be developed and applied to those patients with malignancy.

J WAXMAN
G WILLIAMS
1991

Contents

Contributors List

Paul D Abel

Senior Lecturer and Honorary Consultant Urologist, Department of Surgery, Royal Postgraduate Medical School, Hammersmith Hospital, London.

Wadih Arap

Genitourinary Oncology Service, Division of Solid Tumor Oncology, Memorial Sloan-Kettering Cancer Center, New York.

David F Badenoch

Consultant Urological Surgeon, The Royal London Hospital, London.

JP Blandy

Professor of Urology, The Royal London Hospital Medical College, London

Timothy Crook

Senior Scientist, Ludwig Institute for Cancer Research, St. Mary's Hospital Medical School, London.

Angus Dalgleish

Professor of Oncology, St George's Hospital Medical School, Tooting, London.

Christopher S Foster

Senior Lecturer and Honorary Consultant, Department of Histopathology, Royal Postgraduate Medical School, Hammersmith Hospital, London.

CJ Gallagher

Senior Lecturer in Medical Oncology, The Royal London Hospital, London.

WF Hendry

Consultant Urologist, Royal Marsden and St Bartholomew's Hospitals, London.

HF Hope-Stone

Consultant Radiotherapist, The Royal London Hospital, London.

A Horwich

Professor, Department of Radiotherapy, Royal Marsden Hospital, Sutton, Surrey.

Nicholas James

Research Fellow, Ludwig Institute for Cancer Research, St Mary's Hospital Medical School, London.

Philip W Kantoff

Assistant Professor of Medicine, Harvard Medical School, and Director of Genitourinary Oncology, Dana Farber Cancer Institute.

Tetsuro Kato

Associate Professor, Department of Urology, Akita University, School of Medicine, Akita, Japan.

Patrick F Keane

Senior Registrar, Department of Surgery, Royal Postgraduate Medical School, Hammersmith Hospital, London.

David Kirk

Consultant Urologist, Western Infirmary, Glasgow.

Kilian Mellon

Research Fellow in Urological Surgery, Freeman Hospital, Newcastle upon Tyne.

David E Neal

Senior Lecturer in Urological Surgery, Freeman Hospital, Newcastle upon Tyne.

Tim D Oliver

Reader in Medical Oncology, The Royal London Hospital, London.

David F Paulson

Professor and Chief, Division of Urological Surgery, Duke University Medical Centre, Durham, North Carolina, USA.

Jerome P Richie

Elliot C Cutler Professor of Surgery, Harvard Medical School, and Chief Surgeon, Division of Urological Surgery, Brigham and Women's Hospital.

Howard I Scher

Assistant Attending Physician, Genitourinary Oncology Service, Division of Solid Tumor Oncology, Memorial Sloan-Kettering Cancer Center, New York.

Paul Sondel

Professor of Oncology, University of Wisconsin, Clinical Cancer Center, Madison.

UE Studer

Associate Professor of Urology, Department of Urology, University of Berne, Inseltital, Berne, Switzerland.

Jonathan Waxman

Senior Lecturer and Honorary Consultant, Department of Clinical Oncology, Royal Postgraduate Medical School, Hammersmith Hospital, London.

Gordon Williams

Consultant Urologist, Department of Surgery, Royal Postgraduate Medical School, Hammersmith Hospital, London.

EJ Zingg

Professor, Department of Urology, University of Berne, Berne, Inseltital, Switzerland.

Section I

Testicular Cancer

1 Surgical management of advanced testicular cancer

WF Hendry

On completion of chemotherapy, persistence of a mass on CT scanning should not be regarded as failure, for a residual mass is left behind in almost one-quarter of cases.[1] Ever since the introduction of effective chemotherapy in 1976, these masses have been the subject of intense interest in our Testicular Tumour Unit.[2-4] We have demonstrated that CT scanning is more than 95% accurate in defining their site, size and extent.[5] Initially it was hoped that radiotherapy would eliminate any active tumour remaining after chemotherapy. However, comparative studies showed that there was still residual undifferentiated tumour in 20% of teratoma patients after planned chemotherapy and radiotherapy, compared with 24% after chemotherapy alone.[6] Furthermore, side-effects after radiotherapy following chemotherapy were not inconsiderable, and so this treatment modality was abandoned at our centre, although it is still used by others.[7] It became our policy to recommend excision of all substantial residual masses one month or so after completion of chemotherapy for non-seminomatous tumours. Since the likelihood of residual active tumour was shown to be related to the size of the mass,[6] we set a lower limit of 2 cm transverse diameter—only rarely has active tumour been found in nodes smaller than this.[8]

Surgical assessment

It has always been made clear to patients with metastatic teratoma, before commencing chemotherapy, that surgical excision might be necessary for any deposits that did not disappear. As a result, patients coming to the Joint Testicular Tumour Clinic for assessment for surgery arrive with minds well prepared, with no sense of disappointment or feeling that all has not gone as well as expected. This positive approach makes the surgeon's job much easier than it is with patients referred in from some other units, when an air of despondency surrounds the discussion of the forthcoming operation. It is generally only necessary to explain to our patients that the lump has to be removed to get rid of it, and to make sure that the chemotherapy has completely eliminated the cancer. Most testicular tumour patients are young and adapt well psychologically to their disease, provided it is explained adequately,[9] although inevitably a few have long-term psychosocial problems if treatment results in alteration in sexual function.[10]

The surgeon needs to know exactly where the masses are, and their size. Adjacent structures may be at risk of damage, or may have to be removed along with the mass, and this can only be assessed by careful reference to the scans. Not only is this essential for the surgeon to plan the operative approach, but the patient and his relatives *must* be advised of the likely extent of the surgery, and warned of any likely effects on other organs. In particular, failure to warn the patient of potential loss of a major organ such as a kidney, or interference with ejaculation, could be interpreted as negligence. Nonetheless, a positive matter-of-fact approach should be taken, and whilst potential risks should not be ignored or glossed over, they need not be dwelt upon.

In 70% of cases, the residual masses are in the para-aortic lymph nodes in the retroperitoneum, in 18% they are in the chest, and in 12% they are above and below the diaphragm.[1] In the latter group the thoracic surgeon and the urologist should meet to discuss whether it is possible to remove all the tumours at once, through a thoracoabdominal incision, or whether a staged approach is preferable. In general, we have found that it is better not to be overambitious, hoping to remove everything in one operation, since access and hence safety may be compromised. Our approach is that masses above the diaphragm are always best dealt with by a thoracic surgeon, while those in the neck may require a separate operation by a third surgical specialist.

In planning the surgical approach to retroperitoneal or other abdominal masses, it is very helpful indeed to have a 'scanogram'—this is a freehand drawing of the tumour showing its relation to the great vessels, and in particular to the renal vessels and kidneys (Fig. 1.1). The first decision that must be made is whether an anterior, long midline incision will provide adequate access. Analysis of 140 para-aortic lymphadenectomies at the Royal Marsden Hospital over a 10-year period[11,12] indicated that this incision was used in over three-quarters of cases. It has the great advantage that it provides excellent direct access to the great vessels, with equally good exposure on either side. As a result even very large masses can be completely excised, provided they are below the renal vessels. Occasionally the vena cava itself (Fig. 1.2) may be involved;[13-16] this should be recognized in advance so that adequate arrangements can be made for blood transfusion, and a vascular surgeon may be invited to the operation. Similarly, if a liver metastasis is present it may be sensible to involve a surgeon who is experienced at hepatic resection. Particular attention must be paid to the kidneys: the metastatic tumour commonly causes ureteric obstruction, and although some renal function may return after chemotherapy there may be significant postobstructive atrophy of one or even both kidneys. The residual mass may be inseparably stuck on to the kidney, its vessels or the ureter, and in our experience nephrectomy had to be done in 11% of cases. Obviously it was essential in these cases to make sure that the contralateral kidney function was adequate.

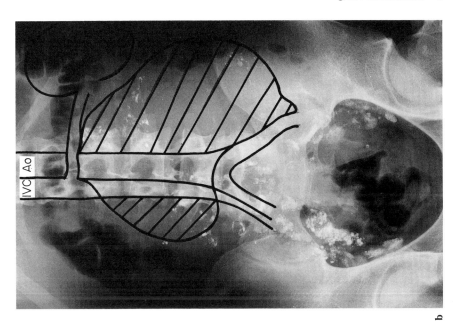

IVC | Ao

b

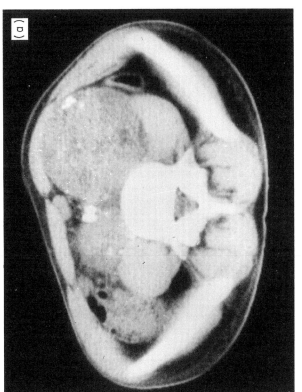

(a)

Fig. 1.1 (*a*) CT scan. (*b*) Scanogram showing extent of residual mass and its relation to the great vessels. Since the tumour lies below the renal vessels, an anterior approach provides adequate access.

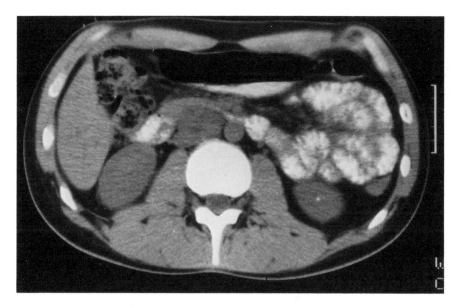

Fig. 1.2   CT scan showing involvement of inferior vena cava.

A thoracoabdominal approach is essential if simultaneous excision of supradiaphragmatic masses is to be carried out. Excellent access is provided to retrocrural nodes (Fig. 1.3), and this incision may be chosen for massive tumours which are predominantly on one side (Fig. 1.4). Perhaps the most difficult decision is to know when the case is inoperable. Tumours below the renal vessels can be excised, as can most nodal deposits above this level, but occasionally a case is encountered in which a tumour encases the coeliac axis and superior mesenteric vessels, extending into the small bowel mesentery (Fig. 1.5). Surgery has little to offer such cases, and these patients should not be subjected to the additional suffering associated with an unnecessary laparotomy.

Occasionally, a residual mass may be present after completion of chemotherapy for pure seminoma. Although rare, these masses may contain active tumour.[17] In our experience, these are much more difficult to excise than metastatic teratomas, lacking a clear-cut plane of cleavage and infiltrating the surrounding tissues deeply. Provided that the primary tumour is seminoma, and serum marker levels are normal, we feel that a CT-guided needle biopsy is preferable to laparotomy to establish whether there is residual active malignancy. If there is, then follow-up radiotherapy is much safer than difficult and hazardous surgical excision.

Tumour may be present in an undescended, abdominal testis. Following chemotherapy, it is usually surprisingly easy to remove the affected testicle.

Results and prognostic factors

Survival following excision of residual masses in the para-aortic area has been calculated for 175 patients treated at the Royal Marsden Hospital between 1976 and

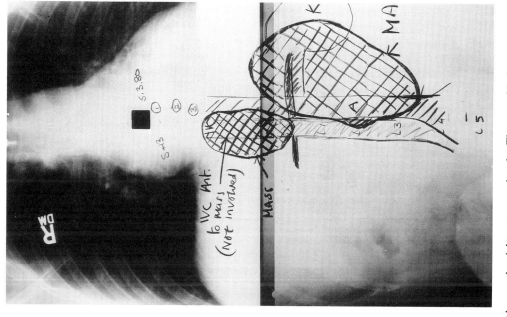

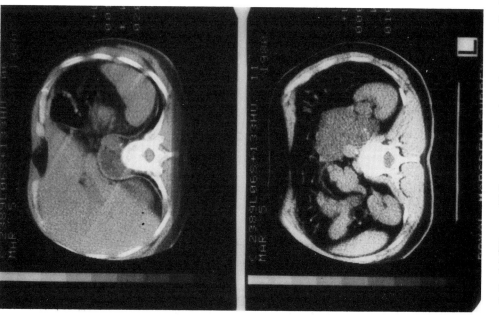

Fig. 1.3 (*a*) CT scan. (*b*) Scanogram showing a large mass displacing the left kidney and a right retrocrural node. These residual masses were removed completely through a left thoracoabdominal incision.

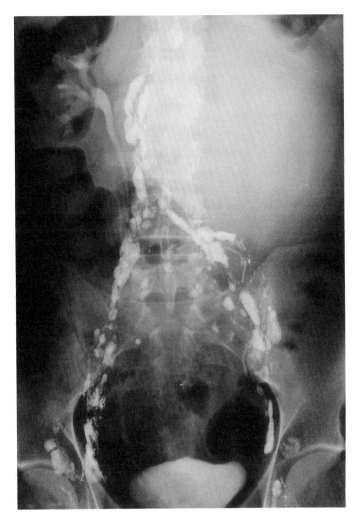

Fig. 1.4 Intravenous urograms (*a*) before and (*b*) after chemotherapy. This residual mass was removed with the left kidney through a left thoracoabdominal incision.

1988 inclusive. The initial stage, and size of the original para-aortic node mass, related to the histology of the primary tumour are shown in Tables 1.1 and 1.2. Roughly equal numbers had intermediate (MTI) and undifferentiated (MTU) tumours. Most (62%) had para-aortic masses greater than 5 cm diameter on presentation. There was residual undifferentiated tumour in 30 (17%), differentiated teratoma in 100 (57%) and only fibrosis/necrosis in 45 (26%). These results are shown related to the size of the excised mass in Table 1.3. It can be seen that residual active cancer is much less common in small masses. However, undifferentiated teratoma was more commonly found if the excision was incomplete (44%), and if markers were raised at the time of surgery (57%). The incidence of residual

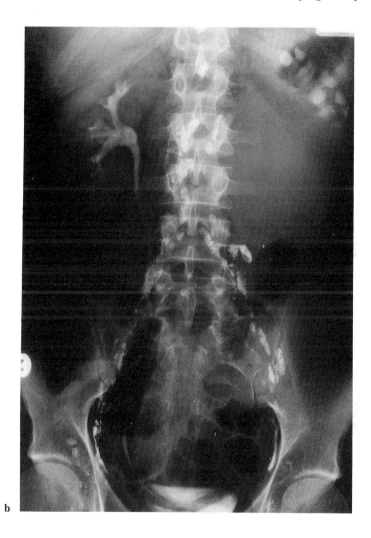

b

active malignancy is rather lower than that reported from other centres (Table 1.4).

Forty-seven patients (27%) had relapsed at between one and 56 months (median 7 months) after chemotherapy and surgery, 18 in the para-aortic area, 12 in the lungs and 7 in both sites; 3 relapsed with brain metastases, and 7 with elevation of markers only. All were treated with further chemotherapy but 28 died. The factors associated with increased likelihood of relapse and ultimately death are listed in descending order of importance in Table 1.5. Heading the list are incomplete excision of the residual mass, and presence of undifferentiated tumour. These two factors are probably not unconnected, in that extensive persistent malignancy is difficult to clear completely. It also indicates that complete clearance of residual

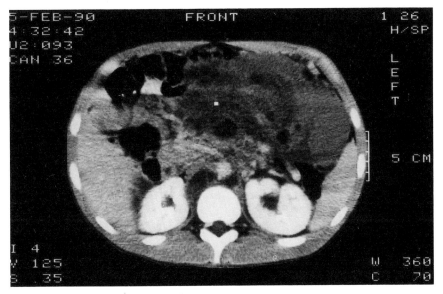

Fig. 1.5   This mass involved the coeliac axis and superior mesenteric artery with invasion of the small bowel mesentery and was therefore inoperable.

masses with active disease in them is of therapeutic benefit, which is not unreasonable. Evidence for the beneficial effect of surgical excision of residual active teratoma was also observed in the pre-chemotherapy era, prior to 1976.[13]

Raised markers at the time of surgery were highly predictive of the presence of active tumour in the residual mass, and of subsequent relapse and death. Nevertheless, it can be seen that 50% of such patients were 'salvaged' by excision of their residual masses, when otherwise their prognosis would have been poor. Widespread or massive disease at presentation were also recognizable as adverse factors in our series (Table 1.5). To these adverse prognostic factors can be added others defined by Donohue[22,23] from clinical experience with over 200 such cases. Undifferentiated tumour was present in 50% of those having chemotherapy for relapse, compared with 10–20% after primary chemotherapy. This reflects the lower complete remission rate after 'salvage' chemotherapy.[24] The presence of sarcoma in the excised tissue was a particularly bad sign.[25,26] On the other hand,

Table 1.1   Histology and stage at presentation in 175 patients who underwent para-aortic lymphadenectomy after chemotherapy at the Royal Marsden Hospital 1976–88

	Number	*TD*	*MTI*	*MTU*	*MTT*
II	79	2	43	32	2
III	22		10	12	
IV	74	3	29	42	
Totals	175	5	82	86	2

Table 1.2   Histology and size of para-aortic mass at presentation in 175 patients who underwent para-aortic lymphadenectomy after chemotherapy at the Royal Marsden Hospital 1976–88

	Number	*TD*	*MTI*	*MTU*	*MTT*
A <2 cm	18		10	8	
B 2–5 cm	49	1	23	24	1
C >5 cm	108	4	49	54	1
Totals	175	5	82	86	2

Table 1.3   Size of residual para-aortic masses after chemotherapy related to histology in excised specimens (Royal Marsden Hospital 1976–88)

	Number	*<3 cm*	*4–8 cm*	*>9 cm*
Necrosis	45	22	21	2
Differentiated teratoma	100	22	52	26
Undifferentiated tumour	30	4(8%)	18(20%)	8(22%)
Totals	175	48	91	36

Table 1.4   Histological findings in metastatic residual masses excised after completion of chemotherapy for advanced stage non-seminoma tumours of testis

Authors	*Number of patients*	*Histology of residual masses*		
		Fibrosis, necrosis	*Differentiated teratoma*	*Active malignancy*
Vugrin *et al.*[18]	37	18(49%)	8(22%)	11(30%)
Bracken *et al.*[19]	60	25(42%)	14(23%)	17(28%)
Donohue and Rowland[20]	123	34(28%)	46(37%)	43(35%)
Staeler *et al.*[21]	65	23(35%)	25(39%)	17(26%)
Royal Marsden (1976–88)	175	45(26%)	100(57%)	30(17%)

Table 1.5   Relapse rate and mortality related to various factors in 175 men who had para-aortic lymphadenectomy after chemotherapy at the Royal Marsden Hospital 1976–88

	Number	*Relapses (%)*	*Deaths (%)*
Incomplete excision	9	89	78
Presence of undifferentiated tumour	30	67	60
Raised markers	30	67	50
>9 cm residual mass	36	53	28
Lung metastases at presentation	60	43	23
Stage IV	74	39	28
Stage III	20	35	20
Stage C	108	35	14

those who had greater than 90% reduction on measured tumour volume in metastases from pure MTU (embryonal carcinoma) all had necrosis/fibrosis in their resected specimens, and this may become recognized as a good prognostic feature that allows surgical excision to be omitted.[22,23]

Complications

Amongst 140 consecutive teratoma cases undergoing para-aortic lymphadenectomy at the Royal Marsden Hospital for residual post-chemotherapy masses, over a 10-year period three died.[11,12] This represents an operation mortality of 2%, similar to that recorded by Donohue in over 200 such cases.[22,23] One patient developed severe respiratory failure 2–3 days after thoraco-laparotomy and died— possibly related to bleomycin lung toxicity; this complication has been observed by others[27] and emphasizes the need for careful preoperative lung function studies. One died of renal failure a year after injury to a renal artery, despite dialysis and kidney transplantation, when the contralateral kidney had postobstructive atrophy. Impairment of renal function, and severe hypertension, have been observed by others,[28] and underline the need for an obsessively careful technique when dissecting around the renal pedicles. The third patient died of secondary haemorrhage 10 days after excision of a huge necrotic mass which was involving the femoral nerve roots. Haemorrhage, primary or secondary, is the greatest risk in this operation. The great vessels were damaged in 12 cases (8.5%) (aorta 5, vena cava 5, renal artery or vein 2). Sometimes what appears to be a simple little node can be inextricably adherent to the aorta, defying all attempts at removal without doing damage; in others, a large mass may have such a well-developed plane of cleavage around it that removal is relatively easy. It is, therefore, imperative that adequate exposure is obtained in all cases, to allow proximal control for repair or grafting of major vessels if necessary.

A kidney was removed in 11% of cases usually because of attachment to the mass or postobstructive atrophy. It is better to remove such a kidney than to risk leaving tumour behind, or to attempt primary repair of a devascularized and damaged ureter.[29]

Chylous ascites or chylothorax has been recorded[15] but has not been seen in this series possibly because drains were not used. Lymphocoele has been seen occasionally, and has been noted by others.[30] Wound infection was not a problem, perhaps because we did not do an incidental appendicectomy.[31] Ejaculation was lost by 22% of 91 patients: analysis showed that this complication was most likely to occur if the initial para-aortic mass was very large (≥ 5 cm diameter) and bilateral (Table 1.6). Loss of ejaculation is caused by division of the sympathetic nerves on both sides of the great vessels,[32] or removal of the hypogastric plexus which lies just below the bifurcation of the aorta. Attempts to modify para-aortic lymphadenectomy to reduce the incidence of this complication have met with limited success.[33–36] Despite optimistic reports of return of ejaculation with the use of drugs such as ephedrine[37] or imipramine,[38,39] we have had no success with treating this complication which should probably be regarded as permanent.

Table 1.6 Incidence of loss of ejaculation related to initial size of para-aortic mass, and extent of para-aortic lymphadenectomy (Royal Marsden Hospital 1976–84)

Size of para-aortic mass on presentation	Number of patients with loss of ejaculation after lymphadenectomy		
	Total	*Unilateral*	*Bilateral*
A (≤2 cm)	0/6	0/5	0/1
B (2–5 cm)	2/14 (14%)	0/11	2/3
C (≥5 cm)	18/71 (25%)	5/40 (12%)	13/31 (42%)
Totals	20/91 (22%)	5/56 (9%)	15/35 (43%)

Conclusions

The number of reports of late relapse in the retroperitoneum after chemotherapy for testicular teratoma is steadily growing.[40–45] The unstable nature of teratomatous metastases, even those composed of apparently adult tissue, was recognized by Logothetis;[46] furthermore Dexeus[8] has recorded carcinoma in a residual para-aortic mass as small as 1.7 cm diameter. The difficulties inherent in treating patients with established relapse make prevention a preferable alternative. Routine excision of residual masses allows early recognition of adverse prognostic features, and elimination of unstable or frankly malignant tissue. We are not alone[21,23] in believing that this policy is preferable to the 'wait-and-see' approach recommended by others.[7,47] Nevertheless, the surgery is difficult and can be dangerous and must be done in specialist cancer centres.

References

1. Tait D, Peckham MJ, Hendry WF, Goldstraw P. Post chemotherapy surgery in advanced nonseminomatous germ cell testicular tumours: the significance of histology with particular reference to differentiated (mature) teratoma. *Br J Cancer* 1984; **50**: 601–9.
2. Hendry WF, Tyrrell CJ, Macdonald JS, McElwain TJ, Peckham MJ. The detection and localisation of abdominal lymph node metastases from testicular teratomas. *Br J Urol* 1977; **49**: 739–45.
3. Boyd PJR, Husband JE, Peckham MJ, Hendry WF. CT scanning and the surgery of metastatic teratoma of the testis: a preliminary report. *Br J Urol* 1978; **50**: 609–11.
4. Husband JE, Peckham MJ, Macdonald JS. The role of computed tomography in the management of testicular teratoma. *Clin Radiol* 1979; **30**: 243–52.
5. Kennedy CL, Husband JE, Bellamy EA, Peckham MJ, Hendry WF. The accuracy of CT scanning prior to paraaortic lymphadenectomy in patients with bulky metastases from testicular teratoma. *Br J Urol* 1985; **57**: 755–8.
6. Hendry WF, Goldstraw P, Husband JE, Barrett, A, McElwain TJ, Peckham MJ. Elective delayed excision of bulky para-aortic lymph node metastases in advanced nonseminomatous germ cell tumour of testis. *Br J Urol* 1981; **53**: 648–53.

7.   Read G, Johnson RJ, Wilkinson PM. The role of radiotherapy after chemotherapy in the management of persistent paraaortic nodal disease in nonseminomatous germ cell tumours. *Br J Cancer* 1986; **53**: 623–8.

8.   Dexeus FH, Shirkhoda A, Logothetis CJ, *et al.* Clinical and radiological correlation of retroperitoneal metastasis from nonseminomatous testicular cancer treated with chemotherapy. *Eur J Cancer Clin Onc* 1989; **25**: 35–43.

9.   Cassileth BR, Steinfeld AD. Psychological preparation of the patient and family. *Cancer* 1987; **60**: 547–52.

10.   Tamburini M, Filiberti A, Barbieri A, *et al.* Psychological aspects of testis cancer therapy: a prospective study. *J Urol* 1989; **142**: 1487–90.

11.   Hendry WF, Goldstraw P, Peckham MJ. The role of surgery in the combined management of metastases from malignant teratomas of testis. *Br J Urol* 1987; **59**: 358.

12.   Hendry WF, Goldstraw P, Horwich A, Peckham MJ. Paraaortic lymphadenectomy after chemotherapy for testicular tumour. *Br J Urol* 1988; **62**: 470–1.

13.   Hendry WF, Barrett A, McElwain TJ, Wallace DM, Peckham MJ. The role of surgery in the combined management of metastases from malignant teratomas of testis. *Br J Urol* 1980; **52**: 38–44.

14.   Maeda O, Yokokawa K, Oka T, *et al.* Inferior vena cava thrombus after retroperitoneal lymphadenectomy for testicular tumour. *Urol Int* 1986; **41**: 318–320.

15.   Jacqmin D, Bertrand P, Ansieau JP, Dufour P, Bollack C. Involvement of the caval vein lumen by a metastasis of a nonseminomatous testicular tumour. *Eur Urol* 1989; **16**: 233–4.

16.   Ahlering TE, Skinner DG. Vena caval resection in bulky metastatic germ cell tumours. *J Urol* 1989; **142**: 1497–9.

17.   Motzer RJ, Bosl GJ, Beller NL, *et al.* Advanced seminoma; the role of chemotherapy and adjunctive surgery. *Am Int Med* 1988; **108**: 513–18.

18.   Vugrin D, Whitmore WF, Sogani PC, Bains M, Herr HW, Golbey RB. Combined chemotherapy and surgery in treatment of advanced germ cell tumours. *Cancer* 1981; **47**: 2228–31.

19.   Bracken BR, Johnson DE, Frazier OH, Logothetis CJ, Trindade A, Samuels ML. The role of surgery following chemotherapy in Stage III germ cell neoplasms. *J Urol* 1983; **129**: 39–43.

20.   Donohue JP, Rowland RG. The role of surgery in advanced testicular cancer. *Cancer* 1984; **54**: 2716–21.

21.   Staehler G, Wiesel M, Clemm C, Gokel JM, Marchner M. Significance of salvage lymphadenectomy in the therapeutic concept of advanced nonseminomatous germ cell tumours. *Urol Int* 1989; **44**: 84–6.

22.   Donohue JP. Indications and results of surgery after chemotherapy of testicular tumours (NSG T and seminoma). *Prog Clin Biol Res* 1988; **269**: 451–9.

23.   Donohue JP. The case for retroperitoneal lymphadenectomy after chemotherapy for selected patients with nonseminomatous tumours of the testis. In: *Controversies in Urology.* Chicago: Year Book Publishers, 1989: 225–9.

24.   Loehrer PJ, Laver R, Roth BJ, Williams SD, Kalasinski LA, Einhorn LH. Salvage therapy in recurrent germ cell cancer: ifosfamide and cisplatinum plus either vinblastine or etoposide. *Am Intern Med* 1988; **109**: 540–6.

25.   Ahlgren AD, Simrell CR, Tricke TJ, Ozols R, Barsky SH. Sarcoma arising in a residual testicular teratoma after cytoreductive chemotherapy. *Cancer* 1984; **54**: 2015–18.

26.   Ulbright TM, Loehrer PJ, Roth LM, Einhorn LH, Williams SD, Clark SA. The

development of non-germ cell tumours within germ cell tumours: a clinico-pathological study of 11 cases. *Cancer* 1984; **54**: 1824–33.

27. Donohue JP, Rowland RG. Complications of retroperitoneal lymph node dissection. *J Urol* 1981; **125**: 338–40.

28. Beck PH, Stutzman RE. Complications of retroperitoneal lymphadenectomy for nonseminomatous tumours of the testis. *Urology* 1979; **13**: 244–7.

29. Skinner DG. Complications of lymph node dissection. In: Smith RB, Skinner DG (eds), *Complications of Urologic Surgery: Prevention and Management*. Philadelphia: WB Saunders, 1976: 422–35.

30. Messing EM, Love RR, Kvols LK. Lymphocele after retroperitoneal node dissection for testis tumour. *Cancer* 1986; **57**: 871–4.

31. Sago AL, Ball TP, Novicki DE. Complications of retroperitoneal lymphadenectomy. *Urology* 1979; **13**: 241–3.

32. Leiter E, Brendler H. Loss of ejaculation following bilateral retroperitoneal lymphadenectomy. *J Urol* 1967; **98**: 375–8.

33. Fossa SD, Ous S, Abyholm T, Loeb M. Post treatment fertility in patients with testicular cancer. I: Influence of retroperitoneal lymph node dissection on ejaculatory potency. *Br J Urol* 1985; **57**: 204–9.

34. Fritz K, Weissbach L. Sperm parameters and ejaculation before and after operative treatment of patients with germ cell testicular cancer. *Fertil Steril* 1985; **43**: 451–4.

35. Jewett MAS, Kong Y-SP, Goldberg SD, *et al.* Retroperitoneal lymphadenectomy for testis tumour with nerve sparing for ejaculation. *J Urol* 1988; **139**: 1220–4.

36. Sherlag AP, O'Brien DP, Graham SD. Use of limited retroperitoneal lymphadenectomy in nonseminomatous germ cell tumours. *Urology* 1989; **33**: 355–7.

37. Lynch JH, Maxted WC. Use of ephedrine in post-lymphadenectomy ejaculatory failure: a case report. *J Urol* 1983; **129**: 379.

38. Nijman JM, Jager S, Boer PW, Kremer J, Oldhoff J, Koops HS. The treatment of ejaculation disorders after retroperitoneal lymph node dissection. *Cancer* 1982; **50**: 2967–71.

39. Nijman JM, Koops HS, Oldhoff J, Kremer J, Jager S. Sexual function after bilateral retroperitoneal lymph node dissection for nonseminomatous testicular cancer. *Arch Androl* 1987; **18**: 255–67.

40. Carr BI, Gilchrist KW, Carbone PP. The variable transformation in metastases from testicular germ cell tumours: the need for selective biopsy. *J Urol* 1981; **126**: 52–4.

41. Chan SYT, Ford G, Sikora K. Late relapse in testicular teratoma after chemotherapy. *Lancet* 1985; **2**: 773–4.

42. Geier LJ, Volk SA, Weldon D, Redmond J. Late relapse in testicular cancer after chemotherapy. *Lancet* 1983; **1**: 1049.

43. Gelderman WA, Oosterhuis JW, Koops HS, Oldhoff J, Sleijfer DT. Late recurrence of mature teratoma in nonseminomatous testicular tumours after PVB chemotherapy and surgery. *Urology* 1989; **33**: 10–14.

44. Kuzmits R, Ludwig H. Late relapse in testicular cancer from a residual tumour. *Lancet* 1986; **1**: 1207–8.

45. Maatman T, Bvkowski RM, Montie JE. Retroperitoneal malignancies several years after initial treatment of germ cell cancer of the testis. *Cancer* 1984; **54**: 1962–5.

46. Logothetis CJ, Samuels ML, Trindale A, Johnson DE. The growing teratoma syndrome. *Cancer* 1982; **50**: 1629–35.

47. Levitt MD, Reynolds PM, Sheiner JH, Byrne MJ. Nonseminomatous germ cell testicular tumours—masses after chemotherapy. *Br J Surg* 1985; **72**: 19–21.

2 New cytotoxic chemotherapy programmes for advanced testicular cancer

A Horwich

The last fifteen to twenty years have witnessed a revolution in the prognosis of patients with advanced testicular cancer. This was stimulated by the development of effective combination chemotherapy for disseminated malignancies. Testicular germ cell tumours were known to be drug-sensitive for many years though responses to single agents were usually transient. The era of combination therapy for testicular cancers was introduced by Li *et al.* [1] using chlorambucil, methotrexate and actinomycin-D. This produced a response rate of 52% in 23 patients, though long-term survivors were uncommon. [2]

A major advance in the chemotherapy of testicular cancers was the development of schedules at the MD Anderson Hospital based on the combination of vinblastine and bleomycin. [3] The VB-1 induction schedule consisted of vinblastine 0.4–0.6 mg/kg divided into two doses on days 1 and 2 of the schedule, with bleomycin 30 units administered by IV injection twice per week for 10 weeks. Cycles of vinblastine and bleomycin were repeated upon recovery of myelosuppression, usually every 4–6 weeks. This schedule was strikingly effective in patients with small-volume metastatic disease, and for the first time significant numbers of long-term survivors were reported. Of 70 patients treated between 1970 and 1974, 22 achieved complete remission and 7 of these subsequently relapsed. The schedule was fairly toxic both because of bleomycin pneumonitis (two deaths) and vinblastine-induced leucopenia (two deaths).

The current era of chemotherapy for germ cell tumours was heralded by the introduction of high-dose cisplatin into the combination of vinblastine and bleomycin (PVB). [4] A recent report from the Indiana University group on 229 patients with metastatic germ cell tumours indicated a 65% probability of survival at 12 years. The rarity of any recurrence more than three years after completion of treatment suggests that this treatment causes cure. Similarly a report from the Royal Marsden Hospital on 320 patients treated between 1976 and 1985, [5] and a review from Charing Cross Hospital on 206 patients treated between 1977 and 1988,[6] suggest that during the 1980s the cure rate rose to approximately 80% with a particularly good prognosis for patients with limited bulk of metastatic disease.

It is important to recognize the group of patients with an excellent prognosis in order to address methods of reducing treatment toxicity, and especially long-term sequelae of treatment. For patients with adverse presentations a number of distinct approaches are being explored to define methods of increasing the efficacy of chemotherapy.[7] The increased morbidity of more intensive treatments has led to the concept of risk-related chemotherapy.

Prognostic groupings

The major factors determining prognosis in patients with metastatic germ cell tumours are volume and extent of metastatic disease, often described by the Royal Marsden Hospital staging system (Table 2.1) and by the serum concentration of tumour markers alphafetoprotein (AFP) and human chorionic gonadotrophin (HCG). Other factors which have been shown to influence prognosis are the histology, level of serum lactate dehydrogenase (LDH), and the age of the patient.[8] The Medical Research Council Testicular Tumour Working Party analysed, retrospectively, prognostic factors in 458 patients treated with chemotherapy between 1976 and 1982. Disease extent and serum marker concentrations were both found to be important prognostic variables, as illustrated in Table 2.2. The three-year survival probability for all patients was 75%, but two-year survivals had risen successively during the period of study from 68% in 1976/78 to 89% in 1981/82. In the latter period the survival of patients in the three prognostic groups were 95%, 85% and 54% respectively, leading to the present perception of two major prognostic groups with the majority of patients in the good-risk category. The

Table 2.1 Testicular tumours (RMH staging)

I   Testicular involvement alone, no evidence of metastases

II Infradiaphragmatic lymph node involvement
    A   Maximum diameter <2 cm
    B   Maximum diameter 2–5 cm
    C   Maximum diameter >5 cm

III Supradiaphragmatic node involvement

IV Extranodal metastases (A, B, C as for stage II)
    Lung substaging:
        $L_1 \leqslant 3$ metastases
        $L_2 > 3$ metastases, all <2 cm diameter
        $L_3 > 3$ metastases, one or more $\geqslant$2 cm diameter
    Liver status:
        H + liver involvement
    High markers:
        AFP > 500 IU/litre
        HCG > 1000 IU/litre

Table 2.2 Prognostic factors in non-seminomatous germ cell tumours

Factor	Number of patients	Three-year survival rate (%)
Clinical stage:		
IM	18	83
II, III A, B	106	87
II, III C	70	75
IV, L1, L2, A, B	104	85
IV, L1, L2 C	43	77
IV, L3, H+	117	54

Source: MRC (1985)[8]

improvement in prognosis was ascribed to increased experience in the use of chemotherapy and post-chemotherapy surgery.[8,9] In keeping with this, the Medical Research Council have recently performed a further prognostic factor analysis based on just under 800 patients with metastatic non-seminoma treated between 1982 and 1988.[10] From this, the adverse presentations of non-seminoma are defined in Table 2.3 with the remaining patients forming the good prognosis group.

There is no international agreement on the definition of good- and poor-risk patients, and this causes problems in the interpretation of single-arm studies based on local classifications since a broader definition of the poor-risk group will apparently lead to improved treatment results in both good-risk and poor-risk categories by the 'stage drift' mechanism. Bajorin *et al.*[11] have compared four definitions of poor-risk, applying published criteria to 118 patients whose chemo- therapy response was already known. There was marked discordance between prognostic systems in allocation of patients to different risk groups; thus, on the same set of patients, different centres would have reported the median survival of a poor-risk subgroup to be 11.5 months (Sloan-Kettering Cancer Center), 15 months (Indiana University), or 23.5 months (EORTC), and two-year survivals to be respectively 21%, 37% and 45%.

At a consensus workshop held in Hull (UK) in 1989, the Medical Research Council and EORTC prognostic classifications were compared and the definition of adverse subgroup presented in Table 2.3 was accepted by both groups as reflecting the results of modern chemotherapy.

Table 2.3 Non-seminoma: definition of the adverse group

One of:

1. More than 20 lung metastases
2. High serum markers:
     AFP > 1000 IU/litre
     or
     HCG > 10 000 IU/litre
3. Liver, bone or brain metastases
4. Mediastinal mass > 5 cm

Source: Horwich *et al.* (1990) for MRC[10]

Though testicular seminoma is almost as common as non-seminoma it usually presents at an early stage not requiring chemotherapy, and thus there is relatively little information on prognostic factors. It is apparent that this is an exquisitely drug-sensitive disease and especially sensitive to platinum either in combination or as a single agent.[12–15] It has been suggested that the adverse subgroups would be defined by very large masses (more than 10 cm in diameter) or by extranodal dissemination (stage 4 disease).

Chemotherapy for poor-risk metastatic non-seminoma

Since the seminal report of the efficacy of the PVB combination[4] a number of approaches have been investigated to increase chemotherapy efficacy. Randomized studies did not demonstrate benefit from additional Adriamycin or from maintenance vinblastine.[16] The replacement of vinblastine by etoposide (BEP)[17] is less toxic and, in patients with advanced disease, also appears to be more effective. A randomized comparison of PVB and BEP[18] found that patients classified on the Indiana University staging to have advanced disease had a survival probability at two years of 76% with BEP, compared with 48% with PVB.

The reduced efficacy of lower doses of cisplatin (i.e. 75 mg/m^2)[19] has been used as the rationale to explore dose escalation of cisplatin beyond the standard of 100 mg/m^2 per course. Following the demonstration that cisplatin renal toxicity could be mitigated by hydration with hypertonic saline,[20] this drug was tested at 40 mg/m^2 × 5; i.e. double the usual dose. Severe toxicity of this approach has been demonstrated.[21] A prospective randomized trial performed by the NCI has compared a regimen containing double-dose cisplatin, etoposide, vinblastine and bleomycin with standard PVB in poor-risk patients.[22] Only 52 patients were randomized and the median follow-up at the time of reporting was four years. The complete remission rate and the survival were higher in the schedule containing both double-dose platinum and etoposide; however, it is uncertain whether the benefit was derived from the platinum dose or the inclusion of etoposide. Furthermore, 88% of the patients treated with the intensive schedule had neutropenic sepsis, and 12 patients had such severe ototoxicity that they required hearing aids following treatment.

A trial by the Southeastern Cancer Study Group and the Southwestern Oncology Group compared standard-dose BEP to a regimen containing the same etoposide and bleomycin doses but with cisplatin at the double dose level of 40 mg/m^2 per day for 5 days. Preliminary reports have not indicated evidence of dose response beyond the standard 100 mg/m^2 per course for cisplatin.[23]

The platinum analogue carboplatin carries considerably less risk of neurotoxicity, ototoxicity and renal toxicity even at high doses and is a more logical basis for dose escalation studies. At Indiana University, high doses of carboplatin and etoposide have been investigated in patients who have relapsed following previous chemotherapy. This has defined optimal doses of these drugs to be etoposide 1200 mg/m^2 and carboplatin 1500 mg/m^2 given in divided doses and followed by autologous bone marrow transplantation.[24] Despite bone marrow support the treatment carried considerable toxicity and significant risk of mortality. Toxicity may be more predictable if carboplatin dose is based on renal clearance rather than on patient size.[25,26]

An alternative approach to intensification of treatment has been to reduce the interval between courses of chemotherapy. In a rapidly proliferating tumour, growth between treatment cycles may be a cause of failure. Wettlaufer *et al.*[27] demonstrated tolerance of a 7-day cycle of platinum, vincristine and bleomycin and a number of pilot studies have explored this method of intensifying chemotherapy.[28-30] The Royal Marsden study[30] illustrated in Fig. 2.1 has been employed in

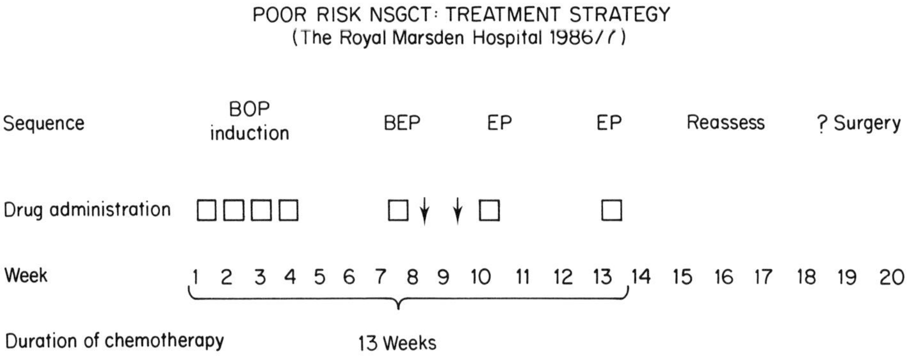

POOR RISK NSGCT: TREATMENT STRATEGY
(The Royal Marsden Hospital 1986//)

Sequence	BOP induction		BEP	EP		EP	Reassess	? Surgery

Drug administration   ☐☐☐☐   ☐↓ ↓☐   ☐

Week   1 2 3 4 5 6 7 8 9 10 11 12 13 14 15 16 17 18 19 20

Duration of chemotherapy   13 Weeks

Fig. 2.1   The intensive induction schedule.[30]

patients in the adverse subgroup identified by the Medical Research Council[8] to have a predicted survival rate of 55%. Sixty-one patients have been treated, and with a median follow-up of 20 months 11 patients have died of malignant disease and 5 of toxicity; the cause-specific survival rate is 74%. Though there appears to be increased antitumour activity there have been significant numbers of treatment-related deaths, including three from sepsis and two from bleomycin lung damage, and these approaches clearly need prospective evaluation in comparison with less intensive regimens.

Results of single-arm studies with alternating regimens have been very impressive.[31,32] The POMB/ACE regimen (cisplatin, vincristine, methotrexate, bleomycin/actinomycin-D, cyclophosphamide, etoposide) was developed in the Charing Cross Hospital in 1977 and has been reported to be particularly effective in adverse subgroups of patients with complete remissions in 14 out of 16 patients with liver metastases and 6 out of 7 with brain metastases.[31] The regimen has been investigated independently by Cullen *et al.*[33] who also found it to be effective in adverse subgroups of patients. Four of 6 patients with liver metastases and 3 of 4 with brain metastases were free from progression at the time of reporting. The MD Anderson schedule alternates CISCA 2 (Adriamycin, cyclophosphamide, cisplatin) with VB-4 (vinblastine, bleomycin). Of 63 patients with advanced stages of metastatic disease (Samuels stage IIIB3–5 or extragonadal primaries) there was an 83% survival.[32]

Although these results may derive from alternating and non-cross resistant schedules, it is noteworthy that the POMB/ACE regimen is also intensive in that the intervals between POMB cycles are usually less than 14 days and this intense scheduling is important for optimal results.[34] In less adverse patients the MSKCC study of alternating EP/VAB6[35] did not suggest that this approach was superior to standard VAB6, and the EORTC randomized trial showed alternating BEP and PVB to be no better than BEP.[36] Although treatment intensification and alternation of drug regimens do appear promising, their benefit remains to be demonstrated in prospective randomized trials.

Toxicity reduction in good-risk metastatic non-seminoma

The range of approaches to reducing toxicity of chemotherapy for metastatic non-seminoma is illustrated in Table 2.4. The major complications of drug regimens employed for germ cell tumours include myelosuppression and bleomycin-induced pneumonitis. Some patients suffer severe nausea and vomiting, abdominal cramps or dermatitis and find it difficult to complete chemotherapy, whereas other side-effects appear following completion of treatment or are chronic. Their full impact may not yet be manifest. These problems include the renal damage and ototoxicity caused by cisplatin[37,38] and the Raynaud's phenomenon caused by bleomycin.[39]

Table 2.4   Reducing toxicity of chemotherapy for germ cell tumours

Mechanisms	*Examples*
1. Reduce number of drugs	Omission of bleomycin
2. Substitute less toxic drugs	Etoposide replacing vinblastine
3. Substitute drug analogues	Carboplatin replacing cisplatin
4. Reducing length of chemotherapy	Three rather than four cycles
5. Omitting maintenance	No vinblastine maintenance
6. Prevent side-effects	Hydration; antiemetics; steroids

The issue of myelosuppression was first addressed in a prospective randomized trial from Indiana University comparing PVB containing vinblastine at 0.4 mg/kg with the same schedule containing vinblastine at 0.3 mg/kg.[16] Although the therapeutic results appeared equivalent and the toxicity lower at the reduced dose, the study was small with only 26 and 27 patients in each arm and only a major difference in efficacy could have been detected. Failure analysis of cisplatin and etoposide dosages[19,40] suggest that dose reduction during remission induction may be hazardous though total drug dose can be reduced by avoiding maintenance therapy.[41]

A second approach to reducing total drug dose has recently been evaluated by the Southeastern Cancer Study Group in patients with less advanced disease. This demonstrated that three courses of BEP chemotherapy were as effective as the standard four-course regimen.[42]

The standard bleomycin schedule from the PVB regimen is 30 mg per week for 12 weeks and is associated with a risk of fatal pneumonitis of approximately 1%.[5] A number of recent trials have suggested that bleomycin may be omitted in the chemotherapy of patients with a good prognosis. An EORTC study[43] of 180 patients compared BEP with EP alone. Complete remission rates were 95.5% and 95.2% respectively and there was no difference in continuous disease-free survivals. A trial from the Australian Germ Cell Trial Group compared PVB with PV in 104 patients.[44] Again no difference in response was found. The Memorial Sloan-Kettering Cancer Center (MSKCC) compared VAB6 to EP.[45] There appeared to be no benefit from the bleomycin-containing schedules.

The problems of toxicity induced by long-term cisplatin may be considerably obviated in the future by replacing it in combination chemotherapy with carboplatin. This drug is, however, more toxic to bone marrow than cisplatin, and pharmacokinetic studies have indicated that dose optimization should be based on renal function rather than on patient size.[25]

A pilot study of the combination of carboplatin, etoposide and bleomycin has been reported in 76 patients with good-prognosis metastatic non-seminomatous tumours.[46] The standard four courses of combination chemotherapy were administered on a 21-day cycle and surgical excision of a residual mass was performed in 27 of these patients. With a median follow-up of 24 months from start of chemotherapy, the two-year cause-specific survival probability was 98.5%, the single cause-related mortality being secondary to bleomycin pneumonitis. Five patients failed CEB chemotherapy but all were successfully salvaged with a combination of surgery and intensive reinduction chemotherapy. A range of doses of carboplatin were employed in this study allowing preliminary analysis of dose/response. The conclusion was that since carboplatin is predominantly detoxified by renal excretion the optimal dose judgement was based on glomerular filtration rate rather than the body surface area of the patient. The pattern of myelosuppression relates to the serum concentration × time of free platinum, and in this combination a serum concentration × time of 5 mg/ml × minutes appears to produce brief and non-problematic periods of bone marrow suppression. Pharmacokinetic data would indicate that this dose level can be achieved using the formula:

$$\text{Dose (mg)} = 5 \times (\text{GFR} + 25)$$

where GFR is the glomerular filtration rate assessed by clearance of chromium-51 EDTA.[25] The regimen is associated with a short sharp fall in granulocytes and platelets usually on day 14 to 16. Though the platelet nadir was less than 50 000 in 16% of treatment cycles, there were no overt problems of bruising or bleeding. Similarly the nadir white blood count was less than 1500 in 11% of cycles but only one cycle was complicated by neutropenic sepsis.

Spermatogenesis appears to recover consistently after CEB chemotherapy in all patients with normal pre-chemotherapy sperm counts.

Chemotherapy for metastatic seminoma

Seminoma is exquisitely sensitive to radiotherapy, and therefore chemotherapy has not been extensively explored in early stages of the disease. Patients with large-volume stage II seminoma had a high recurrence rate after radiotherapy alone in the past, though it has been suggested that careful shrinking-field techniques based on CT evaluation of the tumour volume enables these to be treated with radiotherapy in the modern era. There is little controversy over the use of initial combination chemotherapy for stage III or stage IV seminoma.[47–49] Seminoma is highly sensitive to drug combinations containing cisplatin.[12,50,51] In general, the rarity of these tumours has led to their treatment with schedules developed for the use of non-seminoma, especially PVB and BEP. The results are excellent (Table 2.5), but there is some evidence that the major determinant of these results is cisplatin.[14,52]

Table 2.5   Chemotherapy for advanced metastatic seminoma

Hospital	Drugs	Total patients treated	Survival
Royal Marsden Hospital[12]	PVB or BEP	39	92%
Norwegian Radium Hospital[54]	PVB or BEP	55	78%
MD Anderson Hospital[14]	Cisplatin Cyclophosphamide	62	92%
Royal Marsden Hospital[15]	Carboplatin	33	91%

A problem with comparing different single-centre studies is that the definition of response categories is complicated by the frequency of residual inactive masses after chemotherapy of bulky seminoma.[50] With rigorous CT scanning techniques, residual tissue is found at the site of treated seminoma in approximately two-thirds of patients who do not subsequently relapse, as illustrated in Fig. 2.2. Some authors feel that the size of the residual mass carries prognostic information. Motzer *et al.*[53] analysed the results of surgical excision or biopsy in 19 patients with residual masses, including 13 with a mass of up to 3 cm diameter. All five patients with viable germ cell tumour were in the group whose residual masses measured more than 3 cm diameter. This has not been confirmed in other reports.[15,54] Surgical exploration is complicated by the densely adherent and fibrotic nature of the residual mass in seminoma and by the tendency to haemorrhage. Adjuvant radiotherapy has been used in some centres.[55]

Single-agent chemotherapy has not been investigated extensively in seminoma. Preliminary reports have *not* indicated that this conservative and non-toxic approach is associated with a survival disadvantage.[56,15] The report from the Royal Marsden Hospital on single-agent carboplatin was based on 34 patients treated at least one year prior to analysis.[15] The actuarial chance of remaining alive and free from progressive disease at two years was 80%. Of 6 relapsing patients, 5 have

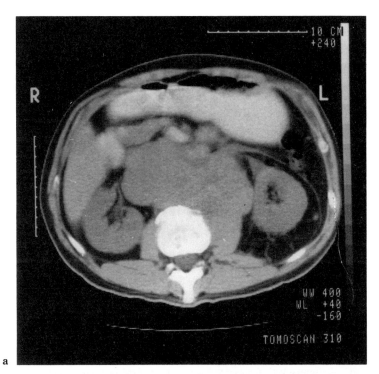

a

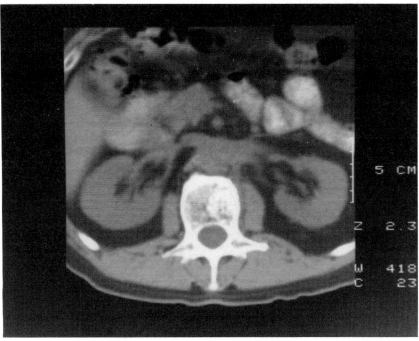

b

Fig. 2.2 (*a*) Mass of retroperitoneal seminoma before chemotherapy in March 1986, and (*b*) response to single agent carboplatin in September 1986.

achieved very prolonged second remission 18–30 months after completion of salvage therapy. The treatment with single-agent carboplatin is extremely well tolerated and is easily administered purely as an out-patient. No patients suffered renal damage, neurotoxicity, ototoxicity or alopecia, and there were no episodes of neutropenic sepsis or thrombocytopenic haemorrhage or bruising. The Medical Research Council has just opened a trial comparing single-agent carboplatin with the more standard combination of etoposide and cisplatin in patients with stage IIC, III and IV seminoma.

Conclusion

Though considerable progress has been made in identifying chemotherapeutic strategies of reduced toxicity, it should be remembered that even in good prognosis subgroups the risk to the patient of dying from progressive malignant disease is far higher than the risk of dying from treatment toxicity, and it is important to ensure that toxicity reduction is not associated with a compromise of efficacy.

References

1. Li MC, Whitmore WF, Golbey R, Grabstald H. Effects of combined drug therapy on metastatic cancer of the testis. *JAMA* 1960; **174**: 1291–9.
2. MacKenzie AR. Chemotherapy of metastatic testis cancer: results in 154 patients. *Cancer* 1966; **19**: 1369–76.
3. Samuels ML. Treatment: chemotherapy. In: Johnson DE (ed.), *Testicular Tumours*. New York: Medical Examination Publishing Co., 1976: 204–22.
4. Einhorn LH, Donohue JP. Cis-diammine-dichloroplatinum, vinblastine and bleomycin combination chemotherapy in disseminated testicular cancer. *Ann Intern Med* 1977; **87**: 292–8.
5. Peckham MJ, Horwich A, Easton D, Hendry WF. The management of advanced testicular teratoma. *Br J Urol* 1988; **62**: 63–8.
6. Hitchins RN, Newlands ES, Smith DB, Begent RHJ, Rustin GJS, Bagshawe K. Long-term outcome in patients with germ cell tumours treated with POMB/ACE chemotherapy: comparison of commonly used classification systems of good and poor prognosis. *Br J Cancer* 1989; **59**: 236–42.
7. Horwich A. Germ cell tumour chemotherapy. *Br J Cancer* 1989; **59**: 156–9.
8. Medical Research Council Working Party on Testicular Tumours. Prognostic factors in advanced non-seminomatous germ-cell testicular tumours: results of a multicentre study. *Lancet* 1985; **1**: 8–11.
9. Einhorn LH. Have new aggressive chemotherapy regimens improved results in advanced germ cell tumours? *Eur J Cancer Clin Onc* 1986; **22**: 1289–93.
10. Horwich A, Stenning S, Mead B, Fossa S, Wilkinson P, Kaye S, Newlands E. Prognostic factors for survival in advanced non-seminomatous germ cell tumours. The Medical Research Council Testicular Tumour Subgroup. *Proceedings of ASCO* 1990; **9**: 513.
11. Bajorin D, Katz A, Chan E, *et al.* Comparison of criteria for assigning germ cell tumour patients to 'good risk' and 'poor risk' studies. *J Clin Onc* 1986; **6**: 786–92.

12. Peckham MJ, Horwich A, Hendry WF. Advanced seminoma: treatment with cis-platinum-based combination chemotherapy or carboplatin (JM8). *Br J Cancer* 1985; **52**: 7–13.

13. Oliver RTD. Surveillance for stage I seminoma and single agent cis-platinum for metastatic seminoma. *Proc Am Soc Clin Onc* 1984; **3**: 162.

14. Logothetis CJ, Samuels ML, Ogden SL. Cyclophosphamide and sequential advanced seminoma: long-term follow-up in 52 patients. *J Urol* 1987; **138**: 789–94.

15. Horwich A, Dearnley DP, Duchesne GM, Williams M, Brada M, Peckham MJ. Simple nontoxic treatment of advanced metastatic seminoma with carboplatin. *J Clin Onc* 1989; **7**: 1150–6.

16. Einhorn LH, Williams SD. Chemotherapy of disseminated testicular cancer: a random prospective study. *Cancer* 1980; **46**: 1339–44.

17. Peckham MJ, Barrett A, Liew KH, *et al.* The treatment of metastatic germ-cell testicular tumours with bleomycin, etoposide and cis-platin (BEP). *Br J Cancer* 1983; **47**: 613–19.

18. Williams SD, Birch R, Einhorn LH, Irwin L, Greco FA, Loehrer PJ. Treatment of disseminated germ-cell tumours with cisplatin, bleomycin, and either vinblastine or etoposide. *N Eng J Med* 1987; **316**: 1435–40.

19. Samson MK, Rivkin SE, Jones SE, *et al.* Dose-response and dose-survival for high versus low dose cisplatin combined with vinblastine and bleomycin in disseminated testicular cancer. *Cancer* 1984; **53**: 1029–35.

20. Ozols RF, Corden BJ, Jacob J, Wesley MN, Ostchega Y, Young RC. High-dose cisplatin in hypertonic saline. *Ann Intern Med* 1984; **100**: 91–4.

21. Daugaard G, Rorth M. High-dose cisplatin and VP-16 with bleomycin, in the management of advanced metastatic germ cell tumours. *Eur J Cancer Clin Onc* 1986; **22**: 477–85.

22. Ozols RF, Ihde DC, Linehan WM, Jacob J, Ostchega Y, Young RC. A randomized trial of standard chemotherapy versus a high-dose chemotherapy regimen in the treatment of poor prognosis non-seminomatous germ-cell tumours. *J Clin Onc* 1988; **6**: 1031–40.

23. Nichols CR, Williams SD, Loehrer PJ, *et al.* Randomized study of cisplatin dose intensity in poor-risk germ cell tumors: a Southeastern Cancer Study Group and Southwest Oncology Group protocol. *J Clin Onc* 1991; **9**: 1163–72.

24. Nichols CR, Tricot G, Williams SD, Besien K, Loehrer PJ, Roth BJ, Akard L, Hoffman R, Goulet R, Wolff SN, Giannone L, Greer J, Einhorn LH, Jansen J. Dose-intensive chemotherapy in refractory germ cell cancer: a phase I/II trial of high-dose carboplatin and etoposide with autologous bone marrow transplantation. *J Clin Onc* 1989; **7**: 932–9.

25. Calvert AH, Newell CR, Gumbrell LA, *et al.* Carboplatin dosage: prospective evaluation of a simple formula based on renal function. *J Clin Onc* 1989; **7**: 1748–56.

26. Newell DR, Eeles RA, Gumbrell LA, *et al.* Carboplatin and etoposide in patients with testicular teratoma. *Cancer Chemother Pharmacol* 1989; **23**: 367–72.

27. Wettlaufer JN, Feiner AS, Robinson WA. Vincristine, cisplatin and bleomycin surgery in the management of advanced metastatic non-seminomatous testis tumours. *Cancer* 1984; **53**: 203–9.

28. Daniels JR, Russell C, Skinner D, *et al.* Malignant germinal neoplasms: intensive chemotherapy with cisplatin, vincristine, bleomycin and etoposide. *Proceedings of ASCO* 1987; **6**: 104.

29. Murray N, Coppin C, Swenerton K. Weekly high intensity cisplatin etoposide for far advanced germ cell cancers (GCC). *Proc Am Soc Clin Onc* 1987; **6**: 394.
30. Horwich A, Brada M, Nicholls J, *et al.* Intensive induction chemotherapy for poor prognosis non-seminomatous germ cell tumours. *Eur J Cancer Clin Onc* 1989; **25**: 177–84.
31. Newlands ES, Bagshawe KD, Begent RHJ, *et al.* Current optimum management of anaplastic germ cell tumours of the testis and other sites. *Br J Urol* 1986; **58**: 307–14.
32. Logothetis CJ, Samuels ML, Selig DE, Swanson D, Johnson DE, von Eschenbach A. Improved survival with cyclic chemotherapy for non-seminomatous germ cell tumours of the testis. *J Clin Onc* 1985; **3**: 326–35.
33. Cullen MH, Harper PG, Woodroffe P, Kirkbridge P, Clarke J. Chemotherapy for poor risk germ cell tumours: an independent evaluation of the POMB/ACE regime. *Br J Urol* 1988; **62**: 454–60.
34. Crawford SM, Newlands ES, Begent RHJ, Rustin GJS, Bagshawe KD. The effect of intensity of administered treatment on the outcome of germ cell tumours treated with POMB/ACE chemotherapy. *Br J Cancer* 1989; **59**: 243–6.
35. Bosl GJ, Geller NL, Vogelzang NJ, *et al.* Alternating cycles of etoposide plus cisplatin and VAB-6 in the treatment of poor-risk patients with germ cell tumours. *J Clin Onc* 1987; **5**: 436–40.
36. Stoter G, Kaye S, Sleyfer D, *et al.* Preliminary results of BEP and PVB (cisplatin, vinblastine, bleomycin) in high volume metastatic (HVM) testicular non-seminomas: an EORTC study. *Proceedings of ASCO* 1986; **5**: 106.
37. Daugaard G, Rossing N, Rorth M. Effects of cisplatin on different measures of glomerular function in the human kidney with special emphasis on high-dose. *Cancer Chemother Pharmacol* 1988; **21**: 163–7.
38. Hamilton CR, Bliss JM, Horwich A. The late effects of cis-platinum on renal function. *Eur J Cancer Clin Onc* 1989; **25**: 185–9.
39. Roth BJ, Greist A, Kubilis PS, Williams SD, Einhorn LH. Cisplatin-based combination chemotherapy for disseminated germ cell tumors: long-term follow-up. *J Clin Onc* 1988; **6**: 1239–47.
40. Brada M, Horwich A, Peckham MJ. Treatment of favourable prognosis non-seminomatous testicular germ cell tumours with etoposide, cisplatin and reduced dose of bleomycin. *Cancer Treat Rep* 1987; **7**: 655–6.
41. Einhorn LH, Williams SD, Troner M, Birch R, Greco FA. The role of maintenance therapy in disseminated testicular cancer. *N Engl J Med* 1981; **305**: 727–31.
42. Einhorn LH, Williams SD, Loehrer PJ, Birch R, Drasga R, Omura G, Greco A. Evaluation of optimal duration of chemotherapy in favorable-prognosis disseminated germ cell tumors: a Southeastern Cancer Study Group protocol. *Clin Onc* 1989; **7**: 387–91.
43. Stoter G, Kaye S, Jones W, *et al.* Cisplatin (P) and VP16 (E) with or without bleomycin (B) (BEP *vs* EP) in good risk patients with disseminated non-seminomatous testicular cancer: a randomized EORTC GU Group study. *Proceedings of ASCO* 1987; **6**: 110.
44. Levi J, Raghavan D, Harvey V, *et al.* Deletion of bleomycin from therapy for good prognosis advanced testicular cancer. *Proc Am Soc Clin Onc* 1986; **5**: 374.
45. Bosl GJ, Geller NL, Bajorin D, *et al.* A randomized trial of etoposide + cisplatin versus vinblastine + bleomycin + cisplatin + cyclophosphamide + dactinomycin in patients with good prognosis germ cell tumours. *J Clin Onc* 1988; **6**: 1231–8.
46. Horwich A, Dearnley D, Harland S, Peckham PM, Hendry WF. Carboplatin–

etoposide–bleomycin (CEB) combination chemotherapy is effective in good prognosis metastatic testicular non-seminomatous germ cell tumours (NSGCT). *Proceedings of ASCO* 1989; **8**: 134.

47.   Ball D, Barrett A, Peckham MJ. The management of metastatic seminoma testis. *Cancer* 1982; **50**: 2289–94.

48.   Gregory C, Peckham MJ. Results of radiotherapy for stage II testicular seminoma. *Radiother Onc* 1986; **6**: 285–92.

49.   Thomas GM, Rider WD, Dembo AJ. Seminoma of the testis: results of treatment and patterns of failure after radiation therapy. *Int Radiat Onc Biol Phys* 1982; **8**: 165–74.

50.   Einhorn LH, Williams SD. Chemotherapy of disseminated seminoma. *Cancer Clin Trials* 1980; **3**: 307–13.

51.   Loehrer PJ, Birch R, Williams SD. Chemotherapy of metastatic seminoma: the Southeastern Cancer Study Group experience. *J Clin Onc* 1987; **5**: 1212–20.

52.   Samuels ML, Logothetis CJ. Follow-up study of sequential weekly pulse dose cis-platinum for far advanced seminoma. *Proc Am Soc Clin Onc* 1983; **2**: 137.

53.   Motzer R, Bosl G, Heelan R, Fair W. Residual mass: an indication for further therapy in patients with advanced seminoma following systemic chemotherapy. *J Clin Onc* 1987; **5**: 1064–70.

54.   Schultz SM, Einhorn LH, Conces DJ, Williams SD, Loehrer PJ. Management of postchemotherapy residual mass in patients with advanced seminoma: Indiana University experience. *J Clin Onc* 1989; **7**: 1497–503.

55.   Fossa S, Borge L, Aass N. (1987). The treatment of advanced metastatic seminoma: experience in 55 cases. *J Clin Onc* 1987; **5**: 1071–7.

56.   Oliver RTD. Long term follow-up of single-agent cisplatin in metastatic seminoma and surveillance for stage I seminoma. *Proceedings of ASCO* 1988; **7**: 120.

3 Management of clinical stage I testicular cancer ‗‗‗

Philip W Kantoff and Jerome P Richie

The markedly improved outlook over the past 15 years for patients with testicular cancer has led to a reassessment of the management options for patients with clinical stage I (CSI) tumours. In the 1990s the cure rate for patients with CSI testicular tumours approaches 100%. A number of different management policies can be used to achieve a successful outcome. The traditional approach practised in the United States has been the retroperitoneal lymph node dissection (RPLND). Outside the USA, lymph node irradiation has been the preferred modality of treatment. However, a significant amount of experience has been acquired in recent years with close surveillance and with chemotherapy used as an adjuvant therapy. The efficacy and relative morbidity of these approaches need to be evaluated.

Staging

Clinical stage I testicular cancer is defined at our institution as the absence of apparent disease following orchiectomy, with normal alphafetoprotein (AFP) and beta human chorionic gonadotrophin (HCG) levels, a normal chest x-ray or chest CT scan, and an abdominal CT scan without evidence of visceral disease where all lymph nodes measure less than 1.5 cm.

Unfortunately, clinical staging is not fully accurate, owing to the poor sensitivity and specificity of the tests currently available. The serum markers AFP and HCG are not produced by 10–15% of non-seminomatous germ cell tumours (NSGCTs) and their serum level may be below the level of detection in very low volume disease. Furthermore, assessment of the retroperitoneum, the site which most frequently harbours occult disease in patients with CSI tumours, is particularly problematic. The difficulty in assessing the retroperitoneum was most clearly demonstrated by Stomper et al.[1] in a study of 51 patients who had undergone abdominal CT scanning as part of their initial evaluation. After CT evaluation, 42 patients underwent RPLND for lymph nodes measuring less than 25 mm on CT and 9 patients received primary chemotherapy for lymph nodes measuring 25–50 mm

Table 3.1 Correlation between CT scan size criteria of retroperitoneal lymph nodes and pathological findings

	Number of patients				
Criteria* for metastases	*Negative predictive value (%)*	*Positive predictive value (%)*	*Sensitivity (%)*	*Specificity (%)*	*Accuracy (%)*
≥ 5 mm	11/14 (79)	23/37 (62)	23/26 (88)	11/25 (44)	34/51 (67)
≥ 10 mm	15/22 (68)	19/29 (66)	19/26 (73)	15/25 (60)	34/51 (67)
≥ 15 mm	19/30 (63)	15/21 (71)	15/26 (58)	19/25 (76)	34/51 (67)
≥ 20 mm	23/37 (62)	12/14 (86)	12/26 (46)	23/25 (92)	35/51 (69)
≥ 25 mm	25/42 (60)	9/9† (100)	9/26 (35)	23/25 (100)	34/51 (67)

* Greatest transaxial diameter of largest node.
† Did not undergo node dissection but demonstrated marked reduction in size of residual teratoma after initial chemotherapy.

on CT. All of the patients had normal markers after orchiectomy. Seventeen of 42 patients undergoing RPLND were found to have lymph node metastases and all of those patients with lymph nodes greater than 25 mm demonstrated tumour regression after chemotherapy. Thus, 26 of 51 patients by pathological or clinical criteria were considered to have lymph node metastases. As demonstrated in Table 3.1, the accuracy for predicting pathological lymph node involvement is only about 67% and is independent of the size criteria used.

The overall sensitivity and specificity of lymphangiography is similar to that of CT scanning.[2] When CT scanning and lymphangiography are combined, the sensitivity of detecting retroperitoneal disease increases 10–15% over CT scanning alone, but the false-positive rate increases proportionately. MRI has thus far failed to increase the accuracy of detecting retroperitoneal disease.

Risk factors for occult disease

Clearly, if a test existed which perfectly discriminated between patients with and without residual disease, the controversies in staging would diminish, but as yet such a test does not exist. However, on the basis of a number of studies, several features have emerged which predict disease at the time of retroperitoneal lymph node dissection or the development of clinically apparent disease while on surveillance.[3–9] Two pathological features of the orchiectomy specimen which increase the likelihood of residual tumour elsewhere are the presence of vascular invasion and a greater proportion of embryonal cell carcinoma versus teratoma. Other features that predict residual tumour in some but not all studies are advanced tumour stage (T2–T4 versus T1) and an elevated preorchiectomy AFP (Table 3.2).

Vascular invasion, the feature most consistently associated with the presence of occult disease, carries a 50% risk as opposed to a 10–20% risk without it. Several studies have demonstrated that having an embryonal component or having pure

Table 3.2 Risk factors for relapse in clinical stage I non-seminomatous germ cell tumours

Series	Embryonal cell cancer (present v. not present)	Teratoma (present v. not present)	Vascular invasion (present v. not present)	T stage (T=1 v. T>1)	Preorchiectomy rising AFP
Surveillance					
MRC[a3]	+	NS	+	NS	+[b]
Auckland Hospital[4]	NS	NS	+	NS	NS
Institute Nazionale Tumore[5]	NE	+	+[c]	+	NS
MD Anderson[a6]	+	+[d]	+	NE	NS[e]
MSKCC[8]	NE	+	NE	NE[f]	NS
RPLND					
DFCI[a9]	NS[d]	+	+	+	NS
SWENOTECA[a7]	NS	+	+	NS	+

+ Statistically significant correlation; NS not significant; NE not examined.
[a] Multivariate analysis performed.
[b] Correlation made in earlier publications, made with absence of yolk sac elements in this publication.
[c] Examined less than one-half of patients.
[d] Correlation made between high percentage of teratoma (>50%) and decreased likelihood of relapse.
[e] Elevated preorchiectomy AFP predictive of relapse.
[f] Patients with T>1 not included in study.

embryonal cell carcinoma (ECC) is associated with an increased risk of occult disease. Biologically, it is likely that ECC has a greater propensity to metastasize than other germ cell components and, when it predominates, the likelihood of occult disease increases. The risks of occult disease in patients whose tumours contained no ECC were 1/31 (3%),[3] 0/12 (0%),[6] and 12/67 (17.9%),[7] in three studies, whereas the risks of occult disease in patients with pure ECC were 4/7 (57%),[8] 9/18 (50%),[5] and 18/46 (39%)[7] respectively. Increasing tumour stage (T2–T4 versus T1) was associated with an increased risk of occult tumour in several studies;[5,9] however, this association was lost in multivariate analysis of two of the larger studies.[3,7] In two studies elevations in the preorchiectomy AFP levels correlated with a reduced risk of occult disease,[3,7] whereas other studies have failed to make this association. Another study demonstrated an increased risk of occult disease, with an elevated preorchiectomy AFP level. The relationship of an elevated preorchiectomy AFP level to occult disease remains uncertain.

Similar pathological correlations have not been made with seminoma owing to the paucity of surveillance and RPLND data. However, in a study correlating clinical stage at presentation with pathological features of the tumour, tumours with vascular invasion were associated with increased clinical stage although this trend did not reach statistical significance.[11]

Management of non-seminomatous germ cell tumours

Nearly all patients with CSI NSGCTs are cured and the current goal of therapy is to maintain this high cure rate while minimizing treatment-related morbidity. Orchiectomy alone will cure approximately 70% of these patients. A variety of methods have been used to effect cure in the remaining 30% of patients.

Retroperitoneal lymph node dissection (RPLND)

The standard approach to the initial management of patients with CSI disease in the United States has been the RPLND. This approach has two purposes: to stage patients more accurately, and to cure those patients with occult disease in retroperitoneal lymph nodes.

The full RPLND routinely performed prior to 1982 included an extensive dissection of retroperitoneal lymph nodes, with consequent loss of ejaculatory function and fertility in the majority of patients. Other complications of the procedure were rare. Over the past 10 years, a better understanding of the pattern of nodal spread and of the neuroanatomy of the retroperitoneal sympathetic chain and its control of ejaculatory function has permitted surgeons to modify the procedure. This has enabled most patients to maintain ejaculatory function and fertility without compromising the procedure.

Donohue *et al.*[12] in 1982 studied the pattern of lymph node involvement in 104 patients with pathological stage II (PSII) NSGCT. They found that when the primary tumour arose in the right testicle, the interaortocaval zone was the most

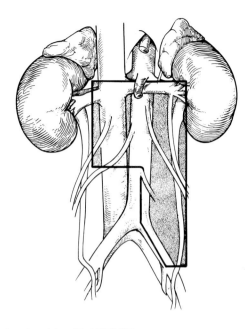

Fig. 3.1   Template for right-sided RPLND.

common site of metastases, followed by the precaval and preaortic zones. For tumours arising in the left testicle, the most common nodal sites were the left para-aortic followed by the preaortic and the interaortocaval zones. Narayan *et al.*[13] in the same year demonstrated that a therapeutically successful procedure could be performed while maintaining ejaculatory function in most patients. Several other groups have developed modified 'nerve sparing' procedures wherein the RPLND may be performed while maintaining ejaculatory function in the majority of patients.[14] In a series of 80 patients with CSI disease, modified RPLND has resulted in preservation of ejaculation in 94% of patients[15] (Fig. 3.1).

Clearly, the RPLND is a more accurate staging procedure than non-invasive staging. Between 20% and 30% of CSI patients will actually be PSII. Conversely, approximately 10% of patients without nodal disease at the time of RPLND (PSI) will relapse, usually owing to hematogenous metastases to the lungs.

In addition to providing staging information, the RPLND is also therapeutic in a proportion of patients. In several studies, patients who were PSII after RPLND received no adjuvant therapy,[16–20] indicating the efficacy of RPLND as the sole therapy (Table 3.3). The earliest study conducted by Staubitz *et al.*[16] demonstrated that 70% of PSII patients remain relapse-free in the long term. Donohue *et al.*[17] noted that 57% (16/28) of patients with nodal disease at RPLND remained disease-free. In a large multicentre trial in which PSII patients were randomized to receive adjuvant chemotherapy or observation, 47/95 (49%) of patients in the observation

Table 3.3 Efficacy of RPLND alone for pathological stage II non-seminomatous germ cell tumours

Reference	Number of patients	Pathological stage	Relapse-free
Staubitz et al.[16]	20	II	14/20 (70%)
Donohue et al.[17]	28	II	16/28 (57%)
Schmoll and Waegener[18]	31	II	14/31 (46%)
Richie[20]	35	IIa	32/35 (91%)
Williams et al.[19]	47	IIa	26/47 (55%)
	48	IIb	21/48 (43%)

IIa Defined as pathological abnormality <2 cm.
IIb Defined as pathological abnormality >2 cm or extending to adjacent tissue with no residual
    disease after surgery.

group remained disease-free in the long term.[19] There was also a trend, not reaching statistical significance, for minimal (<2 cm nodal) disease to be more effectively eradicated than greater volume (>2 cm nodal) disease with RPLND. At the Dana Farber Cancer Institute and Brigham and Women's Hospital, those patients with greater than 2 cm nodal disease removed at RPLND are given the options of receiving adjuvant chemotherapy or being observed, while those patients with less than 2 cm disease and fewer than six positive lymph nodes detected at RPLND are urged to undergo close observation without immediate adjuvant therapy. This is based on the observation that in the selected group of patients with minimal disease (<2 cm abnormalities), 91% remain relapse-free without the need for chemotherapy with a median follow-up of 3.5 years.[20]

It would appear from all the above data that the curability of PSII testicular cancer by RPLND alone depends on the extent of disease found at the time of surgery, but is probably close to 50% overall. Since only 20–30% of patients with CSI NSGCT will have nodal disease detected at RPLND, and 50% of these will be cured with surgery alone, approximately 15% of unselected patients with CSI disease are cured with RPLND. Thus, slightly less than 50% of patients with occult disease– approximately 15 patients in 100–will potentially be spared the morbidity of chemotherapy at the expense of performing surgery on all the patients. This is only true if chemotherapy is withheld in those patients found to have disease at RPLND and only treated at the time of relapse.

If one accepts the debatable premise that RPLND is associated with less morbidity than chemotherapy, can one identify a group of patients with CSI NSGCT who have a high likelihood of harbouring occult disease (high-risk CSI) and a high likelihood of being cured with RPLND alone? The answer to this question is unknown. However, it should be noted that vascular invasion in the orchiectomy specimen (which is associated with an increased risk of having nodal disease at RPLND) is also associated with an increased risk of relapse after RPLND even in PSI patients.[7,9]

Lymph node irradiation

An alternative approach to patients with CSI NSGCTs is lymph node irradiation. This approach had been fairly routine outside the USA prior to the development of effective chemotherapy and routine abdominal CT scanning. The approach was abandoned in most institutions because of a lack of evidence that prophylactic irradiation was effective: no randomized prospective study had been successfully completed comparing radiotherapy with any other modality. It fell into disuse along with the development of effective chemotherapy.

The efficacy of lymph node irradiation still remains in question, although one randomized study has reached maturity.[21] Between 1980 and 1984, 153 patients with CSI NSGCTs were randomized after orchiectomy to either prophylactic XRT or observation. With a minimal follow-up of five years, 23 of 85 (27%) of the patients who were observed relapsed, with 14 of the 23 (61%) relapsing primarily in the retroperitoneum. Only 11/68 (16%) patients treated with XRT relapsed, with 0/11 (0%) relapsing in the retroperitoneum. All patients in both groups who relapsed were salvaged with chemotherapy, with the exception of one patient in the XRT-treated group. These data would suggest that XRT can be an effective modality for CSI NSGCT, and the failure to demonstrate its efficacy previously may be due to a high proportion of understaged patients in historical controls not evaluated by CT scanning. If, however, 'prophylactic' XRT is effective, it would appear that less than 50% of those patients with retroperitoneal disease truly benefit from this therapy. Similarly to RPLND, prophylactic XRT eradicates disease in the retroperitoneum, but there is coexistent disease outside the retroperitoneum in a large proportion of these patients. Unlike RPLND, XRT gives no information regarding nodal status and does not allow a decision to be made regarding the need for adjuvant chemotherapy. Furthermore, many patients are treated unnecessarily, although the morbidity is low, and for those patients who relapse there is potentially a greater likelihood of morbidity from chemotherapy.

Adjuvant chemotherapy

Chemotherapy currently cures approximately 80% of all patients with disseminated NSGCTs and well over 90% of good-risk patients. Because of these outstanding results, several groups have used chemotherapy in patients with CSI NSGCTs.[22–26] Useful data, however, are scarce because of the small numbers of patients, suboptimal chemotherapy regimens, and in some cases the use of RPLND or irradiation in addition to chemotherapy. In one study,[26] patients received adequate chemotherapy after orchiectomy. Eighteen patients with high-risk CSI NSGCTs (because of vascular invasion in the orchiectomy specimen) underwent adjuvant chemotherapy consisting of two cycles of cisplatin, etoposide and bleomycin. After a median follow-up of 30 months, 2/18 (11%) of the patients in the adjuvant chemotherapy group relapsed. One of the two patients developed mature teratoma that was resected, and the other relapsed with testicular cancer which was resistant to chemotherapy. The second patient died of progressive disease. It is not surprising that chemotherapy seemingly reduced the rate of relapse in a population that would be expected to relapse at a rate of approximately 50%. Because there was no control group under observation alone, this study did not show whether or not effective chemotherapy given in the adjuvant setting would cure more people than if given only at the time of relapse. This is critical since, as with RPLND or with XRT, a large proportion of patients will be treated without need. Although chemotherapy is the most effective treatment of testicular cancer, it carries with it greater morbidity than RPLND or XRT, and therefore requires, in this setting of adjuvant therapy, justification for its routine use even in the 'high-risk' group. Furthermore, the optimal type of chemotherapy and number of cycles have not been determined.

Surveillance

Owing to the morbidity of RPLND and XRT, their suboptimal cure rates and the development of effective chemotherapy, a number of institutions have adopted the policy of surveillance for patients with CSI NSGCT and therapy at the time of relapse.[3–8, 26–31] The results of these studies are summarized in Table 3.4. Overall the relapse rate is approximately 29%, which is close to what one would expect based on the incidence of detected PSII at RPLND in addition to the incidence of relapse in patients that are PSI. Relapse rates are lower in groups of observed

Table 3.4   Surveillance programmes for non-seminomatous germ cell tumours

Series	Number of patients	Median follow-up (months)	Relapse no. (%)	Complete[a] response no. (%)	Deaths
MRC Testicular Tumour Subgroup[3]	256	30	70 (27)	69 (99)	2
Princess Margaret Hospital[27]	20	14	8 (40)	8 (100)	0
Auckland Hospital[4]	36	36	12 (33)	11 (92)	2
Institute Nazionale Tumore[5]	85	42	23 (27)	22 (96)	1
MD Anderson Hospital[6]	100	33	31 (31)	30 (97)	4
MSKCC[b8]	102	40	25 (25)	22 (88)	3
DATECA[28]	79	41	24 (30)	24 (100)	2
University Hospital Groningen[34]	54	29	11 (20)	11 (100)	0
Raghavan *et al.*[29]	46	40	13 (28)	11 (85)	2
Stanford[b30]	23	44	3 (13)	3 (100)	0
Pont *et al.*[c26]	22	30	1 (5)	1 (100)	0
Totals	823		221 (27)	212 (96)	16[d]

[a] Patients were treated with chemotherapy, surgery or both.
[b] Patients with T>1 not included.
[c] Patients with vascular invasion not included.
[d] 98% survival for total population and 92% survival of relapsed patients.

patients without high-risk features such as vascular invasion. The median time to relapse on surveillance is approximately 5 months after orchiectomy, with 80% relapsing within the first year. It is very rare for relapses to occur beyond two years after orchiectomy. Most patients who relapse will have elevated markers with or without radiological abnormalities. Since some patients recur with radiological abnormalities alone, close follow-up is mandatory. The majority of patients who relapse will have low-volume disease, so that complete response rates and cure rates are high.

The major concern with surveillance is patient compliance. Clearly, failure to comply to close surveillance increases the likelihood that relapse will be detected with more advanced disease. Moreover, a few patients will relapse and die despite adequate follow-up. Nevertheless, the survival of patients with CSI NSGCT placed on surveillance is equivalent to that of patients treated with RPLND followed by adjuvant chemotherapy. Small differences in survival between these approaches, if they exist at all, would require a large randomized study to detect. Such a trial is not likely to take place because of patient and physician treatment biases and the paucity of eligible patients.

The surveillance approach avoids treating patients unnecessarily; only those patients with disease will receive treatment. Those 30% who relapse will usually have low-volume disease and generally can be cured with 'good-risk' chemotherapy, which consists of three cycles of cisplatin, etoposide and bleomycin, or four cycles of cisplatin (or carboplatin) and etoposide. A subset of approximately 20% of these patients will require post-chemotherapy resection of residual masses. It is likely that more patients will require chemotherapy on surveillance (approximately 30%) than if routine RPLND is performed unless all patients with nodal disease are treated with adjuvant chemotherapy with two cycles of BEP. If, however, patients with nodal disease are observed after RPLND, about 15% will require chemotherapy. This may be a decisive factor in patients in whom the administration of chemotherapy is contraindicated or who have a strong aversion to it. Although surveillance has its appeal, the possibility of relapse makes it psychologically undesirable to some patients. In these patients the follow-up that is adhered to is currently very stringent, and the exact follow-up needs not clearly delineated.

Conclusions

The majority of patients with CSI NSGCTs are cured with orchiectomy alone. A portion of the remainder of patients who harbour occult disease can be cured with RPLND or even possibly XRT, and a further group cured with chemotherapy. The goal of therapy in treating CSI NSGCT is to maintain this high cure rate and minimize treatment-related morbidity. The value of lymph node irradiation in NSGCTs has long been questioned, although recent data have identified a proportion of patients cured with this approach. Routine use, however, exposes many patients unnecessarily to radiation and potentially compromises the ability of some patients to withstand later chemotherapy.

Chemotherapy, although highly effective when used as an adjuvant, is highly toxic. Until the morbidity of chemotherapy is significantly reduced and/or a benefit of adjuvant chemotherapy over chemotherapy given at the time of relapse is demonstrated, routine use of adjuvant chemotherapy even in high-risk groups cannot be justified.

The RPLND is the only therapeutic modality which offers staging information. This additional information reassures some patients and may help physicians devise a treatment strategy particularly for potentially non-compliant patients. Recent modifications in the procedure have minimized the major consequence of surgery, which is loss of fertility. RPLND will cure perhaps 15% and may contribute somewhat to the cure of about another 15% who ultimately receive chemotherapy.

Surveillance is another reasonable alternative to the treatment of selected compliant patients. Enough experience has been gained with it to suggest that if conducted properly nearly all patients will be cured. Furthermore, unnecessary treatment is avoided.

For patients without risk factors for relapse who are compliant and who do not desire staging information, surveillance seems the most reasonable management. For compliant patients with risk factors, it still seems reasonable to offer either surveillance or RPLND. It is difficult to justify routine use of adjuvant chemotherapy until a very high risk group can be identified and the use of adjuvant chemotherapy can be shown to be superior to chemotherapy at the time of relapse.

Management of seminoma

Patients with NSGCTs and patients with CSI seminomas are nearly all cured. Several features set the management of these two entities apart. Firstly, the propensity to metastasize seems to be lower for seminomas; several surveillance protocols for seminoma have demonstrated relapse rates in the 15–20% range rather than 30%. Secondly, seminoma seems to follow a more stepwise pattern of spread. Thus, the high radio-curability of CSI seminomas is due not only to their relative radio-sensitivity, but also to the rarity of occult supradiaphragmatic metastases in CSI patients. Lastly, seminomas tend to disrupt tissue planes making them less amenable to surgical extirpation.

The classic approach to CSI seminoma has been infradiaphragmatic, para-aortic and ipsilateral pelvic node irradiation. Relapse rates in most studies are less than 2% and the majority of these patients can be cured with chemotherapy. Toxicity from infradiaphragmatic irradiation is minimal. Mild nausea and vomiting can occur as well as mild bone marrow suppression. Transient oligospermia may occur but infertility is rare. The incidence of radiation-induced secondary malignancies is unknown but is probably rare if it occurs at all.

Since the majority of patients who are treated with lymph node irradiation for CSI seminoma are being treated unnecessarily, several trials of surveillance for CSI seminoma have been conducted.[32–34] In these trials, most patients who relapse are readily salvaged with XRT and/or chemotherapy. As opposed to NSGCTs, the median time to relapse in the trial by Duchesne *et al.*[34] was 15 months with 3/13 (23%) relapsing beyond three years. Thus, long-term follow-up is needed in these patients. Given the prolonged follow-up necessary and the effectiveness and minimal morbidity of lymph node irradiation, it remains the treatment of choice.

References

1. Stomper PC, Fung CY, Socinski MA, Jochelson MS, Garnick MB, Richie JP. Detection of retroperitoneal metastases in early-stage nonseminomatous testicular cancer: analysis of different CT criteria. *Am J Roentgenol* 1987; **149**: 1187–90.

2. Fung CY, Garnick MB. Clinical stage I carcinoma of the testis: a review. *J Clin Onc* 1988; **6**: 734–50.

3. Freedman LS, Jones WG, Peckham MJ, *et al.* Histopathology in the prediction of relapse of patients with stage I testicular teratoma treated by orchidectomy alone. *Lancet* 1987; **2**: 294–8.

4. Thompson PI, Nixon J, Harvey VJ. Disease relapse in patients with stage I non-seminomatous germ cell tumor of the testis on active surveillance. *J Clin Onc* 1988; **10**: 1597–603.

5. Pizzocaro G, Zanoni F, Milani A, *et al.* Orchiectomy alone in clinical stage I non-seminomatous testis cancer: a critical appraisal. *J Clin Onc* 1986; **4**: 35–40.

6. Wishnow KI, Johnson DE, Swanson DA, *et al.* Identifying patients with low-risk clinical stage I nonseminomatous testicular tumors who should be treated by surveillance. *Urology* 1989; **34**: 339–43.

7. Klepp O, Olsson AM, Henrikson H. *et al.* Prognostic factors in clinical stage I nonseminomatous germ cell tumors of the testis: multivariate analysis of a prospective multicenter study. *J Clin Onc* 1990; **8**: 509–18.

8. Sogani PC, Fair WR. Surveillance alone in the treatment of clinical stage I non-seminomatous germ cell tumor of the testis (NSGCT). *Sem Urol* 1988; **6**: 53–6.

9. Fung CY, Kalish LA, Brodsky GL, Richie JP, Garnick MB. Stage I nonseminomatous germ cell tumor: prediction of metastatic potential by primary histopathology. *J Clin Onc* 1988; **6**: 1467–73.

10. Hoskin P, Dilly S, Easton D, Horwich A, Hendry W, Peckham MF. Prognostic factors in stage I non-seminomatous germ-cell testicular tumors managed by orchiectomy and surveillance: implications for adjuvant chemotherapy. *J Clin Onc* 1986; **4**: 1031–6.

11. Marks LB, Rutgers JL, Shipley WU, *et al.* Testicular seminoma: clinical and pathological features that may predict para-aortic lymph node metastases. *J Urol* 1990; **143**: 524–7.

12. Donohue JP, Zachary JM, Maynard BR. Distribution of nodal metastases in non-seminomatous testis cancer. *J Urol* 1982; **128**: 315–20.

13. Narayan P, Lange PH, Fraley EE. Ejaculation and fertility after extended retro-peritoneal lymph node dissection for testicular cancer. *J Urol* 1982; **127**: 685–8.

14. Pizzocaro G, Salvioni R, Zanoni F. Unilateral lymphadenectomy in intraoperative stage I nonseminomatous germinal testis cancer. *J Urol* 1985; **134**: 485–9.

15. Richie JP. Clinical stage I testicular cancer: the role of modified retroperitoneal lymphadenectomy. *J Urol* 1990; **144**: 1160–3.

16. Staubitz WJ, Early KS, Magoss IV, Murphy GP. Surgical treatment of non-seminomatous germinal testis tumors. *Cancer* 1973; **32**: 1206–11.

17. Donohue JP, Einhorn LH, Perez JM. Improved management of seminomatous testis tumors. *Cancer* 1978; **42**: 2903–8.
18. Schmoll HJ, Waegener W. Adjuvant therapy in resectable stage II nonseminomatous testicular cancer. In: Jones SE, Salmon SE (eds), *Adjuvant Therapy of Cancer IV*. Philadelphia: Grune & Stratton, 1984: 539–48.
19. Williams SD, Stablein DM, Einhorn LH, *et al*. Immediate adjuvant chemotherapy versus observation with treatment at relapse in pathological stage II testicular cancer. *N Engl J Med* 1987; **317**: 1433–8.
20. Richie JP, Kantoff PW. Is adjuvant chemotherapy necessary for patients with stage B1 testicular cancer? *J Clin Onc* 1991; 1393–6.
21. Rorth M, Jacobsen GK, Madsen EL, *et al*. Prediction of relapse in stage I non-seminomatous testicular cancer. *Proceedings of ASCO* 1990; **9**: 131.
22. Skinner DG. Non-seminomatous testis tumors: a plan of management based on 96 patients to improve survival in all stages by combined therapeutic modalities. *J Urol* 1976; **115**: 65–9.
23. Ekman EP, Edsmyr F. Chemotherapy in non-seminomatous testicular tumours stage I. *Br J Urol* 1981; **53**: 184–7.
24. Ansfield FJ, Korbitz BC, Davis HL, Ramirez G. Triple drug therapy in testicular tumors. *Cancer* 1969; **24**: 442–6.
25. Sandeman TF, Yang C. Results of adjuvant chemotherapy for low-stage non-seminomatous germ cell tumours of the testis with vascular invasion. *Cancer* 1988; **62**: 1471–5.
26. Pont J, Holtl W, Kosak D, *et al*. Risk-adapted treatment choice in stage I non-seminomatous testicular germ cell cancer by regarding vascular invasion in the primary tumor: a prospective trial. *J Clin Onc* 1990; **8**: 16–20.
27. Stugeon JFG, Herman JG, Jewett MAS, Alison RE, Gospodarowicz MK, Comisarow R. A policy of surveillance alone after orchiectomy for clinical stage I non-seminomatous testis tumors. *Proc Am Soc Clin Onc* 1983; **2**: 142.
28. Rorth M, von der Maase H, Nielsen ES, Pedersen M, Schultz H. Orchidectomy alone versus orchidectomy plus radiotherapy in stage I non-seminomatous testicular cancer: a randomized study by the Danish Testicular Carcinoma Study Group. *Int J Androl* 1987; **10**: 255–62.
29. Raghavan D, Colls B, Levi J, *et al*. Surveillance for stage I non-seminomatous germ cell tumours of the testis: the optimal protocol has not yet been defined. *Br J Urol* 1988; **61**: 522–6.
30. Freiha F, Torti F. Orchiectomy only for clinical stage I nonseminomatous germ cell testis tumors: comparison with pathologic stage I disease. *Urology* 1989; **34**: 347–8.
31. Gelderman WAH, Koops HS, Sleijter DT, *et al*. Orchidectomy alone in stage I non-seminomatous testicular germ cell tumours. *Cancer* 1987; **59**: 578–80.
32. Thomas G, Gospodarowicz M, Duncan W, *et al*. A preliminary report of surveillance of stage I seminoma post orchidectomy. *Proceedings of ASCO* 1987; **6**: 109.
33. Oliver RTD. Long-term follow-up of single-agent cisplatin in metastatic seminoma and surveillance for stage I seminoma. *Proceedings of ASCO* 1988; **7**: 120.
34. Duschesne GM, Horwich A, Dearnley DP, *et al*. Orchidectomy alone for stage I seminoma of the testis. *Cancer* 1990; **65**: 1115–18.

Section II

Carcinoma of the Penis

4 Viruses and penile cancer

Nicholas James and Timothy Crook

Carcinoma of the penis is uncommon and accounts for less than 1% of adult male cancers in developed countries. In some parts of the world it is more common, accounting for 18% of cancer in areas of the Far East.[1,2] It occurs primarily in the fifth to seventh decades of life and in the uncircumcised, in whom there is a significant correlation with poor hygiene.[3] The predominant histological subtype is squamous cell carcinoma. Other subtypes are uncommon and other malignant lesions such as fibrosarcoma are rare. There is relatively little direct evidence for viral carcinogenesis in penile cancer; most of the evidence is indirect and inferred by analogy with cervical cancer.

There are two indirect lines of evidence that suggest a viral role in the aetiology of carcinoma of the penis. These are, firstly, epidemiological and, secondly, *in vitro* evidence of the transforming potential of viruses with known trophisms for genital tissues, in particular human papillomavirus (HPV) and herpes simplex virus type-2 (HSV-2). However, although the same viruses are implicated in the pathogenesis of cervical cancer,[4] there are significant epidemiological differences. In particular, cervical cancer is much more common, accounting for 4500 cases in England and Wales, compared with 300 cases of penile cancer. In addition, cervical cancer is found from the third decade onwards and is relatively uncommon in later life, the reverse of the pattern of penile cancer. It is clear, therefore, that factors other than a sexually transmissible tumourogenic virus must also be important.

Epidemiology of carcinoma of the penis

Circumcision

The association between circumcision and a low incidence of penile cancer has been long documented. When the evidence was examined in more detail it was discovered that Jews circumcised at birth had a lower incidence than Moslems circumcised in late childhood, who in turn had a lower incidence than uncircumcised men. Further, the wives of uncircumcised men had a higher incidence of cervical carcinoma.[5] This led to the hypothesis that hygiene was an important factor in the pathogenesis of penile cancers and, following from this, that smegma, retained in men with foreskins and poor hygiene, may be carcinogenic. However, more recent studies have shown that Jewish men who follow less 'orthodox' lifestyles have an increased incidence of penile carcinoma compared with their more orthodox counterparts. This suggests that the protective effect of circumcision is mediated via behavioural differences, probably sexual, associated with the strict observance of Jewish and Moslem faiths.[6]

Further evidence for this point of view comes from the inability to demonstrate convincingly that smegma is carcinogenic. For example, prolonged application of smegma to the genital mucous membranes of mice produces only hyperplasia.[7]

Epidemiological evidence for a viral aetiology

There is an increased risk of cervical cancer in the partners of men with penile cancer. There is also an increased risk of cervical cancer in the second wives of men whose first wives died of cervical cancer. Both these observations suggest a transmissible cofactor.[8]

A major component of the evidence that viruses may be aetiologically important in cervical cancer lies in the detection of particular HPV subtypes (16 and 18 in the UK) in association with cervical cancers and cervical intraepithelial neoplasia (CIN) and a lack of association with other subtypes (6 and 11 in the UK) known to cause benign lesions.[4]

Various studies have examined the prevalence of these viruses in a variety of penile lesions, and in the male sexual partners of women with cervical lesions. Studies in this latter group reveal a high incidence of asymptomatic lesions detectable by cytological/brush techniques utilizing peniscopy. HPV DNA was detectable in these lesions and was of the same range of subtypes (6, 11, 16 and 18) as found in the cervical lesions.[9] Up to 50% of male partners of women with abnormal cervical smears have HPV DNA detectable in penile smears.[10] A similar study in asymptomatic men with a history of genital condylomata revealed a 35% incidence of peniscopic lesions.[11]

Herpes simplex type-2 is another candidate for a role in viral carcinogenesis as it is known to be weakly transforming in some *in vitro* systems and can persist in an integrated form in both the male and female genital tracts. It is also associated with the development of cervical cancer, although the present consensus is that this is via its association with sexual promiscuity rather than being directly aetiologically important.

Prevalence of HPV in penile carcinomas and premalignant lesions

There is surprisingly little evidence of detection of HPV in specimens of penile cancer, perhaps because of its relative rarity. Furthermore, the reported incidence is low. For example, a study from Singapore[11] failed to find any evidence of viral structural antigens from either HPV or HSV in 20 men with penile cancers. Other workers have succeeded in isolating HPV DNA at low frequency from penile cancers.[12] These studies can be flawed on methodological grounds, however, as the techniques employed were not sufficiently sensitive to detect integrated DNA reliably (*vide infra*), and expression of structural antigens is not normally found in tissues transformed by viruses so that their absence does not signify absence of the virus. Appropriately controlled studies utilizing the polymerase chain reaction (PCR) to evaluate the prevalence of DNA sequences from the transforming HPV types will allow more definitive conclusions to be drawn concerning the putative role of HPV in penile carcinoma. When carefully controlled and scrupulously executed, PCR allows significantly greater sensitivity in the detection of viral DNA than conventional analytical techniques, and has been used extensively in cervical cancer.[13] No large series of penile cancers studied using PCR has been published.

There is a case report of the detection of HPV in a patient with penile bowenoid papulosis,[14] a premalignant lesion. Further information will be required to assess the potential significance of this finding.

In vitro evidence supporting a viral aetiology

Two obvious leading candidates for a sexually transmissible agent involved in the pathogenesis of anogenital cancers are human papillomavirus (HPV) and herpes simplex virus (HSV) type-2. Human papillomaviruses are associated with proliferative lesions in a variety of tissues and frequently exhibit tight tissue trophisms. Studies examining the ability of HPV to transform various types have shown that penile, cervical and laryngeal tissues are transformable in a high proportion of cases, whereas other epithelial tissues are transformed at low frequency or not at all.

Strong support for a role for HPV, rather than HSV-2, in the aetiology of anogenital cancers is provided by the large body of convincing evidence of the transforming potential of particular HPV types in rodent and human *in vitro* systems, whereas compelling evidence for a transforming effect of HSV-2 has been much more difficult to demonstrate. Preliminary studies performed in established rodent cell lines showed a transforming function for both HPV types 16 and 18, the principal malignantly-associated HPV types. Additional studies, using primary cultures of rodent cells, clearly demonstrated that HPV-16 encodes an immortalizing phenotype, which, in cooperation with an activated *ras* or *fos* oncogene, can malignantly transform cells. Furthermore, maintenance of the transformed phenotype of the cells required continual expression of the E7 open reading frame of HPV-16, clearly showing that HPV encodes a specific transforming function, and does not operate by a 'hit-and-run' mechanism.

The most compelling experimental evidence of a role for HPV rather than HSV in genital cancer has come from analysis of HPV proteins in primary human foreskin and cervical keratinocytes. These cells are very much more recalcitrant than the rodent cells employed in early studies which are easily immortalized. However, DNA from the malignantly-associated HPV types 16, 18, 31 and 33, when transfected into primary keratinocytes, is able to 'immortalize' these cells quite efficiently. Significantly, the immortalized cells show markedly increased resistance to differentiation-inducing signals such as calcium and transforming growth-factor beta. The so-called benign HPV types, 6 and 11, are unable to immortalize these cells, further supporting a specific role for the malignant types in genital cancer. Despite the ability of the malignant HPV types to immortalize primary genital keratinocytes, the cell lines so produced are not fully transformed as they do not have a tumourogenic phenotype. This closely parallels the situation in human anogenital cancers, where it is abundantly clear that factors in addition to HPV are essential for the development of carcinoma, as is the case for smoking and HPV in cervical cancer.

One of the most important areas of HPV research is the identification of the genetic and epigenetic factors which facilitate the progression of HPV-related lesions to carcinoma. In this context HSV-2 is of great interest. This virus has a number of characteristics usually associated with chemical or physical carcinogens. Transfection of HSV-2 DNA into keratinocytes immortalized by HPV-16 confers a tumourogenic phenotype to the cells, although the HSV-2 sequences are lost on subsequent passaging of the cells, suggesting that some form of hit-and-run mechanism might be operative in this system. The clinical significance of this type of *in vitro* data awaits further epidemiological analysis.

Conclusions

In conclusion there is epidemiological evidence for a transmissible agent in the aetiology of penile cancer. The most likely candidates are the human papillomaviruses on the basis of their trophism for genital tissue, their high prevalence and their transforming ability *in vitro*. However, despite the similarities with cervical cancer, the much lower incidence of penile cancer and its later age at onset suggest that other factors must also be important. Definitive evidence of a viral aetiology is still lacking.

References

1. Paulson DF, Perez CA, Anderson T. Cancer of the urethra and penis. In: DeVita VT, Hellman S, Rosenberg SA (eds), *Cancer: Principles and Practice of Oncology*, 2nd edn. Philadelphia: Lippincott, 1985.
2. Harris RE, Hebert JR, Wynder EL. Cancer risk in male veterans utilizing the Veterans Administration medical system. *Cancer* 1989; **64**: 1160–8.
3. American Academy of Pediatrics. Report of the Task Force on circumcision. *Pediatrics* 1989; **84**: 388–91.
4. Vousden KH. Human papillomaviruses and cervical cancer. *Cancer Cells* 1989; **1**: 43–50.
5. Hochman A, Ratzkowski E, Schreiber H. Incidence of carcinoma of the cervix in Jewish women in Israel. *Br J Cancer* 1955; **9**: 358–64.

6. Coppleson M. Carcinoma of the cervix: epidemiology and aetiology. *Br J Hosp Med* 1969; **2**: 961–80.
7. Reddy DG, Baruah IKSM. Carcinogenic action of human smegma. *Arch Pathol (Chicago)* 1963; **75**: 414–20.
8. Cessler I. Human cervix cancer as a venereal disease. *Cancer Res* 1979; **36**: 738–40.
9. Levine RU, Crum CP, Herman E, Silvers D, Ferenczy A, Richart RM. Cervical papillomavirus infection and intraepithelial neoplasia: a study of male sexual partners. *Obstet Gynecol* 1984; **64**: 16–20.
10. Schneider A, Schumann R, De Villiers EM, Knauf W, Gissman L. Klinische Bedeutung von humanen Papilloma-Virus-(HPV)-Infektionen im unteren Genitaltrakt (Clinical significance of human papilloma virus (HPV) infections of the lower genital tract). *Geburtshilfe frauenheilkd* 1986; **46**: 261–6.
11. Rosemburg SK. Subclinical papilloma viral infection of male genitalia. *Urology* 1985; **25**: 554–7.
12. Raju GC, Lee YS. Role of herpes simplex type-2 and human papillomavirus in penile cancers in Singapore. *Ann Acad Med Singapore* 1987; **16**: 550–1.
13. Young LS, Bevan IS, Johnson MA, *et al.* The polymerase chain reaction: a new epidemiological tool for investigating cervical human papillomavirus infection. *Br Med J* 1989; **298**: 14–18.
14. Guillet GY, Braun L, Masse R, Aftimos J, Geniaux M, Texier L. Bowenoid papulosis: demonstration of human papillomavirus (HPV) with anti-HPV immune serum. *Arch Dermatol* 1984; **120**: 514–6.

5 Surgery, radiotherapy and chemotherapy in penile cancer

CJ Gallagher, RTD Oliver, HF Hope-Stone and JP Blandy

Squamous or epidermoid carcinoma of the penis arises in 95% of cases in the prepuce, glans, or coronal sulcus.[1-3] It is a rare malignancy in the western developed world, occurring in 1 in 100000 men and forming 0.5–2% of all malignancies in males. However, the incidence is 5–10 times higher in populations who neither have access to good genital hygiene nor practise neonatal circumcision.[4] While human papillomavirus infection may be a contributory factor in this typical presentation (*qv*), the genital skin has long been known to show increased sensitivity to carcinogens,[5] with more recent evidence for an association between smoking[6] and ultraviolet radiation[7] and an increased incidence of squamous carcinoma of the genital skin compared with other areas of the body. However, these latter factors may be more associated with squamous carcinomas of the shaft of the penis rather than the classical lesions of prepuce or glans. Rarely, the penis may also be the primary site of other tumours such as basal cell carcinoma, melanoma, soft tissue sarcoma, and lymphoma, when their behaviour is governed by a tendency to early dissemination through both haematogenous and lymphatic channels. When Kaposi's sarcoma, in association with human immunodeficiency virus (HIV) infection, involves the genital skin, the other manifestations of the AIDS syndrome make the diagnosis evident. Metastatic involvement of the penis in the later stages of prostate or bladder cancer usually occurs in the presence of advanced pelvic tumour, although at an earlier stage bladder cancer may present as Paget's disease of the glans with intradermal spread of transitional cell carcinoma from the meatus in continuity with the bladder tumour.[4]

Diagnosis and staging

Carcinoma of the penis usually presents in an 'elderly neglected patient with an inflamed irretractable prepuce from which there issues a stinking discharge'.[4] The surrounding cellulitis and reactive lymphadenopathy make clinical staging notoriously inaccurate, and the diagnostic circumcision and biopsy should be performed under antibiotic cover while definitive treatment is planned. Squamous carcinoma of the penis tends to spread locally and via the lymphatic drainage. The skin of the penis and prepuce drain bilaterally to the superficial inguinal nodes while the glans and corpora drain to both the superficial inguinal and to the deep inguinal and iliac nodes.[8] While more than half the patients will present with palpable inguinal lymph nodes, the clinical assessment of the inguinal lymph nodes with respect to metastatic involvement has a false-negative rate of 10–38% and a false-positive rate of 40–60%.[8,10] Biopsy of a sentinel node[11] located medial and proximal to the junction of the superficial epigastric and saphenous veins has been advocated in order to predict metastatic involvement and avoid surgical treatment of those free of metastases. However, this has not been further validated in prospective series and exceptions have been reported[12] with rapid recurrence in inguinal nodes despite a negative sentinel node biopsy.

Staging is most often described according to the system of Jackson[12] in which, in stage 1, the lesion is confined to the foreskin or glans, in stage 2 there is invasion of the shaft, in stage 3 the inguinal nodes are involved but operable, and in stage 4 the disease has invaded the perineum or scrotum, or the lymph nodes are fixed and inoperable, or there are distant metastases. The other clinical staging system of Johnson[14] is more attuned to the surgical management of the disease; stage 1 confined to penis and able to be amputated, stage 2 with operable lymphatic involvement, and stage 3 inoperable. The TNM classification[15] has the advantage of further specifying the degree of nodal involvement or local invasion, but for practical purposes in planning radiotherapeutic and surgical management, Jackson's system is sufficient. Less invasive tests to establish the nodal status have been poorly assessed, however, lymphography is difficult to interpret in the inguinal region in the presence of potentially reactive changes, and enlargement on computed tomographic scanning (CT scan) or magnetic resonance imaging is equally non-specific. CT scan can reduce the number of patients considered for surgical evaluation by demonstrating more distant metastases (e.g. para-aortic lymphadenopathy) and can potentially allow the collection of cytological specimens by CT-scan-guided fine-needle aspirate from enlarged nodes following which the potential benefit of further surgical treatment can be better assessed.

Surgical management

Treatment of the primary lesion by circumcision alone is adequate for small tumours localized to the prepuce, which constitute up to 30% of some series. However, these tumours are still accompanied by the risk of inguinal metastases, and the patients must be observed carefully at follow-up as nodal recurrence may still be fully salvageable by delayed surgery[16] or radiotherapy. Surgery for more extensive lesions by partial penectomy requires the careful examination of frozen sections at the time of operation to ensure a 2 cm margin of normal shaft, as the extension, particularly in the periurethral region, may be more extensive than is macro-scopically apparent.[4] Total penectomy with excision of both corpora and creation of a perineal urethrostomy is required for lesions which approach the base of the shaft. Adequate surgery as defined above is reported to have a less than 10% local failure rate but is necessarily accompanied by loss of normal function and potentially severe psychological morbidity, including the risk of suicide.[17]

Surgery of the regional lymph nodes

Dissection of the inguinal and iliac lymph nodes is the only present means by which an accurate assessment of the extent of lymphatic spread of the penile cancer can be made, though even by this method there may be a 17% false-negative (i.e. subsequent local failure) rate.[18] Prognostication is made more accurate by lymphadenectomy since the risk of relapse increases with the involvement of increasing numbers of nodes[19,20] and with the involvement of the (more distant) iliac nodes.[8] While nodal involvement generally becomes more likely with in-creasingly advanced local disease, 40–60% of those with clinically palpable lymphadenopathy will show evidence of reactive changes associated with infec-tion.[8,10] The only exception is the lymphadenopathy associated with penile lesions restricted to the prepuce or glans, when 80% of the enlarged nodes are likely to contain metastatic carcinoma and are indicative of a poor prognosis.[21]

Impetus for the performance of primary lymphadenectomy as a therapeutic manoeuvre has come from the reported 50–65% five-year disease-free survival following lymphadenectomy for stage 3 disease.[18,22] Others, however, have not had such favourable results, with 17% five-year survival.[23,24] The morbidity of bilateral lymphadenectomy is considerable, with all patients experiencing a degree of lymphoedema which may become severe (i.e. crippling) in 5–25% of patients.[4]

In view of the morbidity and the uncertain benefits, many have attempted to assess retrospectively whether delaying operation until the lymph nodes are obviously clinically involved is associated with as good an outcome as operating at the time of presentation. As a result, opinions both for[16,25] and against[18,20] have been formed, but neither can be substantiated because of the usual problems of small numbers and potential selection bias which limit the degree to which conclusions can be generalized to future patients. The sentinel node biopsy[11] has also been proposed as a means of limiting the use of lymphadenectomy to a therapeutic role and avoiding operation on the 40–60% of patients with clinically palpable but pathologically uninvolved lymph nodes. This, however, has not been prospectively tested and cannot alter the likely morbidity of those operated on.

The great variability of the results of surgery for lymphatic involvement may be due more to variations in patient selection than technique. Surgical cure of such (regionally) disseminated disease must imply a process of relatively limited metastatic potential, and indeed prognosis can be related to the primary tumour characteristics of differentiation and invasiveness.[21] In the context of the typical elderly patient, the variable success but considerable morbidity of lymphadenectomy has led European practice to seek non-operative means of treatment while American centres have continued to pursue the surgical cure of advanced disease.[18,20] Those who benefit most from an operative approach seem to be patients with well-differentiated tumours and minimal inguinal lymph node involvement, since prognosis becomes increasingly worse with the number of nodes involved,[19,20] and surgical cure most unlikely once pelvic nodes are involved.[8] Such a patient, though necessarily difficult to select, may still be offered bilateral lymphadenectomy with a high possibility of cure, particularly if he is of a relatively younger age group and well motivated to overcome the problems that lymphoedema may bring. For the remainder it is to be hoped that advances in the use of radiotherapy and chemotherapy will lead to higher rates of cure or control for the remainder of their life.

Radiotherapy

Early series on the radiotherapy of carcinoma of the penis reported variable but low success rates with a high incidence of stricture and other complications. Modern high-energy external-beam treatment[22,26,27] or the iridium mould[28] with its urethra-sparing characteristics, achieve considerably better results equivalent to those of surgery in stage 1 with preservation of function (Table 5.1). The mould technique requires a cooperative patient and a tumour that is not too advanced to be encompassed by the mould. Either technique achieves complete local disease control in 80–90% of stage 1 patients.[21,29,30] Up to 20% of patients may still require a salvage penectomy if the disease is not completely ablated, and urethral stricture may occur in a further 20%; thus careful surveillance following treatment is

Table 5.1 Comparison of surgery and radiotherapy for stage I disease

Number	Local recurrence (%)	Five-year survival (%)	Authors
Surgery for stage I			
27	19	70	Jackson (1966)[13]
33	9	60	Gursel *et al.* (1973)[49]
7	0	86	Kreig and Luke (1981)[50]
129	–	57	Narayana *et al.* (1982)[23]
Radiotherapy for stage I with salvage surgery			
36	–	89	Engelstad (1948)[51]
63	38	46	Murrell and Williams (1965)[52]
58	14	66	Jackson (1966)[13]
29	41	90	Almgard and Edsmyr (1973)[53]
29	–	66	Johnson *et al.* (1973)[54]
65	49	70	Pointin (1975)[29]
10	10	90	Grabstald (1980)[9]
6	10	83	Kreig and Luke (1981)[50]
33	36	85	El-Demiry *et al.* (1984)[21]

mandatory but the majority may avoid mutilating surgery. Late sequelae of treatment may include some degree of telangectasia, and in long-term survivors there is the possibility of second tumour induction as at any other site in the body.[31] Thus for the younger patient follow-up should be life-long.

Radiotherapy for more advanced stage 2 disease is associated with a much higher rate of local recurrence of 70–80%.[21] The impact on survival may be lessened somewhat by the higher proportion dying of metastatic disease (20–30%), so that for palliation in the frail and/or elderly patient local radiation may be all that is required for symptom control and (temporary) relief from the distress of a fungating lesion.

If radical radiotherapy is administered by external-beam therapy to include the regional lymphatics, it may be successful in up to 67% of those with biopsy-proven nodal involvement.[21,29] Such treatment is not without its problems, however, with acute moist desquamation and ulceration in the perineum and later lymphoedema especially in those with extensive nodal involvement. Bulky disease here as elsewhere is less likely to respond well, and there may be some advantage in chemotherapeutic down-staging before irradiation. Cure can still be achieved in some patients with the most advanced local disease with radical external-beam therapy and should remain the aim in those free of other debilitating disease.[32,33]

Chemotherapy

The greatest experience has been gained with bleomycin in the treatment of advanced or recurrent disease. Bleomycin has been given to large numbers of patients. Ichikawa[34] in Japan reported a 12/24 response rate across all stages of the disease and 123/164 responses in patients given combined therapy with either surgery and/or radiotherapy. Other smaller series with patients with stage 3 or 4 disease report a 21–25% response for a median duration of three months (Table 5.2).[35,36]

Methotrexate has been the subject of many anecdotal case reports.[37] One series of 13 patients demonstrated a 62% response for both low and intermediate dose treatment.[38]

Cisplatinum in two small series achieved a 50% response for 1–8 months,[38–40] although a recent multicentre trial failed to confirm this with 4/26 (15%) partial remissions of only 1–3 months duration.[41] This experience may be a more accurate estimate of the response or reflect the large proportion who had recurrent disease following radiotherapy.

Combination chemotherapy has not been tested against single-agent treatment to demonstrate that it is necessarily superior and there are few reported trials. Chemotherapy with methotrexate, vincristine and bleomycin in five patients produced three partial remissions,[42] and cisplatinum and 5-fluorouracil achieved 5/5 partial remissions for 1–12 months[43] though at greater toxicity. In the experience of the authors the combination of cisplatinum, vinblastine and methotrexate has produced responses in 4/6 patients with advanced nodal metastases and may be

Table 5.2 Chemotherapy for advanced carcinoma of the penis

Drug	Number	Dose	Response	Duration	Authors
Bleomycin	14	Various	3CR (21%)	3mo (med)	Ahmed *et al.* (1984)[38]
Bleomycin	4	Various	1PR (25%)	–	Matreev and Gotsadze (1981)[35]
Bleomycin	15	30–60 mg	3CR+11PR (93%)	–	Kyalwazi *et al.* (1974)[55]
Bleomycin	24	15 mg	12CR+PR (50%)	–	Ichikawa (1977)[34]
Methotrexate	5	250–1500 mg/m²	3CR (60%)	–	Ahmed *et al.* (1984)[38]
Methotrexate	8	30–40 mg/m²	5CR (63%)	–	Ahmed *et al.* (1984)[38]
Cisplatin	6	120 mg/m²	3PR (50%)	1–7mo	Yagoda (1979)[39]
Cisplatin	6	120 mg/m²	1CR+2PR (50%)	2–8mo	Sklaroff and Yagoda (1979)[40]
Cisplatin	26	50 mg/m²×2	4PR (15%)	1–3mo	Gagliano *et al.* (1989)[41]
Combinations					
Cisplatin + 5-fluorouracil	5	100 mg/m² 960 mg/m²×5	5PR (100%)	1–12mo	Hussein *et al.* (1990)[43]
Cisplatin + vinblastine + methotrexate	6	60 mg/m² 6 mg/m² 60 mg/m²	4PR (66%)	2–18mo	Oliver (unpublished)
Methotrexate + vincristine + bleomycin	5	30 mg 1 mg 15 mg×2	3PR (60%)	–	Pizzocarro and Piva (1988)[42]

combined with subsequent radiotherapy for remissions lasting up to 18 months and with marked symptomatic relief from fungating and painful disease for the remainder.

Several of the series report on the use of preoperative chemotherapy to render previously fixed inguinal nodes smaller and more mobile, thus converting previously unresectable disease to a state more readily removed.[44] Not surprisingly in view of the short durations of response in most chemotherapy series, all these surgical specimens have contained residual tumour. Present combination chemotherapy may find a role in the future as an adjunct to local therapy with surgery or radiotherapy, as has been successfully demonstrated in the combined therapy of squamous carcinomas elsewhere.[45,46]

Immunotherapy

While there is no evidence that any biological agent is active in squamous cancer of the penis, there is evidence of interferon activity against the papillomavirus associated condylomata[47,48] and recent dramatic responses with low doses of interleukin-2 in squamous cancers of the head and neck.[49] Combination of chemotherapeutic cytoreduction with immunotherapy for the treatment of residual tumour may yet prove successful in this group of slow-growing epithelial malignancies. Answers to this and other problems in the management of carcinoma of the penis in the future will require the collaboration of the individual centres in group studies to place the treatment of such a relatively rare disease on a more scientific basis.

Conclusions

Stage 1 disease may be equally well treated by local surgery or radiotherapy alone with the balance being tipped in favour of radiotherapy by the possibility of preserving normal function in 80% of patients.

In stage 2 and 3 disease, surgery will provide superior local control for the otherwise fit patient at the expense of partial or complete amputation. On the basis of tumour histology and clinical investigations, it is possible to select a minority of patients with well-differentiated disease limited to the inguinal region for whom bilateral lymphadenectomy will be both appropriate and curative. For most, radiotherapy with, in the setting of a clinical trial, the addition of chemotherapy can still be curative in up to two-thirds of patients, and avoids the morbidity of extensive surgical resection. The latter is particularly relevant for the majority of patients who will be elderly, frail and subject to other concurrent illness of greater relevance to their long-term survival.

Palliation of advanced disease may be satisfactorily achieved in the elderly patient by radiotherapy alone; but in the younger patient, more experimental approaches combining chemotherapy and the use of biological agents such as interleukin and interferon offer hope for future improvements in the management of advanced carcinoma of the penis.

References

1. Bassett JW. Carcinoma of the penis. *Cancer* 1952; **5**: 530–5.
2. Jensen MS. Cancer of the penis in Denmark 1942 to 1962 (511 cases). *Danish Med Bull* 1977; **24**: 66–72.
3. Yu HHY, Lam P, Leong CN, Ong GB. Carcinoma of the penis: report of 52 cases with reference to lymphography and ilioinguinal block dissection. *Clin Onc* 1978; **4**: 47–53.
4. Blandy JP, Hope-Stone HF, Oliver RTD. Carcinoma of the penis and urethra. In: Oliver RTD, Blandy JP, Hope-Stone HF (eds), *Urological and Genital Cancer*. Oxford: Blackwell Scientific, 1989: 258–71.

5. Pott P. *Chirurgical Observations Relative to the Cataract, the Polypus of the Nose, the Cancer of the Scrotum, the Different Kinds of Ruptures and the Mortifications of the Toes and Feet.* London: L Hawes, W Clarke & R Collins, 1775.

6. Hellberg D, Valentin J, Eklund T, Nilsson. Penile cancer: is there an epidemiological role for smoking and sexual behaviour? *Br Med J* 1987; **295**: 1306–8.

7. Stern RS. Genital tumours among men with psoriasis exposed to psoralens and ultraviolet A radiation (PUVA) and ultraviolet B radiation. *N Eng J Med* 1990; **322**: 1093–7.

8. Skinner DG, Leadbetter WF, Kelley SB. The surgical management of squamous cell carcinoma of the penis. *J Urol* 1972; **107**: 273–7.

9. Grabstald H. Controversies concerning lymph node dissection for cancer of the penis. *Urol Clin – Am* 1980; **7**: 793–9.

10. Kossow JH, Hotchkiss RS, Morales PA. Carcinoma of the penis treated surgically: analysis of 100 cases. *Urology* 1973; **2**: 169–72.

11. Cabanas RM. An approach for the treatment of penile carcinoma. *Cancer* 1977; **39**: 456–66.

12. Perinetti E, Crane DB, Catalona WJ. Unreliability of sentinel lymph node biopsy for staging penile carcinoma. *J Urol* 1980; **124**: 734–5.

13. Jackson SM. The treatment of carcinoma of the penis. *Br J Surg* 1966; **53**: 33–5.

14. Johnson DE. Carcinoma of the penis—overview. In: Johnson DE, Boileau MA (eds), *Genitourinary Tumours: Fundamental Principles and Surgical Technique.* New York: Grune & Stratton, 1982: 181–209.

15. Spiessl B, Scheibe O, Wagner G (eds). Penis. In: *UICC TNM Atlas: Illustrated Guide to the Classification of Malignant Tumours.* Berlin: Springer-Verlag, 1982: 166–9.

16. Ekstrom T, Edsmyr F. Cancer of the penis: a clinical study of 229 cases. *Acta Chir Scand* 1958; **115**: 25–45.

17. Hanash KA, Furlow WL, Utz DC, Harrison EG. Carcinoma of the penis: a clinico-pathological study. *J Urol* 1970; **104**: 291–7.

18. McDougal WS, Kirchner FK, Edwards RH, Killion LT. Treatment of carcinoma of the penis: the case for primary lymphadenectomy. *J Urol* 1986; **136**: 38–41.

19. Baker BH. Carcinoma of the penis. *Urology* 1976; **116**: 458–64.

20. Johnson DE, Lo RK. Management of regional lymph nodes in penile carcinoma. *Urology* 1984; **24**: 308–311.

21. El-Demiry MIM, Oliver RTD, Hope-Stone HF, Blandy JP. Reappraisal of the role of radiotherapy and surgery in the management of carcinoma of the penis. *Br J Urol* 1984; **56**: 724–8.

22. Hardner GJ, Bhanalaph T, Murphy GP, Albert DJ, Moore RH. Carcinoma of the penis: analysis of therapy in 100 consecutive cases. *J Urol* 1972; **108**: 428–30.

23. Narayana AS, Olney LE, Leoning SA, Weimar GW, Culp DA. Carcinoma of the penis: analysis of 219 cases. *Cancer* 1982; **49**: 2185–91.

24. Nelson RP, Derrick FC, Allen WR. Epidermoid carcinoma of the penis. *Br J Urol* 1982; **54**: 172–5.

25. Lesser JH, Schwarz H. External genital cancer: results of treatment at Ellis Fischel State Cancer Hospital. *Cancer* 1955; **8**: 1021–5.

26. Lederman M. Radiotherapy of cancer of the penis. *Br J Urol* 1953; **25**: 224–32.

27. Knudsen OS, Brennhovd IO. Radiotherapy in the treatment of the primary tumour in penile cancer. *Acta Chir Scand* 1967; **133**: 69–71.

28. Hope-Stone HF. Carcinoma of the penis. *Proc R Soc Med* 1975; **68**: 777–9.

29. Pointin RCS. External beam therapy. *Proc R Soc Med* 1975; **68**: 779–81.

30. Haile K, Delclos L. The place of radiation therapy in the treatment of carcinoma of the distal end of the penis. *Cancer* 1980; **45**: 1980–4.
31. Wells AD, Pryor JP. Radiation-induced carcinoma of the penis. *Br J Urol* 1986; **58**: 325–6.
32. Sagerman RH, Yu WS, Chung CT, Puranik A. External beam irradiation of carcinoma of the penis. *Radiology* 1984; **152**: 183–5.
33. Kearsley JH, Roberts SJ, Kynaston B. Curative radiotherapy for stage 4 carcinoma of the penis. *Med J Aus* 1986; **3**: 474–5.
34. Ichikawa T. Chemotherapy of penis carcinoma. *Rec Results Cancer Res* 1977; **60**: 140–56.
35. Matreev BP, Gotsadze DT. Chemotherapy of penile carcinoma. *Urol Nefrol (Mosk)* 1981; **4**: 39–42.
36. Ahmed T, Sklaroff R, Yagoda A. An appraisal of the efficacy of bleomycin in epidermoid carcinoma of the penis. *Anticancer Res* 1984; **4**: 289–92.
37. Garnick MB, Skarin AT, Steele GD. Metastatic carcinoma of the penis: complete remission after high-dose methotrexate chemotherapy. *J Urol* 1979; **122**: 265–6.
38. Ahmed T, Sklaroff R, Yagoda A. Sequential trials of methotrexate, cisplatin and bleomycin for penile cancer. *J Urol* 1984; **132**: 465–8.
39. Yagoda A. Phase 2 trials with cis-dichlorodiammine platinum (2) in the treatment of urothelial cancer. *Cancer Treat Rep* 1979; **63**: 1656–60.
40. Sklaroff RB, Yagoda A. Cis-diamminedichloride platinum 2(DDP) in the treatment of penile carcinoma. *Cancer* 1979; **44**: 1563–7.
41. Gagliano RG, Blumenstein BA, Crawford EE, Stephens RL, Coltman CA, Costanzi JJ. Cis-diamminedichloroplatinum in the treatment of advanced epidermoid carcinoma of the penis: a Southwest Oncology Group study. *J Urol* 1989; **141**: 66–7.
42. Pizzocaro G, Piva I. Adjuvant and neoadjuvant vincristine, bleomycin and methotrexate for the inguinal metastases from squamous cell carcinoma of the penis. *Acta Onc* 1988; **27**: 823–4.
43. Hussein AM, Benedetto P, Sridhar KS. Chemotherapy with cisplatin and 5-fluorouracil for penile and urethral squamous cell carcinomas. *Cancer* 1990; **65**: 433–8.
44. Abratt RP, Barnes RD, Pontin AR. The treatment of clinically fixed inguinal lymph node metastases from carcinoma of the penis by chemotherapy and surgery. *Eur J Surg Onc* 1989; **15**: 285–6.
45. Cummings B, Keane T, Thomas G, Harwood A, Rider W. Results and toxicity of the treatment of anal canal carcinoma by radiation therapy or radiation therapy and chemotherapy. *Cancer* 1984; **54**: 2062–8.
46. Weisberg JB, Son YH, Papac RJ, Sasaki C, Fischer DB, Lawrence R, Rockwell S, Sartorelli AC, Fischer JJ. Randomized clinical trial of mitomycin C as an adjunct to radiotherapy in head and neck cancer. *Int J Rad Onc Biol Phys* 1989; **17**: 3–9.
47. Scott GM, Csonka GW. Effect of small doses of human fibroblast interferon into genital warts. *Ven Dis* 1979; **55**: 442–5.
48. Schonfield A, Schattner A, Crespi M. Intramuscular human interferon B injections in treatment of condylomata acuminata. *Lancet* 1984; **i**: 1038–42.
49. Gursel EO, Georgountzos C, Uson AC, Melicow MM, Veenema RJ. Penile cancer: a clinicopathologic study of 64 cases. *Urology* 1973; **1**: 569–78.
50. Krieg RM, Luk KH. Carcinoma of the penis: review of cases treated by surgery and radiation therapy 1960–1977. *Urology* 1981; **18**: 149–54.
51. Englestad RB. Treatment of cancer of the penis at the Norwegian Radium Hospital. *AJR* 1948; **60**: 801–6.

52. Murrell DS, Williams JL. Radiotherapy in the treatment of carcinoma of the penis. *Br J Urol* 1965; **37**: 211–21.
53. Almgard LE, Edsmyr F. Radiotherapy in treatment of patients with carcinoma of the penis. *Scand J Urol Nephrol* 1973; **7**: 1–5.
54. Johnson DE, Fuerst EE, Ayala AC. Carcinoma of the penis: experience with 153 cases. *Urology* 1973; **1**: 404–6.
55. Kyalwazi SK, Bhana D, Harrison NW. Carcinoma of the penis and bleomycin chemotherapy in Uganda. *Br J Urol* 1974; **46**: 689–96.

6 Surgery in the management of lymph nodes in penile cancer

David F Badenoch

The management of inguinal lymph nodes in carcinoma of the penis remains the greatest area of controversy in this disease. This is in part due to the relative rarity of carcinoma of the penis which, in the UK, represents less than 1% of all male cancers. In addition, the inability to evaluate regional lymph nodes satisfactorily and the differing and firmly held philosophical positions in treating the condition radically or conservatively add to the difficulties in management. Its low incidence has led to a lack of controlled prospective studies, and a number of controversial questions need to be answered.

Anatomy and pathology of penile cancer

Lymphatic drainage

The lymphatic anatomy of the penis has been studied in detail by Rouvière.[1,2] It has been shown that the lymphatics of the prepuce and penile skin converge on the dorsum of the penis and coalesce into several trunks. These course together towards the base of the penis and then separate to end bilaterally at the superficial inguinal lymph nodes, particularly the superomedial group. The superficial group of lymph nodes is composed of between 4 and 25 glands (average 8) located in the deep membranous layer of the superficial fascia of the thigh (Camper's fascia). This group then drains into the deep inguinal lymph nodes lying along the femoral vessels within the femoral sheath. There is an extension into the extraperitoneal fatty area through which the external iliac vessels run.

The lymphatics arising from the glans penis are somewhat more complicated. All lymphatics of the glans initially converge on the frenulum and then ascend around the corona to pass on to the dorsum of the penis as between one and four layers of lymphatic trunks. In the region of the suspensory ligament of the penis, these trunks are said to anastomose to form the pre-symphysial lymphatic plexus. From this pre-symphysial area, Rouvière described different pathways that end in the nodes of the superficial and deep inguinal, external iliac and hypogastric regions. The corpora cavernosa are also drained by lymphatic trunks that run beside the dorsal vein of the penis in the region of the pre-symphysial plexus and then anastomose to join the same pathways. They additionally drain directly to deep inguinal and external iliac lymph nodes. Other authors have disputed some of Rouvière's description; in particular, Riveros *et al.*,[3] studying penile lymphangiograms, have never found an iliac lymph node involvement in carcinoma of the penis without inguinal involvement or pre-symphysial involvement. Whitmore questions the possibility of pre-symphysial relay or a direct iliac and hypogastric pathway.[4]

Cabanas, studying 100 penile lymphograms, demonstrated that the superomedial group of superficial inguinal lymph nodes on either side acted as the first lymph node pathway for lymphatics originating in the glans penis.[5] This he called the 'sentinel lymph node' and it is frequently located at the anterior or medial aspect of the superficial epigastric vein, medial to and above the epigastric–saphenous junction. Cabanas did not find that the so-called pre-pubic lymph node or any lymphatic vessels drained directly to the iliac lymph nodes, and he felt that no metastases invaded other inguinal lymph nodes when the sentinel node was disease-free. Thus some controversy in the anatomy of the lymphatic drainage of the penis remains.

Patterns of metastatic spread

Fraley *et al.* have looked into the importance of histological differentiation of the primary penile tumour and the frequency of lymphatic spread in sqaumous cell carcinoma of the penis.[6] They found in a group of 58 patients that, in the 23 cases having a carcinoma-in-situ or well-differentiated disease, only one became metastatic to the lymph nodes; while of the remaining 35 cases of moderately to poorly differentiated disease, 31 metastasized at the groin. Where there was shown to be vascular invasion of the cancer in the primary tumour, this indicated a particularly high correlation with lymphatic metastases.

Patients with carcinoma of the penis having inguinal metastases who do not undergo treatment of the metastases rarely survive two years and almost never survive five years. No spontaneous regression of penile carcinoma has been reported, but 20–50% of patients with inguinal node mestastases who are treated by inguinal lymphadenectomy achieve a five-year disease-free survival.[7–9] The presence of palpable lymphadenopathy at initial presentation of carcinoma of the penis does not inevitably indicate the presence of tumour. Indeed, a false-positive rate of up to 50% has been recorded by many authors and is related to enlargement caused by inflammation and secondary infection. The persistence of inguinal lymphadenopathy after treatment of the primary tumour and a course of antibiotics, or the appearance of lymphadenopathy during follow-up (or both of these possibilities), is much more likely to be due to metastases than an inflammatory reaction. Conversely, from information gathered on those practising radical lymphadenectomy routinely as part of the surgery for early carcinoma of the penis, it has been found that lymph nodes may be histologically positive for malignancy when clinically impalpable in an incidence ranging from 2% to 25%.[7,9–11]

Surgical management of penile cancer

There are a number of controversies that need resolution. Should inguinal lymphadenectomy be performed only in those patients having carcinoma of the penis with palpable lymph nodes after treatment of the primary lesion, or should such surgery be performed on a prophylactic basis and carried out at the time of the primary treatment whether these lymph nodes are palpable or not? Should bilateral or unilateral lymphadenectomy be carried out, or should this depend on the presence of positive sentinel lymph node biopsy? Should lymphadenectomy be extended to include the pelvic lymph nodes?

The case for an initially conservative approach

Although the incidence of palpable inguinal lymph nodes in patients presenting with carcinoma of the penis ranges from 25% to 60%, approximately one-third to one-half of this group will have negative findings on histological examination of the resected lymph nodes; but as has been stated above, approximately 20% of patients with lymph nodes not clinically suspicious will contain metastases. Thus, as Richie points out,[12] the decision for inguinal lymphadenectomy should be based on several factors: the likelihood of metastatic spread to the lymph nodes, the potential benefit gained from regional lymphadenectomy in terms of survival, and the morbidity associated with the surgical procedure. Because enlarged lymph nodes are common in carcinoma of the penis and generally reflect an inflammatory response to the primary tumour, adequate treatment of the primary tumour should be followed by antibiotic therapy and a period of 4–6 weeks before reassessing the inguinal lymph nodes. Infection at the site of the primary lesion would also make regional lymphadenectomy at the time of the primary surgery potentially hazardous by increasing the risk of skin flap necrosis. Where at 4–6 weeks after treatment of the primary lesion there remains clinical lymphadenopathy, then bilateral inguinal with or without iliac lymphadenectomy is logical since approximately 50% of these patients with node-positive disease will have control after this.

Central to the argument of delayed inguinal lymphadenectomy is the ability to follow-up these patients adequately, and this will vary from centre to centre; but where an expectant policy is adopted then clearly regular follow-up visits bimonthly in the first 18 months and possibly tuition in self-examination are necessary. One argument against this policy is that in carcinoma of the penis there are included patients who delay seeking medical attention either for reasons of fear, the dislike of the prospect of an unpleasant operation or because of religious attitudes towards the genitalia.

The significant morbidity that is associated with groin dissections includes not only problems of healing of the skin flaps, especially over the groin crease, but also oedema of the lower limb, thrombophlebitis, pulmonary emboli and lymphocoele. Lymphoedema remains the commonest long term complication and may on occasion be severe enough to greatly disable the patient.

Early lymphadenectomy

Several surgeons have advocated that lymphadenectomy be carried out early in the management of carcinoma of the penis whether lymph nodes are palpable or not. However, most pursuing a more aggressive policy of routine lymphadenectomy now wait some 4–6 weeks to allow any infective changes to have resolved.[13]

A compromise

Another way of trying to limit lymph node excision to those patients who really need it is to perform routine sentinel lymph node biopsy and only go on to complete bilateral lymphadenectomy where the sentinel lymph nodes are positive. These sentinel lymph nodes are said to be situated superomedially to the junction of the superficial epigastric and saphenous veins.[14] However, not all authors believe in the reliability of these lymph node biopsies.[15] Additionally, post-biopsy scarring makes subsequent clinical examination of groins more difficult to interpret.

The modified technique of lymphadenectomy

Until recently, the standard method of inguinal lymphadenectomy was that described by Daseler *et al.* in 1948.[16] This was applicable to a variety of tumours including melanoma of the lower extremity and squamous cell carcinoma of the penis. Daseler *et al.* defined the boundaries of the lymphadenectomy as a quadrilateral area bounded superiorly by a line drawn from the anterior superoiliac spine to the superior margin of the external inguinal ring; laterally by a line drawn inferiorly from the anterior superoiliac spine for approximately 20 cm; and medially by a line drawn inferiorly from the pubic tubercle for approximately 15 cm and inferiorly by a horizontal line joining the medial lateral boundaries. This included excision of the entire lymph node field and overlying subcutaneous tissue. Catalona[13] believes that this operation represents a therapeutic overkill for the majority of patients with carcinoma of the penis in whom lymph node involvement is limited to a small region medial to the femoral vessel, and he has modified the operation. He begins with a 12–15 cm incision, 2 cm below the groin skin crease deepened to the level of Scarpa's fascia. A superior flap is then developed in a plane parallel to Scarpa's fascia and a funiculus of adipose tissue is identified coursing from the base of the penis into the superficial inguinal lymph nodes. The superior flap is dissected approximately 8 cm superior to the groin incision and a dissection deep into the fascia of the external oblique muscle proceeds. This allows exposure of the external inguinal ring and the spermatic cord as the cord passes into the superior aspect of the scrotum. The lymphatic tissue deep to the Scarpa's fascia is then dissected from the external oblique muscle and the spermatic cord as it passes into the scrotum. Similarly, the inferior flap is developed 8 cm below the incision and the incision is deepened into the fascia of the thigh muscles. The saphenous vein is identified and mobilized and its tributaries entering from medial, lateral, superior and inferior directions are ligated and divided, preserving the main trunk of the saphenous vein and the saphenofemoral junction. This lymphatic tissue is then dissected off the anterior surface of the saphenofemoral junction. Deep inguinal lymph nodes are then dissected out and can consist of one to three lymph nodes located deep to the fascia lata immediately medial to the femoral vein. This lymphatic package passes upwards under the inguinal ligament, the most superior of the deep inguinal lymph nodes being called the node of Cloquet. The deep inguinal lymph nodes are dissected to the level of the inguinal ligament and excised as a separate specimen, and the dissection is then continued to the lateral surface of the femoral vein where the deep inguinal lymph nodes between the femoral vein and artery are dissected out and excised. The fatty tissue is dissected off the femoral artery up to the inguinal ligament where the femoral artery passes underneath the ligament. This completes the modified inguinal lymphadenectomy.

Applying these surgical principles, Catalona has reduced the morbidity associated with the more radical dissection.

Survival

What, therefore, are the differences in outcome between those in whom lymphadenectomy is delayed until inguinal lymph nodes become palpable and those in whom it is carried out routinely some 4–6 weeks after treatment of the primary cancer? It is difficult to compare the various published series, although all show a worse prognosis with histologically proven inguinal metastases. In those not undergoing treatment by lymphadenectomy, few survive for two years, whereas 20–50% achieve a five-year disease-free survival following inguinal lymphadenectomy.

Radiotherapy

Radiotherapy for inguinal metastases has been shown to be of less benefit than surgery, though it has its advocates.[17,18] Furthermore, should it be used prophylactically at the time of treatment of the primary lesion, or where lymph node biopsy has proven inguinal metastases, it will provide increased risk of surgical flap necrosis, lymphoedema and vascular breakdown when subsequent surgery is employed. The main role of radiotherapy is in palliating those patients with inoperable lymphadenopathy.

Conclusions

In patients with clinically stage 1 or stage 2 carcinoma of the penis, a wait-and-see policy would appear acceptable provided that suitable follow-up is ensured at regular bimonthly intervals for the first 18 months. A proviso to this is where the primary tumour is poorly differentiated. Even where lymph nodes are impalpable, early bilateral lymphadenectomy should be considered. The role of sentinel lymph node biopsy remains controversial; its theoretical benefit of more accurate staging would seem to be less than that of its disadvantages: a false-negative biopsy and making subsequent lymph node assessment more difficult.

Where lymph nodes are palpable at the time of treatment of the primary tumour, then six weeks should be allowed to elapse with adequate antibiotic treatment to give any inflammatory lymphadenopathy adequate time to resolve, and then bilateral lymphadenectomy performed in those with nodes still palpable. The morbidity of lymphadenectomy is not inconsiderable, and despite modifications of the original technique it should certainly be bilateral where lymphadenopathy has persisted from the time of the primary tumour presentation. However, there is some logic in performing unilateral lymphadenectomy in those patients where lymphadenopathy develops on one side only at subsequent follow-up.

Clearly such a radical policy must be modified in the very elderly, those with established leg oedema or those who are very obese, and here palliative radiotherapy may then be considered. As to whether prophylactic pelvic lymphadenectomy should be performed, there remains great controversy. This is because where pelvic lymph nodes are positive then survival figures are extremely poor. In these cases it may be logical to perform iliac exploration with biopsy and if this is positive then not to go on to perform inguinal lymphadenectomy. In patients with inguinal metastases and without pelvic lymphadenectomy, bilateral inguinal lymphadenectomy has been shown to improve clinical survival, with five-year disease-free survival rates ranging from 20% to 50%.

References

1. Rouvière H. Anatomie des lymphatiques de l'homme. In *Anatomie*, vol. 4. Paris: Masson, 1932.
2. Bouchot O, Auvigne J, Peuvrel P, Glemain P, Buzelin JM. Management of regional lymph nodes in carcinoma of the penis. *Europ Urol* 1989; **16**: 410–15.
3. Riveros M, Garcia R, Cabanas R. Lymphadenography of the dorsal lymphatic of penis. *Cancer* 1967; **20**: 2026–31.
4. Whitmore WF. Tumors of the penis, urethra, scrotum and testis. In: Campbell MF, Harrison HH (eds), *Urology* 3rd edn. Philadelphia: WB Saunders, 1970: 1190–229.
5. Cabanas RM. An approach for the treatment of penile carcinoma. *Cancer* 1977; **39**: 456–66.
6. Fraley EE, Zhang G, Manivel C, Neihans GA. The role of ilio-inguinal lymphadenectomy and significance of histological differentiation in treatment of carcinoma of the penis. *J Urol* 1989; **142**: 1478–80.

7.   De Kernion TB. Carcinoma of the penis. *Cancer* 1973; **32**: 1256–62.
8.   Johnson DE, Lo RK. Management of regional lymph nodes in penile carcinoma: five-year results following therapeutic groin dissections. *Urology* 1984; **24**: 308–14.
9.   Schellhammer PF, Grabstald H. Tumours of the penis. In: Walsh PC, Gittes RE, Perlmutter AD, Stamey TA (eds), *Campbell's Urology* vol 2. Philadelphia: WB Saunders, 1986: 1583–606.
10. Fraley EE, Zhang G, Sazamar R, Lange PH. Cancer of the penis: prognosis and treatment plans. *Cancer* 1985; **55**: 1618–24.
11. Grabstald H. Controversies concerning lymph node dissection for carcinoma of the penis. *Urol Clin N Am* 1980; **7**: 793–9.
12. Richie JP. Delayed inguinal lymphadenectomy in the management of carcinoma of the penis. In: Carlton CE (ed.), *Controversies in Urology*. Chicago: Year Book Medical Publishers, 1989: 314–16.
13. Catalona WJ. Lymphadenectomy in the management of carcinoma of the penis. In: Carlton CE (ed.), *Controversies in Urology*. Chicago: Year Book Medical Publishers, 1989: 311–13.
14. Fowler JE. Sentinel node biopsy for staging penile carcinoma. *Urology* 1984; **23**: 353–4.
15. Perinetti E, Crane DB, Catalona WJ. Unreliability of sentinel lymph node biopsy for staging penile carcinoma. *J Urol* 1980; **124**: 734–5.
16. Daseler GH, Anson BH, Reiman AF. Radical excision of the inguinal and iliac lymph glands: a study based upon 450 anatomical dissections and upon supportive clinical observations. *Surg Gynaecol Obstet* 1948; **87**: 679.
17. Ekstrom T, Edsmyr F. Cancer of the penis: a clinical study of 229 cases. *Acta Chir Scand* 1958; **115**: 25–45.
18. Murrell DS, Williams JL. Radiotherapy in treatment of carcinoma of the penis. *Br J Urol* 1965; **37**: 211.

Section III

Prostatic Cancer

7 Pathological grading systems for prostatic cancer

Christopher S Foster

Identification of cellular features which accurately predict the behaviour of a specific patient's tumour is a major challenge facing contemporary pathology. Prostate cancer is presently the third leading cause of male death from malignant disease in Europe and the United States of America, following only cancers of lung and of skin. [1] Post mortem studies of patients dying from other causes have shown that this disease is the most common human malignancy. [2] Despite its rising prevalence, little progress has been made in identifying parameters which accurately predict the behaviour of individual prostatic cancers. [3] Anatomically localized prostate cancer is not a benign disease and although progression might be slow it is inexorable. However, it is paradoxical that not all primary prostatic carcinomas discovered incidentally exhibit a similar lethal potential. Unfortunately, conventional therapy is of little value in controlling the phenotypically malignant primary tumours. Hence, the therapeutic dilemma is that not all prostatic cancers require aggressive treatment, with its associated morbidity and mortality.

Traditionally, diagnostic histopathologists have attempted to forecast the behaviour of carcinomas by comparing morphological features of normal and neoplastic tissues. Although this approach has identified some features common to prostate cancers *as a group*, it has been of limited value in predicting future behaviour of individual tumours. During recent years, unassisted morphological criteria have been supported by the concomitant use of techniques which include immunohistochemistry, flow-cytometry and *in situ* nucleic acid hybridization. This multiparametric approach to classifying and grading prostate cancer is presently receiving detailed evaluation in many laboratories worldwide.

The majority of prostatic malignancies are adenocarcinomas derived from tubuloalveolar glands of the outer prostatic zone. Non-acinar carcinomas are rare tumours apparently originating from prostatic ducts in the region of the urethra, or from the utricle (Table 7.1). Methods of grading prostatic cancer apply only to the adenocarcinomas, uncommon tumours being assessed by independent criteria.

Table 7.1   Histological classification of prostatic malignant tumours

---

Malignant epithelial tumours
1. Acinic cell carcinomas
2. Non-acinar carcinomas:
    Endometrial
    Mucinous
    Neuroendocrine
    Salivary gland type
    Signet ring carcinomas
    Squamous cell
3. Carcinosarcomas

Non-epithelial malignant tumours
Leiomyosarcomas
Rhabdomyosarcomas
Lymphomas

Morphological appearances

Normal histology

The normal prostate is composed of complex tubular alveolar glands within a fibromuscular stroma. The glandular epithelium is either of low cuboidal or tall columnar secretory type which is frequently arranged into papillary folds. Acini drain by individual intralobular ducts which unite into interlobular ducts. Ducts may be lined by cuboidal or by columnar epithelium. Surrounding the acinar and ductular epithelium is an incomplete layer of 'reserve' cells, the prostatic homologue of human breast myoepithelial cells.

Anatomically, human prostate is comprised of two main groups of glands: inner and outer. Although controversy remains as to their exact distribution,[4,5] it is now accepted that benign enlargement of the prostate arises from the inner group whereas prostatic cancer generally arises from the outer.[6] Owing to the structural arrangement of the glands, biopsy confirmation of early prostate cancer is frequently difficult to obtain since per-urethral biopsy is unlikely to provide neoplastic tissue until the tumour is extensive. Significant tumour enlargement usually occurs before involvement of adjacent structures causes symptoms. Invasion of the prostatic capsule is an early phenomenon which frequently results in periprostatic lymphatic and vascular invasion prior to development of symptoms by a significantly enlarged tumour.

Atypical hyperplasia

Alterations to normal morphology suggestive of malignancy are frequently encountered in prostatic biopsy specimens. Such changes have been variously described as atypical prostatic hyperplasia, dysplasia and adenosis.[7,8] The most important criteria employed to differentiate foci of morphological abnormality are cytological changes accompanying structural acinar change. These latter include formation of

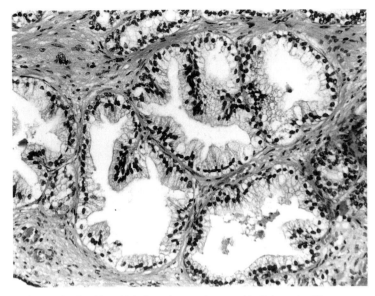

Fig. 7.1 Prostatic gland in which there is prominent epithelial atypia. The appearances fall just short of *in-situ* malignancy. Papillary epithelial projections and cross-bridging without a stromal component are present. Basal or 'reserve' cells are absent from parts of the glands. No intraglandular (Pagetoid) spread is seen. (× 180)

cribriform, papillary or microacinar patterns (Fig. 7.1). In these areas, acini are lined by cuboidal or columnar cells with increased nuclear/cytoplasmic ratio and prominent nucleoli. The basal or 'reserve' layer of cells is maintained. The biological significance of such structural changes remains controversial.[9] Most frequently observed in operative specimens removed for carcinoma, the suggestion has been made that they are pre-malignant and represent early generalized 'field change' within the gland.[10] When encountered, differentiation of benign from well-differentiated adenocarcinoma rests with cytological criteria.

Two morphological features formerly considered of assistance in distinguishing benign from malignant prostatic tissue are: perineural invasion and the presence of apparently specific crystalline structures within malignant acini and/or in adjacent benign glands. Unfortunately, infiltration of perineural spaces by benign prostatic glandular tissue has been reported,[11] an observation analogous to that of benign sclerosing adenosis in the human breast.

Studies of prostatic adenocarcinoma have revealed characteristic, sharply angular crystalline structures in approximately 10% of cases.[12] In a series of 431 cases of nodular hyperplasia, crystalloids were present in only 3.5%.[13] Although found in benign prostates, the crystals were frequently associated with atypical epithelial proliferation, as in the case of microcalcification in breast tissue. The finding of angular microcrystalloids in human prostatic tissues, whilst not pathognomonic of cancer, is an indication that additional microscopic sections should be examined or re-biopsy performed.

Morphological methods of grading

Histological grade

Many systems have been proposed to assess morphological features of prostatic acinar carcinomas and hence derive a histological grade indicative of malignancy (Table 7.2). Such attempts have employed a classical approach by making comparisons between specific cyto-architectural features of normal and malignant tissues. The consequence has been a series of semi-quantitative evaluation techniques, the most frequently adopted being those of Gleason[22] and Gaeta.[29] In an attempt to predict the behaviour of prostate cancer, a variety of different architectural and cytological features have been considered. Unfortunately, these different methods are empirical since they neither employ identical criteria nor attribute similar importance to the same features. Although retrospective analyses have demonstrated good correlation between defined populations of prostatic cancer and patient prognosis, none has been able to predict accurately those potentially lethal early primary carcinomas. Gleason's system is presently employed by the Veterans Administration Cooperative Urological Research Group (VACURG) and is the preferred morphological method of grading prostatic carcinomas throughout the world. The classification devised by Gaeta has been used by the National Prostatic Cancer Project (NPCP).

Gleason's system

The system derived by Gleason is based upon glandular differentiation and growth patterns of the neoplastic glands in relation to prostatic stroma (Table 7.3). Observed glandular patterns may vary from well-differentiated (grade 1) to anaplastic (grade 5). Since most tumours show more than one pattern, to account for this variability Gleason assigned a primary grade to the predominant pattern and a secondary grade to the lesser pattern of prostatic cancer. Both grades are scored as digits which are summated to give the histological score. The method is unique in that cytological characteristics are specifically excluded. Although some inter-observer and intra-observer variations have been reported on repeated grading of the same slides, reproducibility is high.

The three features distinguishing Gleason's system of grading from other morphological methods are: (1) emphasis on pattern recognition; (2) assignation of a secondary grade to each tumour, thus accounting for morphological heterogeneity found in the majority of prostatic cancers; and (3) specific exclusion of cytological characteristics of individual tumours.

Grade 1: Very well differentiated   The architecture of the prostate gland and of the tumour are little distorted. Neoplastic glands are closely packed, round, uniform in shape and diameter and sharply delineated from surrounding, scanty, fibrovascular stroma (Fig. 7.2). Cytologically these acini comprise low columnar cells with clear

Table 7.2 Morphological methods of grading prostate cancer

Authors	System criteria
Broders (1926)[14]	Histological patterns of tumour differentiation
Young and Davis (1926)[15]	Histological patterns of tumour growth
Muir (1934)[16]	Tubule formation, cytomorphology and mitoses
Kahler (1938)[17]	Distinction of squamous and adenocarcinoma
Evans *et al.* (1942)[18]	Gland morphology, cell shape, fibrosis and inflammation
Edwards *et al.* (1953)[19]	Morphological differentiation of neoplastic glands
Shelley *et al.* (1958)[20]	Cytomorphology, tubule formation and nuclear morphology
Vickery and Kerr (1963)[21]	Two morphological categories: well and poorly differentiated
Gleason (1966)[22]	Glandular architecture and stromal involvement
Jewett *et al.* (1968)[23]	Morphological, grades 1–3
Mobley and Frank (1968)[24]	Acinar architecture and nuclear morphology
Utz and Farrow (1969)[25] (Mayo Clinic System)	Seven morphological and cytological criteria
Corriere *et al.* (1970)[26]	Modified Gleason's classification
Mostofi (AFIP) (1975)[27]	Nuclear anaplasia and glandular differentiation
Muller *et al.* (1980)[28]	Glandular differentiation and nuclear anaplasia
Gaeta (1981)[29]	Combination of glandular pattern and nuclear morphology
Brawn *et al.* (1982)[30]	Percentage of tumour containing glandular and solid components

Table 7.3 Gleason's system of grading prostate cancer

Grade	Glandular architecture	Tumour–stromal boundary
Gland formation distinct		
Grade 1	Distinct glands; uniform shape and size; closely packed	Sharply defined glands with no stromal infiltration
Grade 2	Distinct glands; irregular sizes; interglandular spaces present	Less defined than grade 1; some infiltration along major stromal planes
Grade 3A	Distinct glands; increased irregularities in gland size and interglandular spacing	Ragged borders to neoplastic glands with infiltration along major and minor stromal planes
Grade 3B	Tiny abortive glands and individual cell clusters	Poorly defined and ragged margins with extensive infiltration of all stromal planes
Uncohesive growth patterns		
Grade 3C	Rounded masses; cribriform or papillary	Sharply defined borders to expansile masses
Grade 4A	Fused glandular tumour masses	Poorly defined tumour boundaries with extensive infiltration throughout stroma
Grade 4B	Hypernephroid appearance	Poorly defined tumour boundaries with extensive infiltration throughout stroma
Grade 5A	Solid tumours	Sharply defined, expansile edges; single-cell infiltration not significant
Grade 5B	Diffusely infiltrating anaplastic carcinoma	Poorly defined and ragged edges to indistinct glands with widespread diffuse stromal infiltration

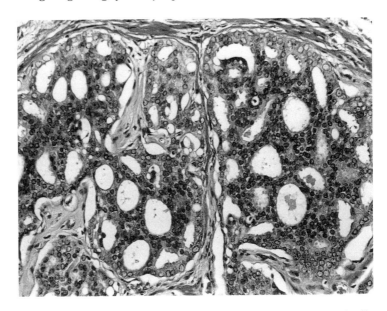

Fig. 7.2 Gleason grade 1: closely-packed prostatic glands filled by masses of uniform small tumour cells exhibiting multiple luminal cross-bridges. There is no extension beyond the limits of the glands, which appear sharp. No basal reserve cells are present. (× 180)

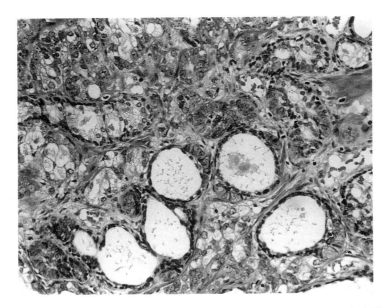

Fig. 7.3 Well-differentiated prostatic adenocarcinoma (Gleason grade 2) infiltrating adjacent glands and undermining non-neoplastic epithelium in a Pagetoid manner.

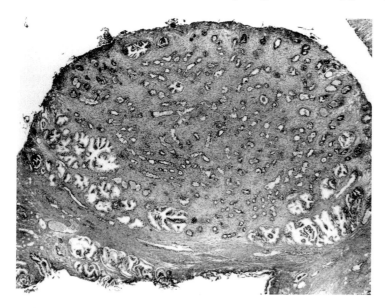

Fig. 7.4   Single prostatic chipping containing an expanding focus of proliferating neoplastic tubules. The edges of the lesion are ragged and poorly defined. (Gleason grade 3). (× 22)

cytoplasm and basally located nuclei containing uniformly dense chromatin. Nucleoli and mitotic figures are not seen. Basal epithelial cells are absent.

Grade 2: Well differentiated   Tumour glands are well-defined although variation in size and shape is present. Spacing between glands is increased. Glandular epithelium is usually more than one cell thick. Cross-acinar bridging results in a cribriform pattern. Gland margins are less defined than are those in grade 1 tumours. Neoplastic glands surround or replace adjacent normal lobules (Fig. 7.3). There is no infiltration of surrounding fibrovascular stroma by neoplastic glands or single tumour cells. Cytologically, cells of grade 1 and grade 2 prostate cancers appear similar with basal nuclei and a uniformly dense chromatin network. Nucleoli and mitotic figures are rarely seen. Hence, features distinguishing grade 1 and grade 2 tumours are architectural and glandular, not cytological.

Grade 3: Glands with variable and distorted architecture   A variety of cribriform structures, together with occasional cords and masses of cells, some showing evidence of aborted glandular differentiation, are found. In grade 3 tumours, the margins are ragged (Fig. 7.4). Absence of well-delineated glandular margins characteristic of grades 1 and 2 carcinomas is the diagnostic hallmark of grade 3 prostatic cancer. Diffuse penetration of adjacent stroma by small aborted glands and single cells is a common feature. Throughout the tumour, there is intermixing of small, medium and large glandular elements with irregular spacing between glands. The cribriform pattern appearing as a feature of grade 2 tumours is now commonly

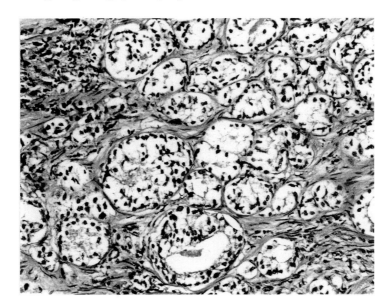

Fig. 7.5 Poorly differentiated prostatic carcinoma of clear-cell 'hypernephroid' type. This tumour comprised masses of fused glands formed entirely of this cell-type. (× 180)

observed. Cytologically, acinar cells are low-cuboidal and contain granular cytoplasm. Nuclei are variable in appearance but typically larger than those of grades 1 and 2 carcinomas. Nuclei display a vesicular appearance with an open and irregularly distributed chromatin pattern. Nucleoli are generally present.

Grade 4: Poorly differentiated   The characteristics of these tumours are masses of fused glands comprising large polygonal and clear 'hypernephroid' cells resembling clear cell carcinomas of renal origin (Fig. 7.5). Prostatic cancers are specifically assigned to this group only when the clear cell pattern is extensive and well-developed. Tumours grow with extremely ragged and infiltrative margins throughout the stroma.

Grade 5: Anaplastic   In these tumours, cells grow either in an infiltrative trabecular pattern or as non-glandular solid tumour masses. Typically, the margins of these solid masses are well-defined, although there is frequently infiltration of the surrounding stroma by single cells and groups of tumour cells occur at the periphery. There is extensive diversity of cytological appearances in grades 4 and 5 carcinomas with prominent nuclear pleomorphism (Figs 7.6 and 7.7). Many nuclei contain an open chromatin network and prominent nucleoli.

Gaeta's system

This is a four-grade system based upon a combination of glandular and nuclear cytological features of the tumour (Table 7.4). The system has been demonstrated

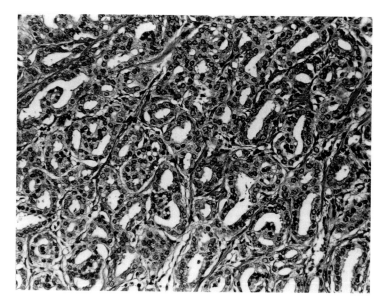

Fig. 7.6 Undifferentiated prostatic carcinoma (Gleason grade 5) composed of masses of small tubules. There are no definite glandular outlines or margins. The tumour obliterates all underlying normal architecture. (× 180)

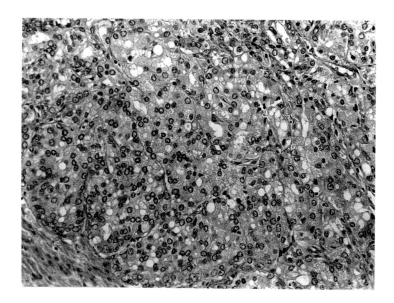

Fig. 7.7 An adjacent region to the carcinoma illustrated in Fig. 7.6. Tumour cells are slightly larger and exhibit a solid arrangement although abortive tubule formation is identified. (× 180)

Table 7.4   Gaeta system of grading prostate cancer

Grade	Glands	Cells
I	Well-defined and separated by scanty stroma	Uniform and normal size; nucleoli conspicuous; chromatin dark and dense
II	Medium and small glands scattered throughout and infiltrating stromal tissues	Some pleomorphism; nucleoli conspicuous, small and basophilic
III	Small, irregular and poorly formed acini without organization; cribriform patterns included	Significant pleomorphism; nuclei vesicular; nucleoli often large and acidiphilic
IV	Round and solid masses of cells or diffuse infiltration of small cells with no glands	Small or large; uniform or pleomorphic; mitotic activity significant

to be straightforward, objective and reproducible. Through incorporation of cytological parameters, it was designed to be more sensitive than the Gleason system. Retrospective studies demonstrated good correlation between tumour grade and death from prostate cancer. Recently, this system has undergone modification from its earlier description by the National Prostatic Cancer Treatment Group (NPCTG) in order to obtain a score which is the sum of the glandular and nuclear grades of the tumour. However, analysis relating progression-free survival to Gleason and Gaeta grading systems has indicated the Gleason score to predict, more successfully than that of Gaeta, the probable biological behaviour of a primary prostatic malignancy.

Other morphological systems

A combined assessment of glandular differentiation and nuclear anaplasia was devised by Müller *et al.*[28] Tumours were graded histologically as highly or poorly differentiated, cribriform and solid. These were scored as 0, 1, 2 and 3 respectively. Nuclear anaplasia was graded as mild, moderate or pronounced and scored 0, 1 and 2. The sum of the scores assigned to glandular differentiation and to nuclear anaplasia was then used to determine the degree of malignancy: grade 1 (score 0 or 1), grade 2 (score 2 or 3) and grade 3 (score 4 or 5). A grading system based on the percentage of a tumour containing differentiated (gland-forming) or undifferentiated (solid) components was proposed by Brawn *et al.*[30] The system extended in four equal steps from grade 1 tumours in which gland formation occurred in between 75% and 100% of the biopsy specimens, to grade 4 tumours in which less than 25% of the specimen showed gland formation. Böcking and Sinagowitz[31] devised a scoring system intended to indicate the probable prognosis of a tumour. Scores of 1 to 3 were assigned to a variety of nuclear and nucleolar characteristics which included area, regularity and size together with the extent of dissociation of tumour cells.

Relative values of morphological criteria

In many of the reported studies, a fundamental assumption is that the morphological grade (such as the Gleason score) remains unaltered throughout the lifespan of a particular tumour. This assumption is not supported by data derived from the natural history of individual prostate cancers, particularly from metastatic sites where the grade may be significantly worse than that of the primary tumour.[32]

Prognostic effects of particular architectural features considered either singly or combined have been analysed by Schroeder *et al.*[33,34] In tumours exhibiting only one pattern, tumour gland architecture and nuclear pleomorphism appeared to influence overall survival. Amounts of tumour, cellular pleomorphism and mitoses were of secondary significance. In tumours containing multiple architectural patterns, prognosis did not reflect the 'worst' part of the tumour. Although survival was poor in carcinomas comprising exclusively grade 3 formations, morphologically similar tumours containing areas of well-differentiated neoplastic glands exhibited significantly better survival. Hence, the anticipated effect of poorly differentiated carcinoma appeared to be modulated by adjacent better-differentiated regions.[34] These and similar analyses support the original concept underlying Gleason's grading system by confirming tumour architecture to be the most important morphological indicator of probable behaviour, only then followed by nuclear anaplasia and the presence or absence of mitoses.

Quantitative methods of grading

Three factors underlie recent efforts to quantify structural features of prostate cancer. First is the concept of tumour progression defined by Foulds[35,36] in which he stated that cancers do not express their full range of malignant biological attributes from the outset but rather progress towards increasing malignancy with time. Support for this hypothesis has come from the recognition of tumour-cell heterogeneity[37,38] and the spontaneous emergence of new biological phenotypes such as metastatic ability and drug resistance. However, Foulds appeared not to appreciate the relationship between tumour morphology, tumour biology and time. McNeal *et al.* subsequently proposed that biological progression of prostate cancer directly correlates with tumour volume and hence identified this parameter to be central to predicting biological behaviour.[39] The third factor is the concept that morphometric information, if sufficiently detailed and suitably analysed, might accurately predict future behaviour of prostatic adenocarcinoma. During recent years, the advent of image-analysis techniques coupled with powerful data-processing computer software has stimulated renewed interest in obtaining morphological grading of human prostate cancer based upon accurately quantified tumour volumes.

Volumetric parameters

Detailed examination of small prostatic tumours found incidentally and large cancers presenting with symptoms indicated a strong correlation between Gleason grade and tumour volume.[40] A further correlation was demonstrated between prevalence of large prostatic neoplasms found at autopsy and clinical incidence and mortality rate of disseminated prostatic cancer. According to McNeal *et al.*, approximately 20% of 'latent' cancers found incidentally at autopsy are sufficiently large to be potentially life-threatening.[39] Although small tumours of grades 1 or 2 are common incidental findings, large prostate cancers invariably contain a mixture of different morphological appearances and are always at least grade 3. Hence, McNeal concluded that the uniquely broad range of histological differentiation seen in prostate cancer is a morphological reflection of biological progression. Unfortunately, these are comparative data obtained between different individuals with morphologically similar tumours, but for which functional and behavioural characteristics are unknown.

Although volumetric parameters are important indices of malignant potential in assessing prostatic cancer, the majority of studies report findings from radical prostatectomies[41] or from autopsy studies. However, Humphrey and Vollmer showed that, in patients undergoing transurethral prostatic resection, the ratio of prostatic chippings containing cancer to the total number of chippings removed may be considered an accurate assessment of tumour stage and volume.[42] Recently, Foucar *et al.* extended this approach by employing a computerized interactive morphometric technique to determine relative areas of cancer in transurethrally-resected prostatic chippings.[43] The two morphometrically determined parameters of *actual area of cancer* and *percentage area of cancer* were compared with the *total number of chippings* and the *percentage of chippings* involved by cancer. Although they identified no statistical value for the *total number* of chippings involved by cancer, the *percentage* of chippings involved by malignancy, the two morphometrically determined parameters and the Gleason score were all found to be significant predictors of survival.

Although these are interesting and valuable observations, the data were collected from a retrospective series of 79 prostatic cancers in whom survival data were already available. In keeping with many different morphological parameters in other malignancies, despite excellent correlation being demonstrated between *groups* of patients and *trends* in the alteration of certain parameters, morphology and morphometry alone are not reliable predictors of behaviour for any individual tumour.

Nuclear morphology

Recent techniques of quantitation and computer-based image analysis have been variously employed as methods of obtaining more detailed and reliable data with which to predict biological behaviour of specific tumours. Diamond *et al.* attempted to relate nuclear roundness to the probability of metastatic potential of human prostate cancer.[44] This same group compared their morphometric data with Gleason grade for the same cohort of 27 patients followed for up to 15 years after radical prostatectomy for stage B1 and stage B2 carcinomas.[45] Computerized image analysis of relative or absolute nuclear roundness in these prostatic tumours could separate accurately the stage B prostate carcinomas into two distinct groups, one with high lethal metastatic potential and one with a benign clinical course. The Gleason grading system could not separate these metastatic and non-metastatic groups without significant overlap.

Nucleolar morphology

The value of nucleolar surface area measurements as objective parameters for predicting the biological behaviour of prostatic carcinomas has been reported by Tannenbaum *et al.*[46] Scanning electron microscopy of at least 100 nucleoli in each specimen were examined from the primary and subsequent prostatic biopsies of 40 stage B and 12 stage D patients. Comparison was made between these data and Gleason grading of the same tumours. Nucleolar surface area measurements appeared to correlate with biological behaviour of individual tumours. Cancers from stage B patients with no evidence of disseminated disease for three or more years contained small nucleoli with values from $0.82\,\mu m^2$ to $3.4\,\mu m^2$. For patients dying of prostate cancer, or developing metastases following radical prostatectomy, values from $4.1\,\mu m^2$ to $5.6\,\mu m^2$ were obtained. Nucleolar surface area values for patients with stage D disease ranged up to $10\,\mu m^2$ with a mean of $5.36\,\mu m^2$. In this cohort of patients, correlation between Gleason's histological grading and disease progression was significantly less accurate. A recent study by Myers *et al.* examined and graded prostate cancer nucleoli according to size (from large and prominent to difficult to identify) following assignment of primary and secondary Gleason patterns.[47] Regardless of Gleason grade, the mean interval from diagnosis to disease progression was shorter in patients with tumour nucleoli designated as prominent or intermediate compared with those with tumour nucleoli graded as non-prominent.

Examination of prostate cancer nucleolar organizer region-associated proteins (AgNORs) has been attempted in several laboratories. Colloidal silver-staining techniques for AgNORs are thought to identify proteins involved in regulating DNA–RNA transcription and hence their presence might be regarded as a measure of cell proliferative activity. Unlike many other malignancies of both epithelial and mesenchymal origin, this technique has not been shown to be of either diagnostic or prognostic value in assessing human prostate cancer.

Fine-needle aspiration cytology

Fine-needle aspiration cytology has proved an extremely valuable modality for diagnosing many different malignant diseases. The technique has recently been compared with core biopsy for diagnosis and monitoring of prostate cancer.[48] In an unselected series of 121 patients undergoing both core biopsy and fine-needle aspiration prior to transurethral resection or radical prostatectomy, diagnostic accuracy was greater for fine-needle aspiration than for core biopsy (82% versus 74%). Except in poorly differentiated cancers, fine-needle aspiration was a poor predictor of final pathological grade. Fine-needle aspiration was not useful in detecting stage A1 prostate cancer. In another controlled study of benign and malignant prostatic disease, significant discordance was found between cytological evaluation of disease and that found on examining conventionally processed tissue blocks from the same prostates.[49] The results of these two studies, performed by competent and practising cytopathologists, cast doubt upon the value of fine-needle aspiration as a routine technique for diagnosing and grading prostatic cancer. It appears probable that those cancers most likely to be missed by this technique are the stage A1, well-differentiated (grades 1–2) tumours. It is precisely this group of prostate carcinomas which should be identified early.

Objective markers of differentiation

In any malignancy, two principal effects contribute to the behaviour of the particular disease. These are: (1) expression (or absence) of intrinsic properties of the tumour cells, and (2) the local host interaction with that particular tumour. A variety of such features related to the cell biology of individual prostatic carcinomas may be demonstrated in both histological and cytological preparations.

Mucin production

In a variety of different malignancies including breast, pancreas, colon and ovary, mucin production has been regarded as an independent marker of behaviour correlating either with improved prognosis or defining a tumour population with particular attributes. In the breast, true mucinous adenocarcinomas ('colloid carcinomas') are recognized to exhibit a significantly better prognosis than ductal carcinomas containing only some foci of mucin. Ro *et al.* examined 12 cases of prostatic carcinoma in which the primary tumours conformed to the strict diagnostic criteria of 'prostatic mucinous adenocarcinoma'.[50] Although not frequently encountered (only 50 similar cases being previously reported with an overall incidence of 0.4%) examination of unusual variants often provides a unique insight into the pathobiology of common tumours. Despite ensuring a 'true' population of mucinous carcinomas, these tumours exhibited no patterns of behaviour or prognosis different from non-mucin-producing prostatic adenocarcinomas. The findings of this study thus supported previous observations which suggested that, in contrast to their counterparts in female breast cancer, mucin production in prostatic cancer does not appear to be a relevant indicator of differentiation or prognosis.[51]

In these studies of mucinous adenocarcinomas, estimates were made of the volumes occupied by the mucinous component within the tumours. However, there was no information about the comparative overall *size* of the tumours examined, even though this parameter is recognized from McNeal *et al.*'s work to be directly correlated with malignant behaviour.[39] Similarly, no data are given which indicate that nuclear size and contour were examined in these tumours. This feature has now been documented as one of the better morphological indicators of high lethal metastatic potential, particularly when examined by computerized image analysis.[52] Unfortunately, nuclear morphometric analyses were not included in these observations of mucinous prostatic cancers.

Flow-cytometry of nuclear DNA

In many tumours, alterations to chromosomal complement and structure are frequently observed. This parameter has been correlated with disease progression or response to therapy in a variety of different malignancies. Flow cytometric assessment of ploidy status in paraffin-embedded tissues of lymph node metastases from 82 patients with stage D2 prostatic carcinomas confirmed a strongly negative effect of aneuploidy on patient survival.[53] In these tumours, there was no correlation between ploidy and other parameters, including tumour grade. In comparison, grade did not approach significance as a predictor of survival. Some retrospective studies have confirmed an association between aneuploid status and metastatic prostate cancer.[54] Other studies employing multivariate analysis of several different parameters have shown that, with the exception of Gleason grade, no other variables contribute any significant prognostic information.[55]

In addition to analysis of cellular DNA content and ploidy status, the proportion of tumour cells within specific phases of the cell-cycle has been employed as a possible correlate of malignancy. Studies of human prostate cancer have shown that the parameter of S-phase fraction, taken in conjunction with cellular features such as 5-α-reductase activity, may be of value in identifying tumours with particularly good prognosis.[56] Diploid tumours with less than 10% of cells in mitosis exhibited a significantly better prognosis than those with mitotic indices greater than 15%. A different study has demonstrated correlation between a shift in distribution of cells from G_0-G_1 phase to $S+G_2M$ phases and increasing Gleason grade.[57] These parameters were independent of tumour volume and clinical stage of the disease.

A different approach to obtaining similar information from tissue sections of prostatic adenocarcinoma is bromodeoxyuridine labelling identified immunohistochemically using specific antisera. Employing this technique, Nemoto *et al.* showed a correlation between Gleason grade and S-phase fraction and growth pattern.[58] Higher S-phase fractions appeared indicative of biological malignancy. Moreover, the heterogeneity of S-phase fraction distribution within prostate cancer tissues could be directly compared to the morphological appearance. Thus, measurement of bromodeoxyuridine labelling-index might prove to be a valuable adjunct to identifying, at diagnosis, those prostate cancers with very good or with very poor indices, irrespective of tumour size or clinical stage.

Prostate-specific proteins

Several proteins specifically expressed by prostatic epithelium have been examined as potential indicators of differentiation. Presently, there are two principal antigenic markers for prostatic cancer: prostate-specific antigen and prostatic acid phosphatase. Prostate-specific antigen is a 34kD protein belonging to the kallikrein family of serum proteases.[59] It can be detected immunohistochemically in normal prostatic epithelial cells, prostatic hypertrophy and prostatic carcinoma. Apart from its possible application in identifying metastatic adenocarcinoma to be prostatic in origin it is not useful as a marker of differentiation.

Prostatic acid phosphatase is a specific isoenzyme of acid phosphatase found in large amounts in prostatic and seminal fluids. In frozen sections of tissue it can be demonstrated histochemically,[60] but not in conventionally processed tissues.[61] Although conventional antisera have been raised to demonstrate prostatic acid phosphatase in paraffin-embedded tissue sections, cross-reactivity occurs with other tartrate-labile acid phosphatases.[62] Recently, a novel hybridoma-derived monoclonal antibody to prostatic acid phosphatase was reported.[63] The potential advantage of this type of antibody is identification of an epitope unique to the prostatic protein as well as resistance to paraffin-embedding and formalin-fixation. Although presently undergoing evaluation as a diagnostic reagent, its already apparent cross-reactivity with a variety of normal and neoplastic tissues will probably preclude the use of this particular monoclonal antibody as a reliable marker of differentiation in prostate cancer.

Growth-factor receptors

Interaction between neoplastic cells and either humoral or structural components of the surrounding environment is a powerful modulator of tumour biology. Differential expression of specific hormone receptors by particular malignancies is recognized to be associated with disease progression. Epidermal growth factor (EGF) receptor expression has been examined in prostatic hyperplasia and neoplasia.[64] Concentrations of EGF receptor in hyperplastic tissues were significantly higher than were those in prostatic carcinomas. Furthermore, within the cancers, expression of EGF receptors appeared to be a function of Gleason histological grade. Thus, EGF receptor status might be employed as an adjunct marker of prostate cancer differentiation.

Androgen-receptor binding activity has been investigated as a possible predictor of response by primary and metastatic prostate carcinomas to endocrine therapy, and hence as a marker of tissue differentiation. Tissues removed by conventional transurethral resection were assessed for androgen binding activity and the data correlated with time to disease progression, clinical stage and Gleason grade. No association was demonstrated between time to progression and clinical stage. However, a correlation was demonstrated between time to progression and histological grade. When grade 4 carcinomas were excluded from the analysis, androgen binding activity became predictive of disease progression independently of histological grade and clinical stage.[65]

Whereas cytoplasmic androgen receptors are labile molecules, prostatic membrane prolactin binding sites are relatively stable. Expression of prolactin receptors has been examined in a range of hyperplastic and neoplastic prostatic tissues removed by transurethral resection.[66] Using a histological grading system of G1–G3, free prolactin receptors were found in none of the poorly differentiated (G3) carcinomas. While only 62.5% of G2 carcinomas were positive, all G1 tumours and benign hyperplastic tissues contained measurable levels of free prolactin membrane binding components. When treated with combined chemotherapy and hormonal manipulation, subsequent tumour-biopsy specimens revealed increased expression of prolactin receptors in those tumours which responded.

Normal and neoplastic prostatic tissues contain proteins that bind androgens with high affinity. These proteins include the androgen receptor, testosterone-binding protein derived from blood plasma and progestin-binding protein. Dihydro-testosterone (DHTS) binds with all androphilic proteins whereas the analogue R1881 and mibolerone bind only with the androgen receptor and progestin-binding protein.[67] Histochemical detection of these proteins has been examined in a series of prostate cancers using fluorescent DHTS, mibolerone and R1881 as ligands.[68] A population of 62 patients with androgen-binding protein-positive stage D2 prostate carcinomas were treated with endocrine therapy. No correlation between expression of the protein and tumour grade was identified. However, a relationship between expression of these proteins and response to treatment became apparent at six months after therapy started. Using fluorescent R1881 as ligand, the fluorescence-positive patients showed better survival characteristics than the fluorescence-negative patients.

Estramustine-binding protein is another receptor which has received interest as a possible marker of prostatic cancer cell differentiation. This protein was originally identified in cytosols from rat ventral prostate.[69] It is present in human prostate and specifically binds estramustine and estromustine, the cytotoxically active metabolites of the microtubule inhibitor estramustine phosphate. In a study of primary prostatic carcinoma biopsies, expression of estramustine-binding protein was examined histochemically both before and after treatment. All prostatic carcinomas expressed this protein prior to treatment. However, staining intensity was greater in morphologically poorly differentiated than in the well-differentiated tumours. Two types of staining pattern were apparent in different tumours: diffuse throughout the cytoplasm of all cells in 70% of cases and focal in the remaining 30%. Irrespective of the type of treatment employed, expression of estramustine-binding protein diminished rapidly in all cases in which cytological and clinical regression occurred. The renewed appearance of estramustine-binding protein in these tumours was found to be an accurate predictor of refractory disease.[70] Hence, decreased estramustine-binding protein correlated with favourable cytological and clinical regression, whereas unchanged staining was indicative of clinical progression and poor cytological regression.

Prostate-associated enzymes

In addition to prostate-specific acid phosphatase, 5-α-reductase has been assessed as a potential marker of prostatic carcinoma differentiation. ▲⁴-5-α-reductase is an endoplasmic reticulum enzyme which rate-limits metabolic reduction of the 4,5 double bond at the A:B ring junction of neutral steroids, including testosterone.[71] A recent study has evaluated the expression of 5-α-reductase by a series of primary prostatic carcinomas.[56] Following division of tumours into three groups on the basis of their 5-α-reductase activity, comparison with their Gleason score was made. This study identified one group of tumours in which none formed metastases (diploid tumours with 5-α-reductase activity greater than 20 pmole/mg of protein per 30 minutes and with less than 10% of cells undergoing mitosis) and a second group of which 78% had metastasized at the time of presentation (diploid tumours with 5-α-reductase activity less than 10 pmole/mg of protein per 30 minutes and with more than 15% of the cells undergoing mitosis). These data suggest that a novel and independent prognostic indicator of prostatic cancer progression might be obtained as a multifactorial discriminant by combining DNA ploidy with 5-α-reductase activity.

Matrix proteins of prostate cancer cells

In all epithelial malignancies hitherto examined, failure to construct an intact basement membrane occurs early in the metastatic process. Synthesis of laminin and its subsequent incorporation into basal lamina has been examined histochemically in a series of biopsy specimens from normal prostates, benign prostatic hyperplasia and prostatic carcinomas. Expression of this protein has been considered as a possible index of early tumour dissemination.[72] The results of this study are not surprising. Expression of laminin conforms to a pattern now readily apparent for many plasma-membrane or secreted glycoproteins: normal and hyperplastic prostatic epithelial cells synthesized and secreted the protein as a basal matrix component. However, correlating with increasing tumour Gleason grade, laminin disappeared from basement membranes. As this process occurred, synthesis of laminin continued but was retained as a cytoplasmic protein by the tumour cells. Although expression of this molecule shows correlation with Gleason grade, and is a good indicator of biological events early in the metastatic process, it provides no more useful information as a possible predictor of tumour behaviour.

Monoclonal antibody studies

Applications of monoclonal antibodies to human prostate cancer fall into three groups.

In the first group, monoclonals have been generated to a variety of well-characterized protein antigens with the expectation that epitope-specificity of these reagents might provide enhanced sensitivity and selectivity above that of polyclonal antibodies. Examples include monoclonal antibodies to human prostatic acid phosphatase[63,73] as well as to oncogene products such as the p21 *ras* protein.[74] Unfortunately, as already indicated, expression of the identified epitope structures in a wide variety of normal and neoplastic tissues[63] imposes identical limitations to those of the polyclonal antisera on the value of these reagents.

The second group of monoclonal antibody reagents are those which have been identified by random selection after generating hybridomas using lymphocytes from animals immunized with prostate cancer cells or their membrane fractions. Since Kohler and Milstein first reported the technique of generating monoclonal antibodies,[75] immunization of animals with whole cells or with non-characterized antigens has been repeatedly shown to be an inappropriate method of producing selective reagents. Nevertheless, several monoclonal antibodies obtained following such immunization have been employed to assess human prostate cancer.[76-78] All these antibodies are either non-specific or they do not identify epitopes expressed in a manner which correlates with tumour grade or patient prognosis.

The third group of monoclonal antibodies reflect cell-biological aspects of cancer and hence exhibit some prognostic value. Nevertheless, these reagents also react with malignancies other than prostatic neoplasms. With respect to prostate cancer, monoclonal antibody Ki-67 has proven to be the most important, even though it stains only frozen tissues which have not been fixed in formalin. Hence, it is of limited value as a routine diagnostic reagent. Ki-67 is a murine monoclonal antibody raised to a nuclear protein only present in proliferating cells.[79] In one study, using this antibody, the mean growth fraction of human prostate carcinomas was found to be 16.3%.[80] This figure was in the same range as that reported from flow-cytometric studies[56,57] and significantly less than the 4% found in benign prostatic glands. For individual tumours, correlation was shown between the tumour growth fraction assessed by Ki-67 staining and histological grade. A recent report has confirmed the ability to differentiate benign and malignant prostatic specimens using Ki-67 immunohistochemical staining.[81] Although the absolute figures from this laboratory were different from those reported earlier, correlation was demonstrated with data previously reported from the same centre using [³H]-thymidine labelling and bromodeoxyuridine incorporation. A relationship between Ki-67 staining and growth pattern of individual prostatic cancers was found. However, data relating to grading were not shown.

Oncogene expression

The role of cellular oncogenes in human prostatic cancer is presently poorly defined. Searches for transforming sequences of DNA homologous to those of known oncogenes, using the 3T3-transfection assay, have been generally unsuccessful.[82] Data from several sources indicate that no known oncogenes are specifically or consistently activated in prostate cancer. In one study, heterogeneous expression of *ras* oncogene p21 protein was present in 25% of primary prostatic cancer cells in one case.[83] In one other case, activation of Ki-*ras* has been described.[82] In all other prostate cancers hitherto reported, amplification of genomic sequences of Ki-*ras*, Ha-*ras*, c-*myc*, N-*myc*, c-*sis*, or c-*fos* has not been found. Considering the consensus finding of a consistently elevated growth fraction in all prostatic carcinomas examined, absence of activated c-*myc* is surprising. Similar findings also have been reported from studies of the Dunning R3327 rat prostatic adenocarcinoma model.[84]

All these studies indicate that there is presently no oncogene-marker with which to enhance detection of prostatic malignancy or identify prostate cancers which will behave in a particular phenotypical manner.

Problems of grading

General problems of grading

The fundamental concept underlying tumour grading is that within any tumour there are specific features which relate to the biology of that disease. Such features may be either architectural or morphological or they may be the expression (or non-expression) of specific cell-associated molecules and hence detectable only using special techniques. These principles have been applied with varying success to a wide variety of neoplasms, particularly carcinomas. However, in no instance has expression of any single parameter been shown to predict the behaviour of any single tumour arising within a particular patient.

It is extraordinary that so great a variety of different morphology-based schemes have been devised to grade and classify human prostate cancer. The fact that they all appear to work in providing some correlation with group behaviour has contributed to the continued survival of such disparate systems. Despite retrospective correlation between aspects of tumour architecture and group behaviour, no structural features, either alone or in combination, accurately predict functional aspects (e. g. invasive potential or drug resistance) of an individual prostate cancer. Furthermore, without objective parameters that can be determined independently of observer variation, morphological grading systems are entirely subjective so that it becomes impossible to compare the interpretations of different pathologists. This is the major weakness of any grading system based entirely on qualitative morphology.

Specific problems of grading prostate cancer

Prostate cancer is a slowly growing tumour. Microscopic examination frequently reveals a wide range of cytological and histological appearances. Behaviour of any individual tumour is unpredictable. Mostofi has suggested that the basic problem in grading carcinoma of the prostate lies in confusion over the criteria for 'anaplasia' and 'differentiation'.[85] He has suggested that detailed evaluation of cell shape would result in an accurate assessment of 'anaplasia'. Similarly, strict criteria should be applied to identifying gland formation within prostatic cancers, and for such formations the term 'differentiation' should be reserved. Unfortunately, it is now clearly apparent from recently published literature that unassisted morphological observations, however detailed these might be, are inadequate at predicting the behaviour of an individual prostate cancer. There is no doubt that identification of several different objective biological parameters, probably analysed in combination, will be required before a reliable system of grading prostatic cancer can be achieved.

Conclusions

The ability to identify cancers which will behave in a particular manner is one of the most sought goals of present-day pathology. All the morphological grading systems are, in this respect, clearly inadequate despite the application of sophisticated computer-based image-analysis systems with which to obtain more precise information. However, carefully applied grading systems have confirmed that, within all prostate cancers, there are *groups* of patients with different prognostic indices but that unassisted histological examination of those tumours will not identify *individual* patients with a good or bad prognosis. This failure of detailed histology has served to stimulate the search for independent markers with which to identify specific and functional aspects of cancer biology.

At present, the most useful parameters with which to assess primary prostatic malignancies appear to be growth-fraction (either by flow-cytometry or Ki-67 immunohistochemistry), ploidy status and 5-α-reductase activity. Other features of prostatic cancer cells should be sought, particularly cell-surface determinants relating to behavioural features such as metastatic ability and drug resistance. Current information also suggests that there is no apparent role for molecular probes to oncogenes in the assessment of prostate cancer histology. Nevertheless, investigation of these tumours for gene rearrangements and/or deletions might reveal regions of the genome important in prostate cancer.

Although there has been little progress in identifying reliable markers of prognosis for prostate cancer since 1926 when Broders first examined histological patterns of tumour differentiation,[14] the types of reagents which are required have been defined. Since the directions in which research should be concentrated to identify those reagents have become apparent, and the techniques to develop them are now available, the future for accurately assessing and grading prostate cancer now appears more optimistic than previously.

References

1. Scardino PT. Early detection of prostate cancer. *Urol Clin N Am* 1989; **16**: 635–55.
2. Dhom G. Epidemiologic aspects of latent and clinically manifest carcinoma of the prostate. *J Cancer Res Clin Onc* 1983; **106**: 210–18.
3. Foster CS. Predictive factors in prostatic hyperplasia and neoplasia. *Hum Path* 1990; **21**: 575–7.
4. Franks LM. Benign nodular hyperplasia of the prostate: a review. *Ann R Coll Surg Engl* 1954; **14**: 92–106.
5. McNeal JE. Normal histology of the prostate. *Am J Surg Pathol* 1988; **12**: 619–33.

6. Price H, McNeal JE, Stamey TA. Evolving patterns of tissue composition in benign prostatic hyperplasia as a function of specimen size. *Hum Path* 1990; **21**: 578–85.
7. Tannenbaum M. Atypical epithelial hyperplasia or carcinoma of the prostate gland: the surgical pathologist at an impasse? *Urology* 1974; **4**: 758–60.
8. Kastendieck H. Correlations between atypical hyperplasia and carcinoma of the prostate. *Path Res Pract* 1980; **169**: 366–78.
9. Helpap B. The biological significance of atypical hyperplasia of the prostate. *Virchows Arch Path Anat* 1980; **387**: 307–17.
10. McNeal JE. Origin and development of carcinoma in the prostate. *Cancer* 1969; **23**: 24–34.
11. Carstens PHB. Perineural glands in normal and hyperplastic prostates. *J Urol* 1980; **123**: 686–8.
12. Jensen PE, Gardner WA, Piserchia PV. Prostatic crystalloids: associations with adenocarcinoma. *Prostate* 1980; **1**: 25–30.
13. Bennett BD, Gardner WA. Crystalloids in prostatic hyperplasia. *Prostate* 1980; **1**: 31–5.
14. Broders AC. Carcinoma: grading and practical application. *Arch Path* 1926; **2**: 376–81.
15. Young HH, Davis DM. *Young's Practice of Urology*. Philadelphia: WB Saunders, 1926.
16. Muir EG. Carcinoma of the prostate. *Lancet* 1934; **i**: 667–72.
17. Kahler JE. Carcinoma of the prostate gland. *Mayo Clinic Proc* 1938; **13**: 589–92.
18. Evans N, Barnes RW, Brown AF. Carcinoma of the prostate: correlation between the histologic observations and the clinical course. *Arch Path* 1942; **34**: 473–83.
19. Edwards CN, Steinthorssen E, Nicholson D. An autopsy study of latent prostatic cancer. *Cancer* 1953; **6**: 531–54.
20. Shelley HS, Auerbach SH, Classen KL, *et al.* Carcinoma of the prostate: a new system of classification. *Arch Surg* 1958; **77**: 751–6.
21. Vickery AL, Kerr WS. Carcinoma of the prostate treated by radical prostatectomy. *Cancer* 1963; **16**: 1598–608.
22. Gleason DF. Classification of prostatic carcinoma. *Cancer Chemother Rep* 1966; **50**: 125–8.
23. Jewett HJ, Bridges RW, Gray GF, *et al.* The palpable nodule of prostatic cancer; results 15 years after radical excision. *J Am Med Ass* 1968; **203**: 403–6.
24. Mobley TL, Frank IN. Influence of tumor grade on survival and on serum acid phosphatase levels in metastatic cancer of prostate. *J Urol* 1968; **99**: 321–3.
25. Utz DC, Farrow GM. Pathological differentiation and prognosis of prostatic carcinoma. *J Am Med Ass* 1969; **209**: 1701–3.
26. Corriere JN, Cornog JL, Murphy JJ. Prognosis in patients with carcinoma of the prostate. *Cancer* 1970; **25**: 911–18.
27. Mostofi FK. Grading of prostatic carcinoma. *Cancer Chemother Rep* 1975; **59**: 111–17.
28. Müller H-A, Ackermann R, Frohmüller HGW, *et al.* The value of perineal punch biopsy in estimating histological grade of carcinoma of the prostate. *Prostate* 1980; **1**: 303–9.
29. Gaeta JF. Glandular profiles and cellular patterns in prostatic cancer grading. *Urology* 1981; **17** (Suppl): 33–7.
30. Brawn PM, Ayala AG, Von Eschenbach AC, *et al.* Histologic grading study of prostate adenocarcinoma: the development of a new system and comparison with other methods—a preliminary study. *Cancer* 1982; **49**: 525–32.
31. Böcking A, Sinagowitz E. Histologic grading of prostatic carcinoma. *Path Res Pract* 1980; **168**: 115–25.

32. Fan K, Peng CF. Predicting the probability of bone metastasis through histopathological grading of prostatic carcinoma: a retrospective correlative analysis of 81 autopsy cases with antemortem transurethral resection specimens. *J Urol* 1983; **130**: 708–11.

33. Schroeder FH, Blom JHM, Hop WCJ, Mostofi FK. Grading of prostatic cancer. I: An analysis of the prognostic significance of single characteristics. *Prostate* 1985; **6**: 81–100.

34. Schroeder FH, Blom JHM, Hop WCJ, Mostofi FK. Grading of prostatic cancer. II: The prognostic significance of the presence of multiple architectural patterns. *Prostate* 1985; **6**: 403–15.

35. Foulds L. The experimental study of tumour progression: a review. *Cancer Res* 1954; **14**: 327–39.

36. Foulds L. *Neoplastic Development*. New York: Academic Press, 1975.

37. Poste G, Grieg R. On the genesis and regulation of cellular heterogeneity in malignant tumours. *Invas Metast* 1982; **2**: 137–76.

38. Fidler IJ, Hart R. Biologic diversity in metastatic neoplasms: origins and implications. *Science* 1982; **217**: 998–1003.

39. McNeal JE, Bostwick DG, Kindrachuk RA, Redwine EA, Freiha FS, Stamey TA. Patterns of progression in prostate cancer. *Lancet* 1986; **1**: 60–3.

40. McNeal JE. Morphologic indices of progression in prostatic carcinoma. In: Coffey DS, Gardner WA, Bruchovsky N, Resnick MI, Karr JP, *Current Concepts and Approaches to the Study of Prostate Cancer*. New York: Alan Liss, 1987: 779–82.

41. Partin AW, Epstein JI, Cho KR, *et al.* Morphometric measurement of tumour volume and per cent of gland involvement as predictors of pathological stage in clinical stage B prostate cancer. *J Urol* 1989; **141**: 341–5.

42. Humphrey P, Vollmer RT. The ratio of prostate chips with cancer: a new measure of tumour extent and its relationship to grade and prognosis. *Hum Path* 1988; **19**: 411–18.

43. Foucar E, Haake G, Dalton L, Pathak DR, Lujan JP. The area of cancer in transurethral resection specimens as a prognostic indicator in carcinoma of the prostate: a computer-assisted morphometric study. *Hum Path* 1990; **21**: 586–92.

44. Diamond DA, Berry SJ, Jewett HJ, *et al.* A new method to assess metastatic potential of human prostate cancer: relative nuclear roundness. *J Urol* 1982; **128**: 729–34.

45. Epstein JI, Berry SJ, Eggleston JC. Nuclear roundness factor: a predictor of progression in untreated state A$_2$ prostate cancer. *Cancer* 1984; **54**; 1666–71.

46. Tannenbaum M, Tannenbaum S, DeSanctis PN, *et al.* Prognostic significance of nucleolar surface area in prostatic cancer. *Urology* 1982; **19**: 546–51.

47. Myers RP, Neves RJ, Farrow GM, Utz DC. Nucleolar grading of prostatic adenocarcinoma: light microscopic correlation with disease progression. *Prostate* 1982; **3**: 423–32.

48. Narayan P, Jajodia P, Stein R, Tanahgo EA. A comparison of fine needle aspiration and core biopsy in diagnosis and preoperative grading of prostate cancer. *J Urol* 1989; **141**: 560–3.

49. Mohler JL, Erozan YS, Walsh PC, Epstein JI. Fine needle core and aspiration biopsy: a new method for diagnosis of prostatic carcinoma. *Cancer* 1989; **63**: 1846–55.

50. Ro JY, Grignon DJ, Ayala AG, *et al.* Mucinous adenocarcinoma of the prostate: histochemical and immunohistochemical studies. *Hum Path* 1990; **21**: 593–600.

51. Epstein JI, Leiberman PH. Mucinous adenocarcinoma of the prostate gland. *Am J Surg Path* 1985; **9**: 299–308.

52. Diamond DA, Berry SJ, Umbrecht C, *et al*. Computerized image analysis of nuclear shape as a prognostic factor for prostatic cancer. *Prostate* 1982; **3**: 321–32.
53. Stephenson RA, James BC, Gay H, Fair WR, Whitmore WF, Melamed MR. Flow cytometry of prostate cancer: relationship of DNA content to survival. *Cancer Res* 1987; **47**: 2504–7.
54. Dejter SW, Cunningham RE, Noguchi PD, *et al*. Prognostic significance of DNA ploidy in carcinoma of the prostate. *Urology* 1989; **33**: 361–6.
55. Richie AW, Dorey F, Layfield LJ, Hannah J, Lovrekovich H, deKernion JB. Relationship of DNA content to conventional prognostic factors in clinically localised carcinoma of the prostate. *Br J Urol* 1988; **62**: 245–60.
56. Habib FK, Bissas A, Neill WA, Busuttil A, Chisholm GD. Flow cytometric analysis of cellular DNA in human prostate cancer: relationship to 5 alpha-reductase activity of the tissue. *Urol Res* 1989; **17**: 239 43.
57. Neill WA, Norval M, Habib FK. Nuclear DNA analysis of prostate tissues: correlation with stage and grade of tumour. *Urol Int* 1989; **44**: 141–6.
58. Nemoto R, Uchida K, Shimazui T, *et al*. Immunocytochemical demonstration of S phase cells by anti-bromodeoxyuridine monoclonal antibody in human prostate adenocarcinoma. *J Urol* 1989; **141**: 337–40.
59. Watt KWK, Lee PJ, M'Timkulu T, Chan WP, Loor R. Human prostate specific antigen: structural and functional similarity with serum proteases. *Proc Natl Acad Sci* 1986; **83**: 3166–70.
60. Barka T. A simple azo method for histochemical demonstration of acid phosphatase. *Nature* 1960; **187**: 248.
61. Abdul-Fadl MAM, King EJ. Properties of the acid phosphatases of erythrocytes and of the human prostate gland. *Biochem J* 1949; **45**: 51.
62. Waheed A, van Etten RL, Gieselmann V, von Figura K. Immunological characterisation of human acid phosphatase gene products. *Biochem Genet* 1985; **23**: 309–19.
63. Haines AMR, Larkin SE, Richardson AP, Stirling RW, Heyderman E. A novel hybridoma antibody (PASE/4LJ) to human prostatic acid phosphatase suitable for immunohistochemistry. *Br J Cancer* 1989; **60**: 887–92.
64. Maddy SQ, Chisholm GD, Busuttil A, Habib FK. Epidermal growth factor receptors in human prostate cancer: correlation with histological differentiation of the tumour. *Br J Cancer* 1989; **60**: 41–4.
65. Benson RC, Gorman PA, O'Brien PC, Holicky EL, Veneziale CM. Relationship between androgen receptor binding activity in human prostate cancer and clinical response to endocrine therapy. *Cancer* 1987; **59**: 1599–606.
66. Tarle M, Culig Z, Kokic I. Unoccupied prolactin binding components of the benign and malignant human prostate in a subclinical and clinical procedure. *Int J Rad Appl Instrum B* 1989; **16**: 461–7.
67. Akimoto S, Fuse H, Sato R, Zama S, Shimazaki J. Binding of mibolerone to androgen receptor of benign hypertrophic human prostates: comparison with R1881. *Endocrinol Japn* 1985; **32**: 141–52.
68. Yamaguchi K, Sumiya H, Fuse H, Matsuzaki O, Ito H, Ki JS. Androphilic protein studied histochemically in stage D2 prostatic cancer. *Cancer* 1988; **61**: 1425–9.
69. Forsgren B, Gustafsson J-Å, Pousette Å, Högberg B. Binding characteristics of a major protein in rat ventral prostate cytosol that interacts with estramustine, a nitrogen mustard derivative of 17β-estradiol. *Cancer Res* 1979; **39**: 5155–64.
70. Fluchter SH, Nelde HJ, Bjork P, Muntzing J, Bichler KH. Effect of treatment on the

expression of estramustine-binding protein (EMBP) in prostatic cancer patients: an immunohistochemical study. *Prostate* 1989; **14**: 27–43.

71. Peterson RE. Metabolism of adrenal cortical steroids. In: Christy N (ed.), *The Human Adrenal Cortex*. New York: Harper & Row, 1971.

72. Sinah AA, Gleason DF, Wilson MJ, *et al*. Immunohistochemical localization of laminin in the basement membranes of normal, hyperplastic and neoplastic human prostate. *Prostate* 1989; **15**: 299–313.

73. Lam KW, Li CY, Yam LT, Sun T, Lee G, Ziesmer S. Improved immunohistochemical detection of prostatic acid phosphatase by a monoclonal antibody. *Prostate* 1989; **15**: 13–21.

74. Fan K. Heterogeneous subpopulations of human prostatic adenocarcinoma cells: potential usefulness of P21 protein as a predictor for bone metastasis. *J Urol* 1988; **139**: 318–22.

75. Kohler G, Milstein C. Continuous cultures of fused cells secreting antibody of predefined specificity. *Nature* 1975; **256**: 495–7.

76. Bazinet M, Cote RJ, Cordon-Cardo C, Myc A, Fair WR, Old LJ. Immunohistochemical characterization of two monoclonal antibodies, P25.48 and P25.91, which define a new prostate-specific antigen. *Cancer Res* 1988; **48**: 6938–42.

77. Kim YD, Robinson DY, Tomita JT. Monoclonal antibody PR92 with restricted specificity for tumour-associated antigen of prostate and breast carcinoma. *Cancer Res* 1988; **48**: 4543–8.

78. Donn F, Bruns T, von Meyerinck L, *et al*. Monoclonal antibody that defines the prostate specific antigen. *Prostate* 1989; **14**: 237–49.

79. Gerdes J, Schwab U, Lemke H, Stein H. Production of a mouse monoclonal antibody reactive with a human nuclear antigen associated with cell proliferation. *Int J Cancer* 1983; **31**: 13–20.

80. Raymond WA, Leong AS, Bolt JW, Milios J, Jose JS. Growth fractions in human prostatic carcinoma determined by Ki-67 immunostaining. *J Pathol* 1988; **156**: 161–7.

81. Gallee MP, Visser de Jong E, ten Kate FJ, Schroeder FH, Van der Kwast TH. Monoclonal antibody Ki-67 defined growth fraction in prostatic hyperplasia and prostatic cancer. *J Urol* 1989; **142**: 1342–6.

82. Peehl DM, Wehner N, Stamey TA. Activated Ki-ras oncogene in human prostatic adenocarcinoma. *Prostate* 1987; **10**: 281–9.

83. Fan K. Heterogeneous subpopulations of human prostatic adenocarcinoma cells: potential usefulness of P21 protein as a predictor of bone metastasis. *J Urol* 1988; **139**: 318–22.

84. Cooke DB, Quarmby VE, Mickey DD, Isaacs JT, French FS. Oncogene expression in prostate cancer: Dunning R3327 rat dorsal prostatic adenocarcinoma system. *Prostate* 1988; **13**: 263–72.

85. Mostofi FK. Problems of grading carcinoma of the prostate. *Sem Onc* 1976; **3**: 161–9.

8 Radical prostatectomy in localized prostatic cancer

Gordon Williams

Radical prostatectomy should still be considered experimental. Its continued use is probably one of the longest running phase I investigations in cancer. In the only clinical trial comparing radical prostatectomy to placebo, no advantage was found for surgery.[1]

If the natural history of localized prostate cancer is examined in detail it becomes possible to recognize the minimal impact that radical surgery has on the overall mortality from prostatic cancer.

The advent of transrectal ultrasound and ultrasound-guided biopsy has increased the detection rate of early prostate cancer. But what is the optimal treatment once such a cancer has been found? If it were possible to stage prostatic cancer accurately to confirm that it was organ-confined, and if it could be shown that there was a high likelihood of cancer progression or cancer death within the life expectancy of that man, then radical prostatectomy to remove the tumour *in toto* would be justified. Unfortunately radical prostatectomy does not achieve its objective because current staging techniques understage 40% of patients.[2] In addition, the vast majority of patients with untreated disease do not have disease progression. As a result radical prostatectomy must be considered to be gross over-treatment for the majority of men with so-called localized prostate cancer. Additionally the operation which has an associated mortality and morbidity cannot be justified in those patients who have extracapsular or metastatic spread.

Such dogmatic views will be hotly disputed by many overseas urologists and the few British urologists who are now beginning to perform radical prostatectomies. This chapter tries to identify a group of men in whom this operation might be justified, but does not succeed in that effort. This group would include men in whom one can guarantee that surgical excision will remove all tumour, and that the removed tumour would have led to the demise of those men during their expected lifetime.

Incidence and natural history

Estimates for 1988 suggest that approximately 99 000 new cases of cancer of the prostate were diagnosed in the United States, and 28 000 died from the disease.[3] Twenty-five per cent of the newly diagnosed patients will have metastatic disease and at least 15% extra prostatic spread.[4]

Ninety-five per cent of prostate cancers are diagnosed in men between the ages of 45 and 89 years with a median age of 72 years.[5] Over 40% of men who died after the age of 90 years will have prostate cancer at autopsy.[6]

One of the major problems in detecting cancer of the prostate is defining the prevalence rate. Many early studies did not use systematic stepwise section of the prostate and report an incidence of 8–14% of latent carcinomas at age 50–60 years, and 11% at age 60–70 years. However, several series of patients undergoing radical cystoprostatectomy for cancer of the bladder have used step sections. Using data from these large series, it is possible to estimate the relationship between age and prevalence and determine an average cancer prevalence of approximately 30% between 50 and 60 years and 36% between 60 and 70 years.[7] The worldwide prevalence of incidental prostate cancer as identified from autopsy studies is high.[8,9] A role for race and geographical factors in the natural history of prostate cancer is provided by the wide geographical variations in the clinical incidence of this disease.

As clinically significant prostate cancer occurs predominantly in elderly men, the natural history of the disease is often interrupted by the death of the host from other causes.[10]

With such a high prevalence of latent cancer it is obvious that in the USA with just 100 000 new cases of cancer of the prostate being diagnosed each year, the great majority of patients never develop clinically manifest disease. If all these latent cancers were to be diagnosed and treated then this would be a gross and unnecessary over-treatment for over 90% of them, as just 28 000 patients die from prostatic cancer annually.

However, this does not mean that we should not continue to strive to identify that very small subset of men with potentially aggressive, confined tumours with an otherwise long life expectancy who would undoubtedly benefit from total eradication of their cancer. This is obviously more relevant in the younger man. There is no evidence that the disease behaves any differently in younger age-groups, but metastatic disease is more prevalent at presentation in younger men.[4] No significant influence of age on the progression of prostatic cancer has been found when comparing patients under 60 years with those of 65–74 years.[11]

The tumour phenotypes which determine cell growth and metastatic potential are still poorly understood. A variety of microscopic features of the tumour have been studied, including nuclear roundness, lymphocyte infiltration, perineural and blood vessel invasion, and more recently tumour ploidy, cell surface carbohydrate expression,[12] oncogene expression and growth factor receptor levels. Despite these advances, it is still not possible to predict tumour behaviour in an individual. Some of these markers are undoubtedly associated with a high metastatic potential, but this is of little help to the individual patient when it is not possible reliably to identify spread into the seminal vesicles or the lymph nodes without major surgery.

These new techniques have still not replaced tumour grade and stage for assessing the likelihood of disease progression. Tumour grade and local stage correlate with the microscopic local extent of the tumour,[13] and the presence or absence of nodal or distal metastases;[14] more generally, well-differentiated tumours are associated with lower T categories and vice versa. However, assessment of tumour grade is subjective irrespective of the system used, and the assessment of T category without the pathological specimen is often inaccurate despite advances in imaging techniques. Though useful for distinguishing likely tumour behaviour in groups of patients, they are of less reliable prognostic value for the individual.

Tumour stage and progression

In a study of 20 patients with incidentally diagnosed prostate cancer found during transurethral resection, a normal 15-year life expectancy was found for those with well-differentiated tumours, and a normal 10-year but diminished 15-year survival for those with high-grade lesions.[15] Incidentally diagnosed tumours were later divided into categories, A1 and A2 or T0A or T0B according to tumour grade and percentage of the prostate involved.[16] Extended follow-up of 94 patients with untreated A1 disease with a Gleason score of less than 7 found that 26 (27.6%) died from unrelated causes within four years. None of the 18 followed from four to eight years, nor 42 of 50 followed from eight to eighteen years, developed progression. However, eight did progress at a mean of seven years, and in six of these prostate cancer was the cause of death.[17] In a series of 145 patients with T1–2 N0 M0 tumours the outcome of surgery was related to the anatomical extent of the disease and the Gleason score related to the extent of the disease and the probability of extension of disease beyond the prostate.[18]

Patients with A2 prostatic cancer (i.e. larger volume and/or higher grade tumours) have progression rates of around 25%. Gleason has shown that a patient with a well-differentiated nodule of less than 1.5 cm diameter and a Gleason score of 4 to 8 has very little chance of dying of prostate cancer.[19] Since 25% of patients with clinical A2 lesions have lymph node metastases[20] and should have been categorized as D, the incidence of progression parallels that of lymph node metastases. Data on progression rates for true A2 lesions (i.e. without nodal involvement) are not available.

The recent adoption of a classification similar to the TNM system using the traditional A, B and C categories but adding N and M categories will ensure that in future we are at least describing similar patient groups and not comparing, for example, A2 N0 with A2 N1 or A2 NX when arguing a case for deferred or active treatment by either surgery or radiotherapy.

By definition, A1 and A2 lesions are found in clinically benign prostate glands. In such patients, who are subsequently treated by radical prostatectomy, either no residual tumour will be found in 8% or non-organ-confined tumour in 46% of cases.[21,22] Current staging techniques are still too inaccurate to give a prognosis for an individual patient. However, when considering A1 and A2 N0 tumours, prolonged survival without treatment can be expected; and in those with A1/A2 N1 tumours the rate of progression mirrors the incidence of this disease category. Radical lymphadenectomy in this situation is of prognostic and not therapeutic value.

Category B lesions are often cited as the classical indication for radical therapy. To obtain the natural history of this group of patients is difficult. In particular, B lesions are subdivided into B1, B2 and B3, and are associated with an incidence of lymph node metastases of 25%.[23] One hundred and twenty-nine B category patients (85% of whom were B2 or B3) were treated by transurethral resection alone.[15] Crude survival rates at 5, 10 and 15 years were 19%, 4% and 1% respectively. Overall survival rates of 90%, 55% and 20% were found at 5, 10 and 15 years in a series of patients with B category disease randomized in 1975 to placebo or radical prostatectomy. Unfortunately data for causes of death and a requirement for endocrine therapy were unavailable.[1] An 87.7% actuarial disease-specific survival rate for 170 untreated patients with B category disease has been reported.[24] In the 223 untreated patients with locally confined tumours (lymph node staging was not carried out), the five-year progression-free survival for grade I was 82.9%, grade II 50.3%, and grade III 26.7%. With a mean follow-up of 78 months, prostate cancer was considered to be the cause of death in only 16 patients (7%). Had patients with identified nodal metastases and with grade III disease been excluded, the corrected five-year survival would approach 100% for both stage A and B disease. Stage was a predictor of progression and grade a predictor of both progression and disease-specific death.[24] In another study, 75 patients with stage B disease whose average age was 67 years received no treatment for at least one year. Fifteen-year actuarial survival for B1 disease was 67 ± 12%, B2 42 ± 10%, and B3 67 ± 21%, with an expected fifteen-year survival according to mean age at diagnosis of 45%, 38% and 31% respectively. At the time of last follow-up, only 11 had died from prostate cancer and 18 from other causes. Not all these patients remained untreated: 23 had TURs, 18 endocrine therapy and 5 pelvic lymphadenectomy with ^{125}I implants.[25] This study clearly shows that some patients with stage B disease may have no further symptoms, a low incidence and delayed onset of metastatic disease, and an almost normal life expectancy with a high probability of dying of other causes. Supposedly curative therapy may be unnecessary on a stage for stage basis.

Staging methods

The techniques available for staging prostate carcinoma that are of particular value in assessing the feasibility of curative surgery or radiotherapy include acid phosphatase, prostate specific antigen, ultrasound, CT scanning, MRI and digital rectal examination.

Serum acid phosphatase

If elevated this usually indicates metastatic disease. Sixty per cent of patients with an elevated acid phosphatase and clinically localized cancer have positive pelvic nodes. A further 20% develop bone metastases within two years.[26] Acid phosphatase has been reported to be elevated in 0–48% of organ-confined disease,[27,28] in 35–75% of stage C,[28,29] and in 9–90% of those with lymph node involvement.[27,28] It is undoubtedly too imprecise to provide information of value for the individual.

Ultrasound

This has demonstrated that prostatic malignancies may be hypo, hyper, iso or of mixed echogenicity. Since the tumours are often multifocal, some tumours will be missed and others inaccurately staged. Large cancers can replace all of the normally isogenic peripheral zone, masking any ultrasound reference for normal tissue to contrast with the hypoechogenic tumour.[30] Ultrasound is unable to identify microscopic capsular or extracapsular invasion into periprostatic tissues or seminal vesicles; and even using ultrasound-guided biopsy these areas may be missed, which defeats the object of a radical prostatectomy. Lesions greater than 3 cm usually exhibit capsular or seminal vesicle involvement, whereas those of less than 1 cm are generally confined to the prostate.[31] Of 60 patients with stage B2, B3, or C prostate cancer, 20 had abnormal seminal vesicle appearances and 40 normal. Ultrasound-guided biopsies were positive in only 14 of those with abnormal seminal vesicles, but 7 of those with normal seminal vesicles were found to have histological evidence of tumour invasion after radical prostatectomy.[32] In a further study, only 5 of 13 patients with capsular or seminal vesicle penetration found after surgery were correctly identified preoperatively with ultrasound.[33] A sensitivity of only 29% for seminal vesicle involvement in patients undergoing radical prostatectomy has been reported.[34]

CAT scanning and MRI

CAT scanning can assess the periprostatic area and lymph node size but not involvement. Intraprostatic detail is poor.

Magnetic resonance imaging can demonstrate intraprostatic anatomy and is similar to CAT scanning in assessing the periprostatic area and lymph node size. Normal-sized nodes may, however, contain tumour.

Prostate-specific antigen

PSA has been used both for staging and monitoring progress in prostatic cancer. However, the failure to use appropriate reference groups has led to upper limits of normal ranging from 1.7 to 46 mg/ml.

All subjects within a reference group should be adequately assessed for prostatic disease, urinary symptoms, physical examination, transrectal ultrasonography and histological evaluation.

A failure to demonstrate any significant difference between PSA in benign prostatic hypertrophy and localized cancer (stages A and B) has been reported.[35] These workers also found large variations in the incidence of PSA elevation in the different stages of prostate cancer.

In a detailed analysis, PSA was shown to be the most efficient of twelve tumour markers assessed, but it lacked the sensitivity required to diagnose early prostate cancer.[36]

The prognostic importance of PSA in 70 patients with regionally confined (B2 to D1) tumours has been evaluated and a highly significant association between PSA and disease-free survival found.[37] Twenty-four of 26 patients who had disease progression had an elevated PSA in the preceding 12 months. However, 9 of 44 patients with an elevated PSA within the preceding 12 months did not progress. When PSA is only moderately elevated, its value in predicting prognosis is limited. Using Cox's proportional hazards model to determine the relative importance of PSA, disease stage and type of treatment, PSA predicted progression, and the disease stage and type of treatment were relatively unimportant. Only 43 patients were used for this analysis.[37] The lead time for disease progression depends on the degree of elevation of PSA. The higher the level the shorter the time to progression.

Although the data suggest that it would be difficult to identify patients who were about to progress by means of the pattern of change of their PSA with time,[38] PSA does have a role in determining the success or failure of the complete extirpation of the prostatic cancer. The persistence of PSA in the serum is a clear marker of the failure of radical surgery and is being increasingly reported. Data on the outcome of such patients are awaited.

Comparison of treatment outcomes

Many factors have led to the author's decision not to undertake radical prostatectomies in patients with so-called localized disease: in particular, the subjectivity of current grading criteria, the absence of predictors of progression, the inaccuracies of current staging techniques with regard to both local and distal spread, the possibility that the disease was removed at the original transurethral resection, the mortality and morbidity associated with radical prostatectomy, and a death rate from non-prostatic cancer which exceeds that of the cancer itself. The following discussion deals with the evidence of therapeutic benefit from radical surgery and from expectant treatments, and fails to identify anything but a minimal impact such therapy has on disease outcome.

Deferred treatment

The best results obtained so far in highly selected patients undergoing radical prostatectomy have been five-year survival rates of greater than 90%.[39–41] In the only published controlled trial, of radical prostatectomy versus placebo, no advantage was found in the group treated by radical surgery.[1]

To advocate deferred treatment is not nihilistic nor is it a recent view. In 1959, Scott stated that endocrine therapy should be reserved for those with metastases causing pain.[42] In the placebo arm of the Veterans Administrative Study, only 50% of patients progressed to metastatic disease in five years. In a retrospective study with a minimum follow-up of five years, it was found that in M0 patients there was no difference in time to first or second progression in the treated and untreated groups. In M1 patients, endocrine therapy did not influence overall survival, and 36% of M0 patients needed no anticancer therapy in five years.[43]

The clinician's decision on the need to treat may be based on increase in prostate size, elevation of biochemical markers or the development of symptomatic metastases. Some studies using deferred treatment may give an unwarranted pessimistic outlook with regard to the need for treatment unless the indication is stated. The realization that the true objective response to endocrine therapy is only in the region of 50% and the lack of evidence that immediate treatment is necessary has led to the setting up of two large studies comparing immediate and deferred treatment.

The Medical Research Council and the EORTC are respectively comparing immediate and deferred orchidectomy or GnRH agonist treatment for patients who are M0 or asymptomatic M1, and for patients who are T0–4, N0–2 M0. Patients with locally advanced disease which could cause a fatal outcome if left untreated (e.g. ureteric obstruction) are excluded from these studies.

The outcome of these studies is likely to confirm the view that a policy of active surveillance will spare many patients the trauma, both physical and psychological, of major surgery and will ensure that treatment with its side-effects is given only to those in whom symptomatic progression has been identified.

Radical prostatectomy

Stage A1–A2 disease

Forty-one patients with A1 tumours underwent a staging lymphadenectomy. None had pelvic lymph node involvement. In addition, 51% of patients had no evidence of residual tumour in the resected prostate (step sectioning was not performed).[44] In a further series, 31 patients underwent radical prostatectomy for stage A1 carcinoma. Sixteen had no residual tumour, 11 had only focal residual tumours that the authors considered clinically insignificant, and only 4 had diffuse residual disease.[45] Despite the frequency with which a radical prostatectomy is performed for this category, it is surprisingly difficult to find meaningful long-term cancer progression and cancer death rates. For example, 25% of clinical A2 tumours have lymph node metastases and should therefore be categorized as D1. Paulson *et al.*[46] found that 25% of their patients with A category disease had seminal vesicle involvement and 49% had non-organ-confined tumours. Of 101 patients with stage A prostate cancer treated by radical prostatectomy from four series followed from 0 to 25 years, cancer progression occurred in only 10% and cancer deaths in 1%.[47] The proportion of patients with A disease was not always stated.

A 75% survival at ten years for patients with A2 disease undergoing a radical prostatectomy has been reported. However, of these surviving patients only two-thirds are apparently free of tumour.[45] In addition, 10% of the patients died of cancer.[48] A radical prostatectomy cannot be said to have achieved its objective in those with residual disease and those who died from cancer.

Stage B disease

In Jewett's early series of radical prostatectomy for B1 disease, 27% survived for 15 years free of tumour. Overall, approximately one-third with B1 nodules died from prostatic cancer. No patient with microscopic seminal vesicle involvement survived for 15 years.[49]

A 15-year disease-free survival of 52% was reported by Hodges *et al.*[50] When adjuvant endocrine therapy was used, a 15-year disease-free survival of 75% was obtained.[51] These results are the same as the survival in the general population without overt prostate cancer.

For clinical category B2 patients the problem of defining the extent of the tumour by digital rectal examination or even ultrasound is difficult. One-half to two-thirds may have seminal vesicle involvement making them unsuitable for radical prostatectomy. In addition up to 50% will have lymph node involvement.[52,53] However, when the lymph nodes are free of tumour, 86% of patients with clinical category B2 tumour are histologically confined.[54]

Only 50% of patients with histologically confirmed B2 lesions were alive and free of tumour at 10 years, and 23% had died of prostate cancer.[55] Stage B tumours encompass a wide spectrum of disease which current staging techniques are unable to distinguish between with the degree of accuracy required to advise the individual patient. A radical prostatectomy does not achieve its objective in a high proportion of patients with category B disease.

Complications of radical prostatectomy

Death

In one of the largest series of patients treated by radical prostatectomy a death rate of 2% was reported.[53] No deaths were reported in a series of 207 patients undergoing radical perineal prostatectomy.[56] Wider review of the literature suggests that 0–5% of deaths can be expected following radical prostatectomy.[47,51]

Anastomotic urethral stricture

This has been reported to occur in 2.5–23% of cases. The best approach for the urethrovesicle anastomosis is by the perineal approach. Using this approach, an 18% stricture rate has been reported.[56]

Incontinence

In my experience of talking to urology residents in the USA, the incidence of both mild and severe incontinence tends to be under-reported. At least 6% can be expected to have some significant degree of incontinence.[56–58]

Rectal injury and colostomy

This has been reported in 0.5–7% of cases. An incidence of 5% was reported by Gibbons *et al.*[56] and 3% by Middleton *et al.*[57]

Impotence

Approximately 50% of men undergoing radical prostatectomy are already impotent. Even with the nerve-sparing operation[59] up to 50% of those who are potent preoperatively will be impotent postoperatively.

Conclusions

Information as to whether radical prostatectomy favourably affects the outcome of prostate cancer confined to the gland will only be provided by randomized controlled trials. Despite its widespread use since its first description by Young in 1904,[60] it should still be considered experimental.

The National Institute of Health Consensus Development Conference on the management of clinically localized prostate cancer[61] did not consider deferred treatment an option, and concluded that properly designed and randomized trials to evaluate disease control and quality of life after modern radiation therapy compared with after radical prostatectomy are essential. In addition, the patient should have available the following information when considering with his physician the choice of treatment: the probability of a cure, of death or of complications and side-effects of radical prostatectomy and radiation therapy; the risk of impotence and incontinence from either treatment; psychosocial consequences of either choice; the extent and risk of pre-treatment staging assessment tests; and the economic consequences of each form of treatment. We are a long way from providing this information for the individual patient.

There is no doubt that some patients do have a malignant tumour confined to the gland which, if left, will spread and cause the demise of that man within his normal period of life expectancy. On-going research will, it is hoped, enable us to identify such a patient who is likely to benefit from radical surgery. At present, a radical prostatectomy frequently fails to achieve its objective because of our inability to stage the disease.

Radical prostatectomy is over-treatment for those patients whose disease will not progress, and ineffective treatment for patients who will die anyway of progressive disease.

References

1. Madsen PO, Graversen PH, Gasser TC, Corle DK. Treatment of localised prostate cancer: radical prostatectomy versus placebo: a 15-year follow-up. *Scand J Nephrol* 1988; **110**: 95–100.
2. Lange PH. Controversies in management of apparently localised carcinoma of prostate. *Urology* 1989; **34** (suppl): 13–18.
3. Silverberg E, Lubera J. Cancer statistics. *CA* 1989; **38**: 5–22.
4. Murphy GP, Natarajan N, Pontes JE. The National Survey of Prostate Cancer in the United States by the American College of Surgeons. *J Urol* 1982; **127**: 928–34.
5. Winkelstein W, Ernster VL. Epidemiology and etiology. In: Murphy GP (ed.), *Prostate Cancer*. Littleton, MA: PSG Publishing, 1979: 1–17.
6. Hanash KA. Natural history of prostatic cancer. In: *Prostate Cancer: Imaging Techniques, Radiotherapy, Chemotherapy and Management Issues*. New York: Alan Liss, 1987: 289–320.
7. Optenberg SA, Thompson IM. Economics of screening for carcinoma of the prostate. *Urol Clin N Am* 1990; **17**: 719–37.
8. Meickle AW, Smith JA. Epidemiology of prostate cancer. *Urol Clin N Am* 1990; **17**: 709–18.
9. Breslow N, Chan CW, Dhom G, Drury RAB, Franks LM, Gellei B, Lee YS, Lundberg S, Sparke B, Sternby NH, Tulinus H. Latent carcinoma of prostate at autopsy in seven areas. *Int J Cancer* 1977; **20**: 680–8.
10. George NJR. Natural history of localised prostatic cancer managed by conservative therapy alone. *Lancet* 1988; **ii**: 494–7.
11. Harrison GSM. The prognosis of prostatic cancer in the younger man. *Br J Urol* 1983; **55**: 315–20.
12. Abel PD, Foster CS, Tebbutt S, Williams G. Differences in expression of oligosaccharide determinants by phenotypically distinct sublines of the Dunning 3327 rat. *J Urol* 1990; **144**: 760–5.
13. Stamey TA, McNeal JE, Freiha FS, Redwine E. Morphometric and clinical studies on 68 consecutive radical prostatectomies. *J Urol* 1988; **139**: 1235–41.
14. Donohue RE, Mani JH, Whitesel JA, Moh RS, Scanavino D, Augspurger FR, Biber RJ, Fauver HE, Wettlaufer JN, Pfister RR. Pelvic lymph node dissection: guide to patient management in clinically locally confined adenocarcinoma of the prostate. *Urology* 1982; **20**: 559–65.
15. Hanash KA, Utz D, Cook EN, Taylor WF, Titus JL. Carcinoma of the prostate: a 15-year follow-up. *J Urol* 1972; **107**: 450–3.
16. Jewett HJ. The present status of radical prostatectomy for stages A and B prostatic cancer. *Urol Clin N Am* 1975; **2**: 105–24.
17. Epstein JI, Paull G, Eggleston JC, Walsh PC. Prognosis of untreated stage A1 prostatic carcinoma: a study of 94 cases with extended follow-up. *J Urol* 1986; **136**: 837–9.
18. Paulson DF, Walther PJ. Is grade or stage of primary importance in determining the outcome after radical prostatectomy for disease clinically confined to the prostate? *Br J Urol* 1989; **63**: 301–5.
19. Gleason DF. 1988. Histology grade, clinical stage and patient age in prostate cancer: Consensus Development Conference on the Management of Clinically Localised Prostate Cancer. *NCI Monograph G.R. 7*: 3–6.
20. Smith JA, Cho Y-H. Management of stage A prostate cancer. *Urol Clin N Am* 1990; **17**: 769–77.

21. Epstein JI, Oesterling JE, Walsh PC. The volume and anatomical location of residual tumour in radical prostatectomy specimens removed for stage A1 prostate cancer. *J Urol* 1988; **139**: 975–9.

22. Paulson DF, Robertson JE, Daubert LM, Walther PJ. Radical prostatectomy in stage A prostatic adenocarcinoma. *J Urol* 1988; **140**: 535–9.

23. Austenfeld MS, Davis BE. Treatment of stage D1 adenocarcinoma of the prostate. *Urol Clin N Am* 1990; **17**: 867–84.

24. Johansson JE, Andersson SO, Krusemo UB, Adami HO, Bergstrom R, Kraaz W. Natural history of localised prostatic cancer. *Lancet* 1989; **i**: 799–803.

25. Whitmore WF. Natural history of prostatic cancer. *Urol Clin N Am* 1990; **17**: 689–97.

26. Whitesel JA, Donohue RE, Mani JH, Mohr S, Scanavino DJ, Augspurger RR, Biber RJ, Fauver HE, Wettlaufer JN, Pfister RR. Acid phosphatase: its influence on the management of carcinoma of the prostate. *J Urol* 1984; **131**: 70–2.

27. Killian CS, Vargas FS, Lee CL, Wang MC, Murphy GP, Chu TM. Quantitative counterimmunoelectrophoresis assay for prostate acid phosphatase. *Invest Urol* 1980; **18**: 219–24.

28. Pontes JE, Choe BK, Rose NR, Ercole C, Pierce JM. Clinical evaluation of immunological methods for detection of serum prostatic acid phosphatase. *J Urol* 1981; **126**: 363–5.

29. Lee CL, Chu TM, Wajsman LZS, Man LZ, Slack NH, Murphy GP. Value of new fluorescent immunoassay for human prostate acid phosphatase in prostate cancer. *Urology* 1980; **15**: 338–41.

30. Waterhouse RL, Resnick MI. The use of transrectal prostatic ultrasonography in the evaluation of patients with prostatic carcinoma. *J Urol* 1989; **141**: 233–9.

31. McNeal JE, Kindrachuk RA, Freith FS, Bostwick DG, Redwine EA, Stamey TA. Patterns of progression in prostate cancer. *Lancet* 1986; **ii**: 60–3.

32. Hodge KK, McNeal JE, Stamey TA. Ultrasound guided transrectal core biopsies of the palpably abnormal prostate. *J Urol* 1989; **142**: 66–70.

33. Andriole GI, Catalona WJ. Transrectal ultrasonography in the staging of prostate cancer. In: Resnick MR, Watanabe H, Karr JP (eds), *Diagnostic Ultrasound of the Prostate*. New York: Elsevier Science Publishing, 1989: 25–30.

34. Salo JO, Kivisaari L, Rannikko S, Lehtonen T. Computerised tomography and transrectal ultrasound in the assessment of local extension of prostatic cancer before radical retropubic prostatectomy. *J Urol* 1987; **137**: 435–8.

35. Kuriyama M, Wang MC, Papsidero LD, Killian CS, Shimaro T, Valenzuela L, Nishiura T, Murphy GP, Chu TM. Quantitation of prostate specific antigen in serum by sensitive enzyme immuno assay. *Cancer Res* 1980; **40**: 4568–662.

36. Stromme JH, Haffner F, Johannessen NB, Talseth T, Fredeich P, Theodorsen L. Diagnostic efficiency of biological markers in blood serum on prostate cancer: a comparison of four different markers and 12 different methods. *Scand J Clin Lab Invest* 1986; **46**: 443–50.

37. Killian CS, Yang N, Emrich LJ, Vargas FP, Kuriyama M, Wang MC, Slack NH, Papsidero LD, Murphy GP, Chu TM, and the investigators of the National Prostate Cancer Project. Prognostic importance of prostate-specific antigen for monitoring patients with stage B2–D1 prostate cancer. *Cancer Res* 1985; **45**: 886–91.

38. Siddall JK, Cooper EH, Newling DWW, Robinson MRG, Whelan P. An evaluation of the immunochemical measurement of prostatic acid phosphatase and prostate specific antigen in carcinoma of the prostate. *Eur Urol* 1986; **12**: 123–30.

39. Belt E, Schroeder FH. Total perineal prostatectomy for carcinoma of the prostate. *J Urol* 1972; **107**: 91–6.

40. Correa RJ, Gibbons RP, Cummings KB, Mason JT. Total prostatectomy for stage B carcinoma of the prostate. *J Urol* 1977; **117**: 328–9.

41. Boxer RJ, Kaufman JJ, Goodwin WE. Radical prostatectomy for carcinoma of the prostate, 1951–1976: a review of 329 patients. *J Urol* 1977; **117**: 208–13.

42. Scott WW. Panel discussion on some aspects of urological endocrinology. In: North Central Section of the American Urological Association, Postgraduate Seminar. Cited by Thompson GJ: Longterm control of prostatic cancer. *Surg Clin N Am* 1959; **39**: 963–71.

43. Parker MC, Cook A, Riddle PR, Fryatt I, O'Sullivan J, Shearer RJ. Is delayed treatment justified in carcinoma of the prostate? *Br J Urol* 1985; **57**: 724–8.

44. Smith JA. Stage A carcinoma of the prostate. In: *Clinical Management of Prostatic Cancer*. Chicago: Yearbook Medical Publishers, 1988: 85–96.

45. Smith JA. Patient selection for radical prostatectomy. *Urology* 1989; **33** (suppl): 17–20.

46. Paulson DF, Stone AR, Walther PJ, Tucker JA, Cox EB. Radical prostatectomy: anatomical predictors of success or failure. *J Urol* 1986; **136**: 1041–3.

47. Catalona WJ (ed.). *Radical Prostatectomy in Prostate Cancer*. New York: Grune & Stratton, 1984: 84–116.

48. Middleton RG, Smith JA. Comparison of 5 and 10 year survival following radical prostatectomy (abstract). *J Urol* 1989; **141**: 309A.

49. Jewett HJ, Bridge RW, Gray GF, Shelley WM. The palpable nodule of prostatic cancer. *J Am Med Ass* 1968; **203**: 115–18.

50. Hodges CV, Pearse HD, Stille L. Radical prostatectomy for carcinoma: 30 year experience and 15 year survival. *J Urol* 1979; **122**: 180–2.

51. Cochran JS, Kadesky MC. Private practice experience with radical surgical treatment of cancer of prostate. *Urology* 1981; **17**: 547–9.

52. Walsh PC, Jewett HJ. Radical surgery for prostate cancer. *Cancer* 1980; **45**: 1906–11.

53. Elder JS, Jewett HJ, Walsh PC. Radical perineal prostatectomy for clinical stage B2 carcinoma of the prostate. *J Urol* 1982; **127**: 704–6.

54. Middleton RG, Smith JA. Radical prostatectomy for stage B2 prostatic cancer. *J Urol* 1982; **127**: 702–3.

55. Middleton RG, Larsen RH. Selection of patients with stage B prostate cancer for radical prostatectomy. *Urol Clin N Am* 1990; **17**: 779–85.

56. Gibbons RP, Correa RJ, Branne GE, Mason JT. Total prostatectomy for localised prostatic cancer. *J Urol* 1984; **131**: 73–6.

57. Middleton RG, Smith JA, Melzer RB, Hamilton PE. Patient survival and local recurrence rate following radical prostatectomy for prostatic carcinoma. *J Urol* 1986; **136**: 422–44.

58. Steiner MS, Morton RA, Walsh PC. Impact of anatomical radical prostatectomy on urinary incontinence. *J Urol* 1991; **145**: 512–15.

59. Walsh PC. Radical prostatectomy: preservation of sexual function, cancer control. *Urol Clin N Am* 1987; **14**: 663–73.

60. Young HH. The early diagnosis and radical cure of carcinoma of the prostate; being a study of 40 cases and presentation of a radical operation which was carried out in 4 cases. *Bull Johns Hopkins Hosp* 1905; **16**: 315–18.

61. National Institute of Health Consensus Development Conference. The management of clinically localised prostate cancer. *J Urol* 1987; **138**: 1369–75.

9 Radical surgery, radiotherapy or observation for early-stage prostatic cancer

David F Paulson

Considerable controversy exists over the relative impact of surgery or radiation for the treatment of apparent organ-confined disease. Much of this controversy arises because of the variable biological course of prostatic malignancy and the difficulty in predicting the biological outcome of apparent organ-confined disease. This variable biological course has even promoted concern that observation could be appropriate in certain circumstances. Thus, single institutional trials which examine the impact of a single therapy and attempt to compare that with a non-randomized group of patients alternatively managed either from within that institution or derived from another institution are potentially flawed because of the non-biased segregation of either high biological risk or low biological risk patients in the population under study.

This chapter attempts to discuss in a non-biased way the results of a randomized trial that examines the relative impacts of radical surgery or radiation for patients with organ-confined disease in which both patient populations were staged in an equivalent fashion. It also examines the experience of a single institution wherein radical surgery was preferentially applied to patients with localized prostatic cancer to determine the manner in which this single-institution trial compares with the outcome of surgery in the randomized trial. The influence of the extent of local disease on outcome in patients treated by radical surgery, and the potential of histopathological and flow cytometric analyses to predict outcome, are discussed. Finally, the impact of observation only on patients with apparent localized disease is examined, as is the degree to which the outcome after radiation therapy for apparent localized disease parallels the natural history of patients with prostatic carcinoma.

Analysis of randomized trial data

Early in the 1970s a large multi-institutional study involving investigators at 13 major centres and their associated Veterans Administration Medical Centers set out to determine the accuracy of then current staging studies to assess the anatomical distribution of disease and, upon identification of the anatomical distribution, to compare surgery, radiation or observation in the management of that disease.[1,2] The first patients were entered into the study in February 1975 and the last patient in September 1978.

In this study, 509 men with newly diagnosed, biopsy-proven prostate adenocarcinoma were assigned a preliminary clinical stage based on rectal examination, colorimetric serum acid phosphatase level, a plain chest x-ray, and metastatic bone survey. Staging, designed to determine the anatomical distribution of disease, was sequenced to progress from those studies that showed the most widespread evidence of disease and then focused gradually on the prostate. All men with elevated acid phosphatase were believed to have systemic disease and were excluded from the randomization schema. In accordance with the sequential schema, all men who demonstrated no evidence of osteoblastic disease on skeletal films were subjected to a technetium-99 bone scan. Approximately 25% of all patients with no bony disease identified on routine skeletal x-rays had bony disease on the basis of isotopic bone scanning. The frequency of bone disease increased as the volume of local disease increased (Fig. 9.1).

Following the exclusion of disease in the axial and appendicular skeleton, nodal status was assessed. Patients who demonstrated no evidence of bone metastases underwent bipedal lymphangiography, with the accuracy of the lymphogram determined by pelvic lymphadenectomy. The hypothesis was that prostate carcinoma,

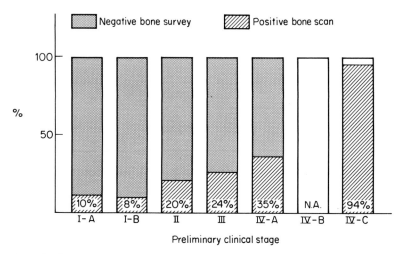

Fig. 9.1 Patients with bone disease detected by radioisotopic scanning who were considered disease-free by skeletal survey. Reproduced with permission from *Genitourinary Cancer Management.*[3]

like most other human solid tumours, had the propensity to metastasize early to the regional lymphatics.

The lymphatics of the prostate exit the posterior aspect of the gland and involve initially the hypogastric (primary), obturator (secondary), external iliac (tertiary), and presacral (quarternary) lymphatics.[4] The anatomical limits of the staging lymphadenectomy were designed not only to encompass the primary and secondary areas of nodal drainage, but also to leave undisturbed tertiary lymphatics lateral to the external iliac artery and vein. Thus the margins of the node dissection were limited to the triangle bordered by the external iliac vasculature, the pelvic floor, and the hypogastric vasculature; all node-bearing tissue in this area was removed, including the node-bearing tissue surrounding the obturator nerve and vessels (Fig. 9.2). As anticipated, the incidence of node-positive disease was found to increase as the volume of local disease increased (Fig. 9.3). When the lymphograms were interpreted by the review radiologist and the results compared with the incidence of node-positive disease as determined by pelvic lymphangiography, it was noted that, when the nodes were called positive, they were positive 90% of the time. However, when they were called negative, there was a 12% false-negative rate. The success of the review radiologist should be contrasted with that of the institutional lymphangiographer who had a 27% false-positive rate and a 44% false-negative rate (Table 9.1).

Table 9.1   Lymphangiogram versus node dissection

	Node dissection	
Lymphangiogram	*Positive*	*Negative*
Positive (Ref)	90%	10%
Positive (Local)	73%	27%
Negative (Ref)	21%	78%
Negative (Local)	44%	56%

In an attempt to determine whether the histopathological characteristics of the tumour tissue biopsied initially to establish the diagnosis of cancer could be used to predict the presence or absence of nodal extension, the investigators analysed the incidence of positive nodes as a function of the Gleason sum. This analysis demonstrated that both high- and low-grade disease (determined by the Gleason sum) functioned as relatively accurate predictors of node-positive disease, equivalent to that of the imaging modalities. Eighty-seven per cent of the patients with a Gleason sum less than 5 had node-negative disease, whereas 100% of those with a Gleason sum of 9 or 10 had node-positive disease (Table 9.2). With some minor variations, this general trend has been substantiated by other investigators.

Patients whose disease was confined to the prostate, determined by digital examination, and who had no evidence of bone- or node-positive disease, were assumed to have organ-confined disease and were randomized to radical prostatectomy or external-beam radiation therapy. These patients with clinical stage A2 or

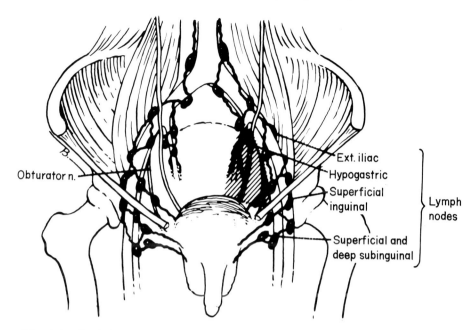

Fig. 9.2   Shaded area indicates area of limited pelvic lymph node dissection for staging of prostate carcinoma. Reproduced with permission from *Genitourinary Cancer Management*.[3]

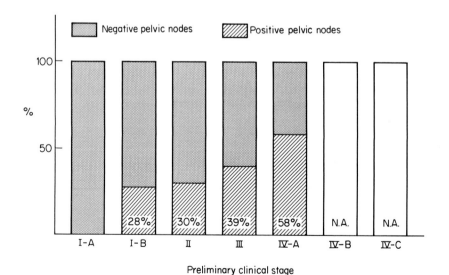

Preliminary clinical stage

Fig. 9.3   Incidence of pelvic node extension as a function of preliminary clinical stage in patients with no bone disease as determined by isotopic bone scan. Reproduced with permission from *Genitourinary Cancer Management*.[3]

Table 9.2   Node biopsy

Gleason sum	Positive	Negative	Number in group	
2–5	13.9%	86.1%	36	
6	32.4%	67.6%	34	
7	49.9%	50.1%	21	$P<0.0005$
8	75.0%	25.0%	12	
9–10	100.0%	0%	7	
Score unknown	33.0%	66.1%	12	

stage B (T1–2 N0 M0) cancers were randomized in balanced groups of four by institution to either radical prostatectomy or megavoltage radiation therapy.[5]

Any patient with an occult focal cancer was excluded from this randomization scheme as were any patients who had clinical stage C (T3 N0 M0) disease. Prostatectomy could be accomplished by a perineal or retropubic route; however, the anatomical limits of the dissection had to include the apex of the prostate and the seminal vesicles (Fig. 9.4). Patients assigned to radiation therapy were treated with megavoltage equipment, i.e. the highest available energy (cobalt-60, linear accelerator, and/or betatron x-ray beam), with a minimum surface-to-axis distance of 80 cm. The field size was to include the prostate, periprostatic region, and pelvic lymph nodes as determined by lymphograms and localization films. The upper margin of the radiation field was at the level of the iliac crest, the lateral margin at least 1 cm beyond the external iliac nodal chains, and the lower margin 1 cm below the inferior prostate. All fields were treated with a total tumour dose of 4500–5000 cGy in 40 days total elapsed time. The dose was specific from the appropriate

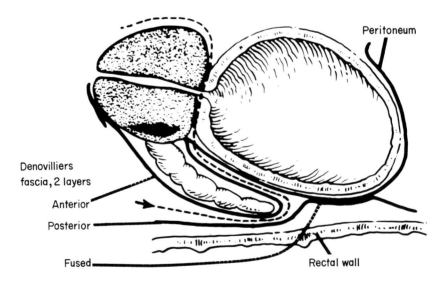

Fig. 9.4   Limits of dissection for a radical prostatectomy. Reproduced with permission from *Genitourinary Cancer Management.*[3]

isodose curve as a minimum dose in the volume of the prostate. An additional treatment boost of 2000 cGy was delivered to the prostate.

Patients were followed at two-month intervals for the first year and at three-month intervals thereafter. Serum biochemical profiles with acid phosphatase determinations, Karnofsky's performance ratings, and a physical examination were obtained at each follow-up; chest x-rays and isotopic bone scans were obtained at six-month intervals. The impact of treatment was determined with 'first evidence of treatment failure' as the endpoint. Investigators chose this criterion rather than survival to avoid confounding the impact of the first therapy by the subsequent application of a second therapy that could alter the survival experience. Survival data were not accrued as funding was withdrawn by the National Cancer Institute, and patient follow-up and data analysis could not be completed as originally projected. Furthermore, lack of funding precluded analysis of morbidity data and follow-up of accrued morbidity data. Treatment failure was identified by acid phosphatase elevation on two consecutive follow-up appointments or by the appearance of bony or parenchymal disease with or without concomitant acid phosphatase elevation. A new appearance of increased isotopic uptake was identified as the presence of bony disease. The appearance of such metastatic bony disease was either progressive on subsequent scans or was accompanied by elevation of serum acid phosphatase levels. Identification of cancer in the prostate on follow-up biopsy after radiation did not signify treatment failure in assessment of relative treatment efficacy. Curves representing non-parametric estimates of 'time to first evidence of treatment failure' were generated according to the Kaplan–Meier method.[6] Censored values representing patients without evidence of treatment failure at the time of the last follow-up are represented by a single vertical tick in Fig. 9.5. Treatment efficacy in pairs of subgroups was assessed for differences by the Cox–Mantel test.[7] Fifty-six patients received external-beam radiation therapy, and 41 underwent radical prostatectomy. An analysis of the time-to-failure curves of the two treatment groups indicated that radical surgery possessed a distinct advantage over radiation therapy in controlling disease and was significant at the 0.037 level (Fig. 9.5). This study was criticized, detractors arguing that patients with more aggressive disease had been assigned to radiation therapy and the length of follow-up was too short. All patients were examined before randomization by both radiotherapist and surgeon and both had to agree that the disease was clinical stage B (T2). Analysis of the relative Gleason grade between the two groups indicated that the average Gleason grade in the radiation therapy arm was 5.1, with an average Gleason sum of 5.5 in the radical surgery arm. If the Gleason sum functions as an indicator of biological aggressiveness, the two groups seem equivalent, although those undergoing surgery had a slightly higher Gleason sum than those treated by radiation. An additional 20 months of follow-up continued to demonstrate a disease control advantage of radical surgery over radiation therapy (Fig. 9.6).

In the original study design, persistent evidence of disease by biopsy after definitive radiation therapy did not constitute failure, even though current information would suggest that this does identify a patient population at increased risk for

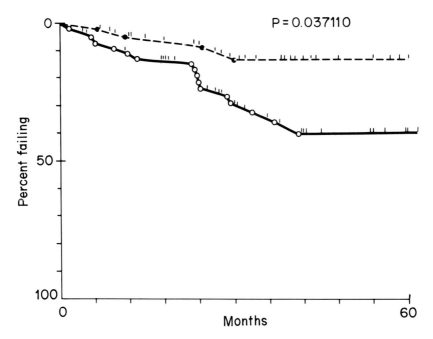

Fig. 9.5 Time to first evidence of treatment failure for patients randomized to radiation therapy (solid line, $N=56$) or radical surgery (broken line, $N=41$) whose disease is confined to the prostate. Reproduced with permission from Paulson *et al.*[5]

progression. If the biopsy-proven patients (7 of 21 who had repeat biopsies at one year were positive) are included as treatment failures, the curves diverge even further (Fig. 9.7). The imbalance that resulted, with respect to the statistical distribution of patients, was not intentional; the study was not weighted in favour of radical prostatectomy. The study was designed for researchers to use balanced groups of four within each of the 13 participating institutions. Patient accession was halted on a specific day, and the randomization scheme was not allowed to go to completion. At the time the study was completed, 42 patients had been randomized for radical prostatectomy and 55 for radiation therapy. Four patients refused radical prostatectomy after they were randomized and demanded radiation therapy. Three patients who had been randomized to radiation therapy demanded radical prostatectomy. As the study analysis was designed to determine the impact of treatment, the final population pool under study encompassed the 41 patients who received radical prostatectomy and the 56 who received radiation therapy.

Examination of the data derived from this randomized trial prompts questions as to the natural history of untreated, apparently localized disease. This question is important in order to evaluate the disease control advantage produced by active treatment. Johannson[8] followed 223 patients who had apparent organ-confined disease but did not therapeutically intervene at the time of diagnosis. Of 223 patients observed only, 72% were without local or systemic progression or local extension at five years (Fig. 9.8). Progress was grade-dependent, with 83% of

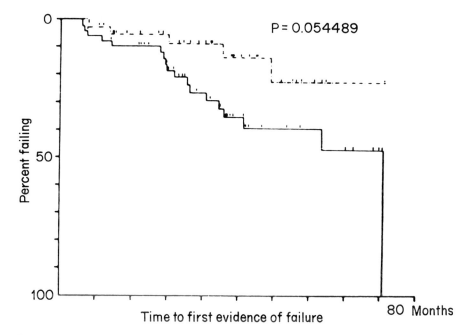

Fig. 9.6 Time to first evidence of treatment failure for patients randomized to radical surgery (broken line, *N*=41) or radiation therapy (solid line, *N*=56) when the analysis is completed with an additional 20 months of follow-up. The difference between the two treatment arms remains distinct. Reproduced with permission from *Genitourinary Cancer Management.*[3]

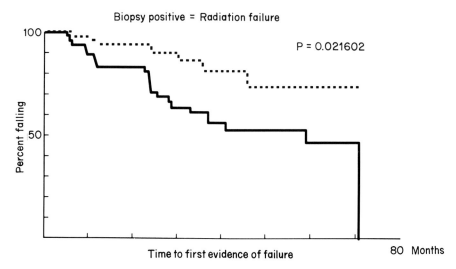

Fig. 9.7 Time to first evidence of treatment failure for patients randomized to either definitive radiation (solid line, *N*=56) or to radical prostatectomy (broken line, *N*=41). Patients failing radiation in this efficacy projection include the 7 of 21 patients who had postradiation positive biopsies.

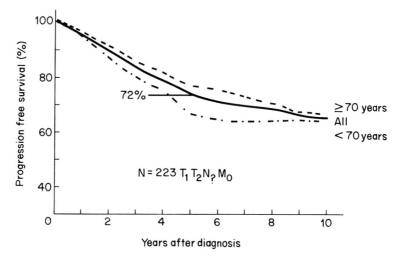

Fig. 9.8 Cumulative proportion of patients without local or systemic progression of disease, in whole groups (All) and by age at diagnosis. Altered and redrawn from Johansson *et al.*[8]

grade I patients being disease-free at five years as opposed to only 27% of grade III patients. The progression which occurs in the clinical patient populations observed by Johannson more closely resembles the apparent disease control produced by radiation therapy in the randomized trial of the Urologic Research Group than those produced by radical surgery in this same trial.

These studies suggest that active surgical intervention may be more important in providing disease control than is observation. Are there, then, randomized trial data to suggest that radiation and observation may be equivalent therapies? The answer would appear to be 'yes'.

An additional interesting aspect of this randomized trial focused on large-volume, node-negative, localized disease (T3); the population was randomized to receive either radiation therapy or delayed hormonal therapy (no immediate treatment). Again, with 'first evidence of treatment failure' as the endpoint, the failure rates for patients actively treated by radiation therapy versus those treated by observation only are superimposed (Fig. 9.9).[9] One may interpret these data as indicating that the purported disease control impact of radiation therapy on large-volume prostate cancer may reflect nothing other than the natural history of the disease.

One may ask whether the randomized trial data purporting the superior impact of radical surgery reflect institutional experience, wherein radical surgery is the primary form of therapy chosen for apparently localized disease. Recent review of 441 patients at Duke University Medical Center who underwent radical prostatectomy demonstrates an overall disease control response (Fig. 9.10) similar to that seen within the randomized trial. However, the population base within this single institutional experience can be manipulated in a retrospective manner to project a most favourable outcome. When the patients were retrospectively analysed to

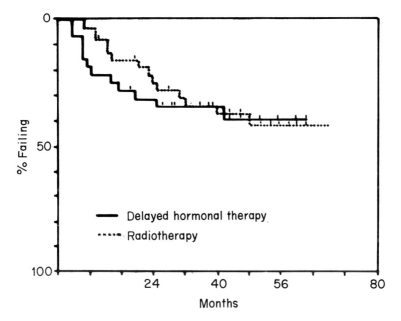

Fig. 9.9 Difference in interval to first evidence of treatment failure between both groups was not statistically significant ($P=0.71$). Reproduced with permission from Paulson *et al.*[9]

reflect the volume of disease in the patients being subjected to radical surgical control, a marked difference in outcome is noted. Patients who had organ-confined disease demonstrated only a 12% failure rate at 10 years. Seventy-four patients with specimen-confined disease demonstrated a 30% failure rate at 10 years, while 123 margin-positive patients presented a failure rate of 60% at 10 years (Fig. 9.11). In addition, analysis by Gleason grade also demonstrated a disease control advantage to those whose Gleason sum was 7 or less (Fig. 9.12). These retrospective data projections document the difficulty any investigator has in providing an unbiased data analysis of non-randomized prospective studies. Any retrospective non-randomized series may be biased if the population is weighted with either high- or low-volume disease or high- or low-grade disease (as scored by Gleason sums); that population weighted with either high-volume or high-grade disease will be destined to fail at a more rapid rate than that which is weighted with low-volume or low-grade disease.

There is an increasing body of data which demonstrates that the clinical course of apparent organ-confined prostatic carcinoma is influenced by biological risk factors, both identified and unidentified. One identified risk factor is nuclear ploidy. Studies conducted at Duke University Medical Center clearly indicate that patients with diploid tumours had a much more favourable outcome than patients with aneuploid tumours if their primary treatment was radical prostatectomy. In fact, the impact of ploidy exceeds the impact of local volume of disease. Patients with diploid tumours who have organ-confined disease and who are subjected to radical prostatectomy

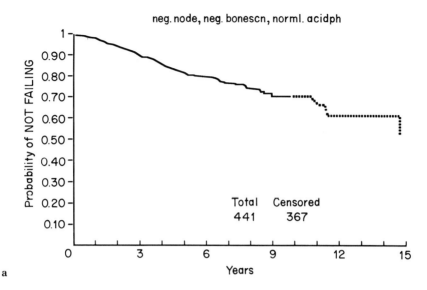

a

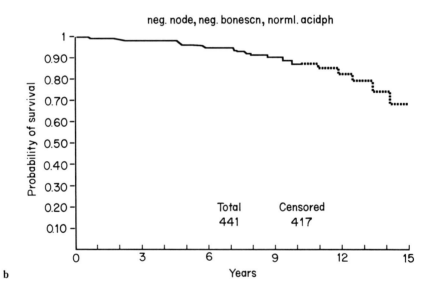

b

Fig. 9.10 (*a*) Probability of not failing and (*b*) probability of survival for the total population undergoing radical prostatectomy.

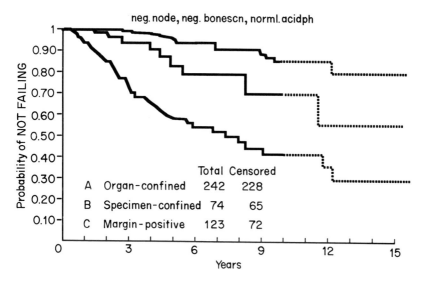

Fig. 9.11 Probability of not failing as a function of organ-confined disease, specimen-confined disease and margin-positive disease (organ *vs* specimen confined *P*<0.002; organ *vs* margin-positive *P*<0.0001; specimen-confined *vs* margin-positive *P*<0.001).

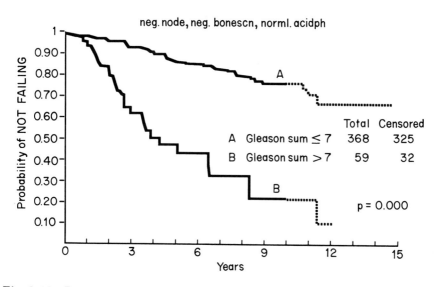

Fig. 9.12 Probability of not failing as a function of the Gleason sum.

will apparently not die of their malignant disease. Whether such outcome would occur had they not been subjected to radical prostatectomy remains undetermined. Patients with diploid tumours who were margin-positive or whose disease extended into the seminal vesicles did less well than patients whose tumours were diploid and organ-confined but did much better than patients whose tumours were aneuploid and organ-confined. Lastly, patients whose tumours were aneuploid and not organ-confined did very poorly after radical prostatectomy. These observations do much to explain the differences which can occur in non-randomized trials.

Conclusion

Although the randomized trial, conducted in the Veterans Administration Medical Center trials, may be flawed, it is an unbiased, randomized prospective trial in which the physicians based treatment selection on the anatomical distribution of disease and used current methodology to determine the local and regional extent of malignant growth. Further, there is presented a considerable body of data which demonstrates that the apparent impact of radiation therapy may be nothing more than an observation of the natural history of the disease. Whether patients selected for radical surgery were further advantaged by other biological characteristics of tumour irradiation remains to be defined.

References

1. Paulson DF, and Uro-Oncology Research Group. The impact of current staging procedures in assessing disease extent of prostatic adenocarcinoma. *J Urol* 1979; **121**: 300–5.
2. Paulson DF, and Uro-Oncology Research Group. Predictors of lymphatic spread in prostatic adenocarcinoma. *J Urol* 1980; **123**: 697–9.
3. deKernion JP, Paulson DF (eds). *Genitourinary Cancer Management*. Philadelphia: Lea & Febiger, 1987.
4. Smith MJV. The lymphatics of the prostate. *Invest Urol* 1966; **3**: 439.
5. Paulson DF, Lin GH, Hinshaw W, *et al.* Radical surgery versus radiotherapy for stage A2 and stage B (T1–2 M0 N0) adenocarcinoma of the prostate. *J Urol* 1982; **128**: 502–4.
6. Kaplan EL, Meier P. Nonparametric estimation for incomplete observations. *J Am Stat Ass* 1958; **53**: 457–81.
7. Cox DR. Regression models and life tables. *J R Stat Soc* 1972; **34**: 187–220.
8. Johansson JE, Andersson SO, Krusemo UB, *et al.*, Natural history of localized prostatic cancer. *Lancet* 1989; **1**: 800.
9. Paulson DF, *et al.* Radiation therapy versus delayed androgen deprivation for stage C carcinoma of the prostate. *J Urol* 1984; **131**: 901.

10 Deferred treatment for advanced prostatic cancer

David Kirk

Androgen withdrawal remains the only real method of controlling prostatic cancer too advanced for local treatment. Although at least a subjective response will occur in a majority of patients,[1] it will be temporary. Unless the patient dies first from other causes, relapse is inevitable, usually within two years in those with metastatic disease. While radiotherapy and other palliative measures may be helpful in relieving symptoms, until significant advances in chemotherapy occur, hormonal therapy will provide the only chance of influencing the patient's disease and its use must be timed to achieve maximum benefit.

Prostatic cancer usually affects elderly men who have a short natural life expectation and probably also suffer from other potentially fatal conditions.[2] Indeed, of those patients dying during the studies of the Veterans Administration Cooperative Urological Group (VACURG) less than 50% did so from prostatic cancer.[3] Although the Veterans' patients were a selected group with a high average age even for men with prostatic cancer, it remains true that many men with the disease will die from other causes. Treatment of their cancer will not increase their life span and many patients with asymptomatic disease may die from other causes before they need treatment on symptomatic grounds. Any advantage to the remainder from instituting early treatment will be at the expense of subjecting the others to treatment from which they may not live to benefit. In addition, the treatment is not without side-effects.

Changing attitudes to hormonal therapy

For some 25 years after discovery of the androgen dependence of prostatic carcinoma,[4] hormonal treatment was prescribed in the confident belief that its use prolonged the patient's life, and that the benefit was greater the earlier it was started. This view largely came from comparing the survival of hormone treated patients[5] with those managed before hormonal therapy was available.[6] We now recognize the deficiencies in historical controls, and much of this improvement in survival may have resulted from the other medical advances occurring at that time, not least the introduction of antibiotics. Publication of the results of the VACURG studies,[3] which included randomized control groups treated initially with a placebo, revealed a somewhat different picture.

While early hormonal treatment in those with localized disease seemed to delay the onset of metastases, this produced no dramatic increase in survival compared with placebo 'treated' patients. Since the protocols allowed those receiving placebo to be started on active treatment once disease progression occurred, these results can be interpreted as showing that deferring hormonal treatment until a definite indication develops may not affect the patient's survival.

Although a review of the records of patients with prostatic carcinoma treated at Johns Hopkins Hospital immediately before and immediately after the introduction of hormonal treatment could not demonstrate any increase in life expectancy attributable to its use,[7] the view that hormonal therapy has no effect on survival should be challenged. Urologists regularly see patients who present with, for example, bilateral ureteric obstruction which is reversed by hormonal treatment. Patients must live longer following treatment of such a life-threatening condition. What is in doubt is whether a further prolongation of life would have resulted if treatment had been started at an earlier stage of the disease.

Once questions were raised about the effect of early hormonal treatment on survival, its use in the management of prostatic cancer required serious re-examination. Should patients be subjected to hormonal manipulation as soon as their prostatic tumour is diagnosed, or can its use be delayed until symptoms or complications occur, as Byar[3] suggested? Very few would now recommend hormonal therapy for all patients with prostatic cancer. It is outside the scope of this chapter to discuss the merits or nature of local treatment designed to cure or control early confined disease. In effect hormonal therapy is 'deferred' in such patients, although this is done in the hope that the success of the primary treatment will make its use unnecessary. Early consideration of hormonal treatment may be appropriate for the patient with a T3–T4 tumour[8] considered incurable, even if metastases cannot be detected, or for the patient known to have metastases.

Which patients should receive hormonal therapy?

Most urologists would agree on the absolute indications for hormonal therapy.[9] Although it can be argued that a solitary painful metastasis might be amenable to radiotherapy, and so treating it might enable further deferment of hormonal treatment, painful metastatic disease is the clearest indication for which few would consider any other option. Subjective response rates are excellent, and can be extremely rapid—it is not unknown for patients undergoing orchiectomy to wake from the anaesthetic free of pain. Less clear-cut is the man not so much in pain but debilitated by his disseminated cancer. Careful assessment is sometimes needed to detect this in an elderly man. Hormonal treatment can again be dramatic, but patients who present in the last stages of the disease not infrequently respond poorly. This tendency for a limited response in more advanced disease is well recognized[5] and is apparent in the VACURG data referred to earlier. (Peeling, personal communication). Response of soft tissue compared with bony metastases may also be poorer.

Pathological fractures and actual or impending cord compression are usually indications for hormonal treatment, but primary surgical treatment, internal fixation or cord decompression will often be necessary as well. Indeed, where such catastrophes are the initial presentation of the disease, the diagnosis of prostatic cancer may be made by biopsies taken at these procedures.

What of hormonal therapy in extensive localized disease? Not only might recurrent outflow obstruction occur, but there is also a risk of obstructive uropathy from direct ureteric invasion. Many of the patients for whom hormonal therapy is considered will have presented with outflow obstruction, and the transurethral resection (TUR) used to relieve this will have provided the confirmatory biopsy material. As will be discussed, the risk of local progression and return of symptoms is one argument in favour of early treatment. Certainly the use of repeated TURs in the man who has recurring obstruction is to be decried. Ultimately his tumour will invade the external sphincter and incontinence will occur, either from the infiltration itself, or by producing retention which can only be relieved by a resection involving the sphincter mechanism. Upward invasion of the ureters also may occur in time. There is no doubt that hormonal therapy will provide excellent if only temporary local control, although radiotherapy will be as effective and might be considered more logical in 'localized' disease. Data, as yet unpublished, from an MRC study of patients with T2–T4 disease has shown radiotherapy, orchiectomy or both together to be equally effective in controlling the *local* tumour, but distant progression was significantly faster in those receiving radiotherapy alone. As in the VACURG studies, this increased distant progression rate was not associated with increased mortality, as progression was an indication for hormonal therapy.

My own inclination is to consider radiotherapy at presentation in those with extensive tumours, especially if the Gleason score is high (see Table 7.3). Other patients in whom the results of a TUR are initially satisfactory will, if the prostatic symptoms recur, become candidates for radiotherapy rather than a further TUR, although enough men may avoid this complication[10] to justify an initial expectant approach. In patients with established metastatic disease, local progression is indicative of disease activity, and if hormonal therapy has not been started it would be the logical choice. If a further TUR *is* necessary, combining it with a subcapsular orchiectomy is sensible in many cases.

Deferred treatment for asymptomatic advanced disease

If these indications for immediate hormonal treatment are clear, what of the man who presents with outflow obstruction readily managed by transurethral prostatic resection with no metastases, or with metastases which are not a source of symptoms? The patient well-pleased with the results of his TUR may not thank the urologist for any side-effects arising from hormonal treatment, especially if he is sexually active. He is, however, suffering from cancer and a moderately effective form of treatment is available. A similar problem is posed by the patient with apparently confined disease in whom a positive pelvic lymph node biopsy has ruled out radical local treatment. Arguments can be advanced either for starting treatment immediately or for its deferment until unquestionable need arises.

This is an important issue much disputed by those managing patients with prostatic cancer. Whilst clear evidence that early treatment is beneficial would resolve the matter, treatment by androgen withdrawal has potential disadvantages to the patient, and with the increasing expense of newer methods of treatment such as the LHRH analogues there are significant economic implications. Paradoxically, although early treatment might seem most important in the younger patient, he is just the one who may be most upset by the resulting loss of sexual function. Thus if no disadvantage could be found from delaying treatment, there would seem to be every reason for so doing.

Early treatment has not been shown conclusively to be without some effect on survival. If there is any chance that early treatment prolongs survival, it is argued that patients should not be deprived of the possibility of longer life. The data from the VACURG study is difficult to interpret,[11] particularly the results for the oestrogen treated patients, where the conflicting effects of reduced cancer mortality and increased cardiovascular deaths have to be resolved. How many of those dying from cardiovascular causes would have died from cancer otherwise? Contrary to what is frequently stated,[12] the VACURG trials, not specifically designed to test this question, only raised the possibility of deferring treatment. In particular, starting treatment in placebo patients was a dispensation rather than a defined part of the protocol, and the indications for and nature of such treatment must have varied. Trials which uncover unexpected results usually ask further questions, rather than producing new solutions. To quote Byar: 'These data *support the concept* that hormonal treatment can be delayed . . . '.[3] In other words, the point had yet to be proved.

The question of survival can only be determined by a prospective controlled study specifically devised to test this question. Such a study is currently being conducted by the Medical Research Council in the UK.[13] This is a major undertaking since, to compensate for the expected high death rate from other causes, a very large trial entry will be needed, and this study is unlikely to produce a meaningful result for some years. Recognized as being an important enterprise,[14] it is supported by many urologists throughout the UK. A similar question is being asked by an EORTC protocol in patients without bony metastases in whom positive lymph node biopsies have ruled out curative local treatment.

Quality of life

Any improvement in survival from early treatment is likely to be small. While for a young woman with breast cancer a few extra months of life might be worthwhile, whatever the price in side-effects, an elderly man with prostatic cancer might present a different balance sheet.

Given the limited life expectation of most men with prostatic cancer, many urologists now feel that treatment should be aimed as much at avoiding complications and symptoms as at prolonging survival. A number of potential problems need consideration.

Local progression

There is little doubt that a significant number of patients with prostatic cancer develop further outflow obstruction requiring a second TUR[15] due to tumour progression. This might be prevented or slowed down by early hormonal treatment. Whether it is sufficiently common to warrant early systemic treatment in all patients is less certain;[10] and, especially in patients without metastases, radiotherapy might be the more logical method of controlling the primary tumour. The need for a second TUR for local tumour progression could be considered an indication for therapy, and if orchiectomy is the treatment indicated it can conveniently be performed at the same time.

General ill-health

In the absence of specific symptoms, more subtle effects such as weight loss or anaemia, resulting from the presence of an uncontrolled tumour, unrecognized by the patient or his doctor, might respond to early treatment with an improvement in general well-being. This is certainly true in some patients and, not infrequently, general malaise is an indication for abandoning deferred treatment. However, some men with untreated prostatic cancer remain in excellent health. Early treatment of *all* patients on these grounds alone does seem hard to justify, but regular careful clinical assessment, and monitoring weight, haemoglobin, etc., should be an essential part of deferred treatment, if not of the management of all men with this disease. Well-being is a mixture of physical and psychological factors. In this context, some men fully aware of their condition might prefer to be receiving treatment while others, when the options are put to them, will opt for deferred treatment, and if persuaded otherwise might not tolerate side-effects such as hot flushes very well.

Avoidance of catastrophes

The risk of a pathological fracture or paraplegia occurring suddenly in the untreated patient causes justifiable concern and certainly demands careful follow-up so that prompt treatment can be given as soon as premonitory symptoms occur. While 'preventive' hormonal therapy will appeal to the cautious, these complications occur in relatively few men. Since the risk will remain in those who do not respond and will return when relapse occurs, vigilance still will be necessary following treatment if these severe complications are to be avoided.

Disadvantages of treatment

Any benefits of early treatment have to be balanced by its potential side-effects, from which no method of androgen deprivation—be it orchiectomy, oestrogens, antiandrogens or LHRH analogues—is free. Unlike much cancer chemotherapy, hormonal therapy for prostatic cancer (at least conventionally) needs to be given continuously, usually for the remainder of the patient's life. This involves not only a continuing cost to the health service in terms of drug bills, but also to the patient in potential side-effects. Supporters of deferred treatment will point out that side-effects will be better accepted by the patient who has had symptoms before treatment is started, and avoided by those who die from other causes before an indication for treatment occurs.

Immediate or deferred treatment?

Clearly, the arguments are finely balanced. The results of the VACURG studies stimulated interest in deferring treatment. It was not their intention to investigate timing of treatment, and until recently the question 'immediate or deferred treatment?' has not been addressed directly in a prospective fashion. Retrospective studies have produced conflicting views. One group in London[16] retrospectively comparing patients who had been managed either by immediate or by deferred treatment (in an uncontrolled manner) could detect no detrimental effects from delaying treatment. However, a report on deferred treatment which has been the preferred policy in Newcastle[15] must raise some doubts about its wisdom, especially as 17% of their patients who died from prostatic cancer did so *before* hormonal therapy could be commenced.

Both these groups concluded that only a prospective controlled study comparing immediate and deferred treatment would resolve this issue. The protocol for the MRC's study acknowledges the arguments outlined above, and in addition to recording survival data, monitors the number of TURs performed, records events such as pathological fractures, and requests regular measurement of the patient's haemoglobin, weight and performance status. Until this study is completed, and perhaps not even then, this will continue to be one of the most controversial topics in urology.

Given the indeterminate effect of the timing of treatment on survival, each of the possible options has something to commend it. Early treatment is perhaps safer—its most extreme exponents will perform an orchiectomy and then discharge the patient on the grounds that he has had the only effective treatment available. The problems avoided in the short term by early treatment are, of course, only delayed and will occur later when the inevitable hormone relapse occurs unless some other condition first kills the patient.

Deferring treatment restricts the period when the patient is prone to the undesirable effects of therapy, and provides the satisfaction of seeing a symptomatic benefit from treatment; but it must be emphasized that it is not the easy option. The risk that irreversible problems could occur, even death, before treatment is started is real, but should be avoidable. Where treatment is deferred careful follow-up is essential, the patient and his general practitioner have to be fully aware of the situation, and the urologist willing and able to respond immediately to new developments. The situation is analogous to surveillance in men with stage 1 testicular teratoma, and when an appropriate level of supervision is not possible, deferred treatment should not be attempted. However, at least in selected patients there does seem to be some advantage in this approach.

Total androgen ablation

Does the advent of total androgen ablation[17] alter the balance of the arguments? Recent evidence that combining standard therapy with a non-steroidal antiandrogen may indeed improve survival[18] has introduced a new argument into the question of the timing of therapy. This results partly from what probably should be considered a misconception, namely that conventional therapy has no effect on survival and that it is for this reason it can be deferred. Thus if total androgen ablation *did* improve on conventional therapy this argument in favour of deferred treatment would be lost. Despite the report from Johns Hopkins[7] it does seem inconceivable that hormonal therapy can have no effect on survival. In reality any increased effect of total androgen ablation must be only a question of degree which might be as readily realized even if it were deferred. Although the differences were not statistically significant, in Crawford and his colleagues' study[18] better response rates were apparent in patients presenting with less advanced disease. This might mean that if treatment is deferred, as the patients' disease will have advanced they likewise will respond less readily than if they had been treated sooner. It is instructive to reread Nesbit and Baum's paper of 1950,[5] where they make the same observation about conventional hormonal treatment and advocate early treatment for this reason. However, a patient with advanced disease at diagnosis is not comparable with one presenting at an earlier stage but whose treatment has been delayed until progression occurs. The patient *presenting* with advanced disease probably has a particularly aggressive tumour, and such tumours may be inherently less sensitive to hormone treatment.

One argument in favour of deferred treatment is that the biological time course of prostatic cancer is so long, and the point at which it is diagnosed is so arbitrary, that to demand treatment be started simply because diagnosis has been made rather than for a more specific indication can be considered illogical. To follow the opposing view to its extreme would imply that even patients with disease potentially curable by local therapy should be started on hormonal therapy lest they relapse later. The lessons from the past must not be forgotten, and it would be a pity if an observation in patients treated by total androgen ablation similar to one made in the 1940s about conventional hormonal therapy took us back to the 'treatment on suspicion' attitude which the VACURG studies swept away.

If total androgen ablation becomes the hormonal treatment of choice, it affects both the positive and the negative sides of the deferred versus immediate treatment argument. While recent investigators do not seem to have encountered the levels of toxicity seen in earlier studies of non-steroidal antiandrogens,[19] their use does introduce an additional range of potential side-effects for the patient. There is also a considerable increase in expense, which will be substantial even if total androgen ablation is confined to those who currently are offered hormonal therapy. What would be the effects on drug bills if all the men at present managed by deferred treatment were suddenly to be commenced on both an LHRH analogue and a non-steroidal antiandrogen? Clearly if this were the right management this expense would have to be borne, but whether this is so is far from certain. The timing of treatment must still be considered a vital topic for investigation, but those of us conducting such studies must be prepared to introduce total androgen ablation into our protocols if the arguments in its favour as a more effective therapy are sustained.

Conclusions

The timing of hormonal treatment may not greatly affect the outcome in prostatic cancer. Some patients have a clear need for immediate treatment on symptomatic grounds. In others, deferment of hormonal treatment would seem to be a valid option, although its practice requires close supervision and will not be suitable for all patients. Since very few urologists would now prescribe hormonal therapy for all men with prostatic cancer, and since a proportion of those receiving 'curative' treatment or not treated on the grounds of good prognosis will in fact develop progressive disease requiring hormonal therapy, there is in one sense a consensus that deferred treatment is appropriate for some patients. However, as with many aspects of managing prostatic cancer, a general consensus on this issue when applied to patients with advanced but asymptomatic disease has not yet been achieved. It can only be hoped that studies to resolve this and other issues receive the support they need.

Currently the matter has to be decided for each individual. Age, health and the patient's expectations and social situation all come into the calculation. Where the correct solution for a patient is not obvious there is much merit in holding a frank discussion of the issues with the patient himself. He, after all, is the person most involved, and may be in the best position to guide the urologist towards the correct decision.

References

1. Resnick MI, Grayhack JT. Treatment of stage IV carcinoma of the prostate. *Urol Clin N Am* 1965; **2**: 141–61.
2. Stamey TA. Cancer of the prostate: an analysis of some important contributions and dilemmas. *Monogr Urol* 1982; **3**: 65–96.

3. Byar DP. The Veterans Administration Cooperative Research Group's studies of cancer of the prostate. *Cancer* 1973; **32**: 1126–30.

4. Huggins C, Hodges CV. Studies on prostate cancer. 1: The effect of castration, of oestrogen and of androgen injection on serum phosphatases in metastatic carcinoma of the prostate. *Cancer Res* 1941; **1**: 293–7.

5. Nesbit RM, Baum WC. Endocrine control of prostatic cancer: clinical survey of 1818 cases. *JAMA* 1950; **143**: 1317–20.

6. Nesbit RM, Plumb RT. Prostatic carcinoma: a follow-up on 795 patients treated prior to the endocrine era and a comparison of survival rates between these and patients treated by endocrine therapy. *Surgery* 1946; **20**: 263–72.

7. Lepor H, Ross A, Walsh PC. The influence of hormonal therapy on survival of men with advanced prostatic cancer. *J Urol* 1982; **128**: 335–40.

8. UICC. *TNM Classification of Malignant Tumours*, 3rd edn. Geneva: Union Internationale Contre le Cancer, 1978.

9. Catalona WJ, Scott WW. Carcinoma of the prostate. In: Walsh PC, Gittes RE, Perlmutter AD, Stamey TA (eds), *Campbell's Urology*. Philadelphia: WB Saunders, 1986: 1463–534.

10. Gee WF, Cole JR. Symptomatic stage C carcinoma of prostate: traditional therapy. *Urology* 1980; **15**: 335–7.

11. Kirk D. Trials and tribulations in prostatic cancer. *Br J Urol* 1987; **59**: 375–9.

12. Fraser KS. Prostatic carcinoma. *Br Med J* 1985; **290**: 1824.

13. Kirk D. Prostatic carcinoma. *Br Med J* 1985; **290**: 875–6.

14. Editorial: Dilemmas in the management of prostatic carcinoma. *Lancet* 1985; **ii**: 1219–20.

15. Handley R, Carr TW, Travis D, Powell PH, Hall RR. Deferred treatment for prostate cancer. *Br J Urol* 1988; **62**: 249–53.

16. Parker MC, Cook A, Riddle PR, Fryatt I, O'Sullivan J, Shearer RJ. Is delayed treatment justified in carcinoma of the prostate? *Br J Urol* 1985; **57**: 724–8.

17. Labrie F, Belanger A, Dupont A, Edmond J, Lacoursiere Y, Monfette G. Combined treatment with LHRH agonist and pure antiandrogen in advanced carcinoma of prostate. *Lancet* 1984; **ii**: 1090.

18. Crawford ED, Eisenberger MA, McLeod DG, Spaulding JT, Benson R, Dorr FA, *et al.* A controlled trial of leuprolide with and without flutamide in prostatic carcinoma. *N Engl J Med* 1989; **321**: 419–24.

19. MacFarlane JR, Tolley DA. Flutamide therapy for advanced prostatic cancer: a phase II study. *Br J Urol* 1985; **57**: 172–4.

11 The molecular basis of prostatic cancer and optimal hormonal treatment

Jonathan Waxman

Prostatic cancer is the second most common cancer in men and is exquisitely sensitive to endocrine therapies. In the last 20 years the complications of conventional treatment have been described and new agents have been developed to take their place. Controversy remains as to whether there is any advantage to the patient from these new treatments compared with orchiectomy. There has been recent interest in the possibility of an increased survival with combination endocrine therapies. However, this benefit has been confirmed in only one randomized study. In the last five years the science of molecular biology has been applied to prostatic cancer, and has provided clues as to the changes that lead to hormone independence. This chapter reviews these clinical developments and the molecular basis of prostatic cancer.

Steroid hormone receptors

Hormone receptor assays are technically difficult in prostatic cancer and this relates to problems in separating stroma from tumour, a high concentration of endogenous steroids, which lead to receptor saturation, and the presence of two non-specific binding proteins, albumin and sex hormone binding globulin. The active tissue metabolite of testosterone is dihydrotestosterone (DHT). There seems to be conflicting evidence for the presence of receptors for DHT in benign hypertrophy. In one series of 23 patients, DHT binding was absent,[1] and this is in contrast with the finding in another study of receptor positivity in 14 of 17 patients.[2] In prostatic cancer the situation is more clear-cut and DHT receptor positivity corresponds with hormonal responsiveness. Receptor concentration correlates with response, and in 23 patients in whom DHT binding was greater than 110 fmol/mg, the mean response was for 17 months and survival 24 months. In patients with binding less than 110 fmol/mg of DNA, mean response was for 7 months and survival 17 months.[3] Oestrogen and progestogen receptor positivity does not correlate with response to treatment. In a series of 22 patients with prostate cancer, only 6 were found to contain 17 beta oestradiol receptors,[4] and in a further series 14 of 26 patients' tumours contained oestrogen receptors and 13 of 15 progesterone receptors.[5]

The gene encoding the androgen receptor has been cloned. The androgen receptor gene has homology with the oestrogen, glucocorticoid and progesterone receptor genes, and is sited on the X chromosome. The androgen receptor has 917 amino acid residues, which are encoded by a 2751 nucleotide sequence. The N-terminus contains sequences which probably activate transcription; DNA binding and steroid binding properties are a function of the C-terminus.[6] A comparison has been made of androgen responsive and unresponsive prostatic cancer cell lines. DU 145 and PC 3, which are unresponsive, do not express androgen receptor protein nor mRNA, which are expressed in LNCaP, the responsive line.[7] These studies are recent, and further analysis is required.

Peptide growth factors and receptors

There have been limited investigations into the importance of growth factors and their receptors in prostatic cancer. A human cell line has been shown to secrete transforming growth factor alpha and epidermal growth factor.[8] Receptors for epidermal growth factor have been demonstrated in 44 of 65 (68%) prostatic tumours but only 3 of 52 (6%) benign hypertrophy specimens. Positivity did not relate to tumour stage nor grade.[9] Expression of epidermal growth factor receptor mRNA is higher in carcinoma than in benign prostatic tissue.[10]

Recently, a new class of peptide receptor for gonadotrophin releasing hormone together with its ligand has been found in a human hormone-sensitive prostatic cancer cell line and tumour biopsy specimens. The receptor is not expressed in hormone-insensitive cell lines although the ligand is present.[11] This finding suggests a direct effect of this group of compounds in carcinoma of the prostate, and is supportive evidence for the autocrine hypothesis of growth regulation. This hypothesis describes the local production of growth factors by malignant cells, and the stimulation of cell growth by these factors. It may be possible to produce peptide analogues of other growth factors such as epidermal growth factor, which are specific enough to have an inhibitory function.

Oncogenes

The p21 protein product of the *ras* oncogene has been assessed by immuno-histochemistry, and 23 of 29 cancers but none of 19 benign hypertrophy specimens expressed p21. The degree of positivity correlated with differentiation.[12] *ras* oncogene mutations are uncommon, and were described in only one of 24 tumours.[13] c-*myc* transcript levels have been shown to distinguish between prostatic cancer and benign hypertrophy and are significantly higher in tumours.[14] There is differential expression of oncogenes in cell culture, in response to an altered hormonal milieu: c-*fos* and h-*ras* mRNA levels dramatically decrease with withdrawal of androgens without change in c-*myc* mRNA.[15]

Tumour suppressor genes

It has recently been shown that cancers may develop as a result of the inactivation by deletion or mutation of genes whose function is the suppression of the development of tumours. These genes are termed 'tumour suppressor genes' or 'antioncogenes'.

The loss of genetic material in association with the development of human tumours was first described for retinoblastoma where there is allelic loss at chromosome 13 q 14. This abnormality has been demonstrated in approximately 70% of all patients with retinoblastoma and in both sporadic and hereditary forms. Tumour suppression is thought to result from the activity of the normal retinoblastoma gene product which is termed RB. This protein interacts with the protein products of oncogenic viruses which are known to be transforming such as the E7 product of human papillomavirus and large T protein of the SV40 virus. Retinoblastoma gene mutations are not restricted to retinoblastoma. They are also seen in other tumours such as osteosarcoma, breast cancer and small-cell lung cancer. Retinoblastoma gene loss has been assessed in human prostatic cancer cell lines. The hormone-sensitive line LNCaP and the hormone-insensitive line PC 3 were shown normally to express retinoblastoma protein products. However, an aberrant protein was expressed by the DU 145 cell line, suggesting that retinoblastoma gene mutation may be important in this hormone-independent malignancy. Normal retinoblastoma gene expression was restored in the DU 145 cell line by gene transfer. These transfected cells were implanted into nude mice and tumour development compared with controls within the same mouse inoculated with these two different DU 145 cell line variants. The tumours resulting from the transfected cells were significantly smaller than those resulting from inoculation of the non-transfected cell.[16]

Clinical developments in prostatic cancer

Hormonal therapies for prostatic cancer were first used in the early part of this century when White performed orchiectomy on patients with prostatic disease.[17] Some of them had benign hypertrophy and some cancer. Treatment was popularized in the mid-1940s by Huggins and Hodges and these treatments included oestrogen therapy, orchiectomy and adrenalectomy.[18] Since that time there has been a proliferation of medical treatments for prostatic cancer, but despite these advances we are still unclear as to the optimal treatment for this condition.

The first significant analysis of the effects of endocrine treatment for prostatic cancer was performed by Nesbitt and Baum in 1953. This retrospective analysis of over 2000 cases showed a significant advantage to treatment.[19] This analysis was flawed because of reference to an inappropriate control group. In 1967, the Veterans Administration Cooperative Urological Research Group published their prospective analysis of a randomized study comparing orchiectomy or oestrogen therapy with placebo. These studies, which involved nearly 2000 patients, found an equivalence of survival in the patients who received placebo treatment when compared with those treated patients.[20] A later analysis showed that many of the patients treated in the placebo arms of the studies did eventually receive hormonal therapies from their primary care physicians; and so the real conclusion of this study is considered by many to be that early and late endocrine therapies have the same effect in terms of survival, treatment only acting to temporarily palliate the condition. The other important finding of this study was the observation of a significant cardiovascular morbidity and mortality with oestrogen therapy. This effect is due to an increased extracellular volume and platelet stickiness secondary to increased antithrombin-III levels.[21] These effects of oestrogens are measurable even with low-dose diethylstilboestrol regimens.

The barbaric nature of orchiectomy and the side-effects of oestrogens have provided an impetus to develop new hormonal therapies for prostatic cancer. A further reason for these pharmaceutical developments is the need to provide treatment that confers a survival advantage where none has been previously shown. There is also a counter-argument against the introduction of new medical treatments by urological oncology Luddites whose argument is that orchiectomy as practised is a safe procedure with minimal morbidity and comparatively little cost. Certainly the average current costs for medical treatment is two to three times that of orchiectomy, but this argument seems remarkably retrogressive.

Cyproterone acetate

Cyproterone acetate is a progestogenic antiandrogen. Its endocrine effects are complicated. It inhibits the production of pituitary gonadotrophins, thereby decreasing testosterone indirectly. It limits the synthesis of androgens within the adrenal and testis, and peripherally it displaces testosterone from its cytoplasmic receptor and decreases the formation of the nuclear androgen complex. It also has weak glucocorticoid properties. It was introduced into clinical practice before the introduction of modern definitions of response, and early trials showed a local response in 68% of 292 patients and a cytological response to a more differentiated form in 18% of 98 patients.[22] The EORTC 30761 trial compared treatment with cyproterone acetate at a dose of 250 mg daily with medroxyprogesterone acetate thrice-weekly intramuscularly at a dose of 500 mg for 8 weeks followed by 100 mg twice-daily orally or 1 mg of diethylstilboestrol thrice-daily. The patient groups were not comparable and 40% of patients objectively responded to treatment. More patients treated with medroxyprogesterone acetate had high-grade tumours, and more had advanced stage tumours and were of poorer performance status than the other treatment groups. There was no difference between the objective response rates comparing diethylstilboestrol or cyproterone acetate but these two agents were more effective than medroxyprogesterone acetate. Progression rates were the same. The cardiovascular toxicity of cyproterone acetate was lower than that for patients treated with diethylstilboestrol.[23]

Flutamide

Flutamide is an antiandrogen which is entirely specific in its effects, competing for the androgen receptor. It was first introduced into clinical practice in 1975 when six responses were reported in 26 patients with refractory prostatic cancer.[24] There has been little enthusiasm for prescribing flutamide as a single agent in the treatment of prostatic cancer; this is because there is a concensus view that as a single agent it is comparatively ineffective in the control of the disease. Additionally, there were reports of depression associated with its use which limited prescribing. Approximately 15% of patients treated with flutamide have gastrointestinal disturbance. Recent studies have investigated the combination of this agent with gonadotrophin-releasing hormone agonists (see below).

Other antiandrogens

There has been continued interest from the pharmaceutical industry in the development of new antiandrogens. Nilutamide competes with testosterone and dihydrotestosterone for their peripheral receptor and also affects the adrenal hydroxylase systems.[25] There have been limited investigations of its use in combination therapy. Casodex is a non-steroidal antiandrogen which has structural similarities to flutamide. It has no central effects, so with treatment serum luteinizing hormone and testosterone levels increase.[26] The advantage of both casodex and nilutamide is that patients treated with these agents maintain potency. Dose-finding studies have been published for casodex, and in preliminary communications a response rate similar to that expected for orchiectomy has been demonstrated.

Gonadotrophin-releasing hormone agonists

Gonadotrophin-releasing hormone agonists act by down-regulating the pituitary gonadal axis, decreasing serum testosterone levels. As described earlier, an alternative mechanism for action has been suggested whereby these compounds are thought to have a direct effect at the level of tumour, down-regulating their own receptors on the cell surface. These compounds were introduced into oncological practice to provide an alternative to orchiectomy and oestrogen therapy. As single agents they are as effective as conventional treatments, and this has been demonstrated in randomized studies comparing analogues to orchiectomy and oestrogen therapy. More specifically they are without some of the disadvantages of castration and oestrogen therapy.[27] A proportion of patients treated with these compounds develop a transient exacerbation of symptoms of their disease.[28] This may be avoided by the concurrent use of antiandrogens.[29] The agonists were initially given as a daily subcutaneous injection or by five or six times daily nasal insufflation. Depot preparations have become available whereby these compounds can be given as a single injection in the form of a rod implant or microcapsules once-monthly. Even longer-acting depot preparations have been manufactured which can be administered once every three months.[30] There has been considerable difficulty concerning the introduction of these very-long-acting depots; their use is limited by litigation over patents, which is to the detriment of the patient.

It has been suggested that in the context of a disease that is androgen-sensitive it is important to eliminate all sources of androgenic steroids. In the normal man, 95% of circulating androgens are of testicular origin and 5% come from the adrenal. In the medically castrate man the situation is different and it is estimated that up to 45% of androgens within the prostate itself are of adrenal origin. Because of this, the use of an antiandrogen in combination with the gonadotrophin-releasing hormone agonist has been strongly advocated.[31] The scientific basis for trials of gonadotrophin-releasing hormone agonists and antiandrogens were not generally considered credible. However, such was the interest in the idea that the National Cancer Institute instigated a study comparing leuprolide with leuprolide and flutamide. In this careful trial in which over 600 patients were randomized, an advantage was found to combination therapy both in terms of median time to progression (16 months compared with 14 months) and median survival (35 months compared with 28 months).[32] Despite this result the controversy remains; and at a recent congress (Second International Symposium on GnRH Analogues in Cancer and Human Reproduction, 1990) ten similar trials were reported which involved 3447 patients. In not all of these studies is the appropriate information available. However, in three of seven trials in which objective response was described there was an advantage to combination therapy, and in three of eight trials an advantage in terms of median time to progression. In just one of nine trials was there prolonged survival, and this trial was the previously reported National Cancer Institute Study; so it would seem that the issue remains controversial.

Conclusion

This chapter has considered whether we have a better understanding of the molecular basis of prostatic cancer, and if optimal hormonal treatment for this condition is available. Scientific investigation of the molecular origins of prostatic cancer has resulted in an understanding of the mechanisms that lead to hormonal independence, and a recognition of the importance of the autocrine hypothesis in the regulation of cell growth. New treatments have been developed to improve the quality of patients' lives. Optimal therapy has not been designed, as we do not have treatment that is curative.

References

1. Nijs M, Hawkins EF, Coune A. Binding of 5 alpha dihydrotestosterone in human prostatic cancer: examination by agar gel electrophoresis. *J Endocrinol* 1976; **69**: 18–19.
2. Geller J, Cantor T, Albert J. Evidence of a specific dihydrotestosterone-binding cytosol receptor in the human prostate. *J Clin Endocrinol Metab* 1975; **41**: 854–62.
3. Trachtenberg T, Walsh PC. Correlation of prostatic nuclear androgen receptor content with duration of response and survival following hormonal therapy in advanced prostatic cancer. *J Urol* 1982; **127**: 466–71.
4. Martelli A, Soli M, Bercovich E, *et al*. Correlation between clinical response to anti-androgenic therapy and occurrence of receptors in human prostatic cancer. *Urology* 1980; **16**: 245–9.
5. Concolino G, Marcocchi A, Margitta G, *et al*. Steroid receptors and hormone responsiveness of human prostatic carcinoma. *Prostate* 1982; **3**: 475–82.
6. MacDonald A, Chisholm GD, Habib FK. Production and response of a human prostatic cancer line to transforming growth factor-like molecules. *Br J Cancer* 1990; **62**: 579–84.
7. Brinkmann AO, Faber PW, van Rooij HCJ, *et al*. The human androgen receptor: domain structure, genomic organization and regulation of expression. *J Steroid Biochem* 1989; **34**: 307–10.
8. Tilley WD, Wilson CM, Marcelli M, McPhaul MJ. Androgen receptor gene expression in human prostate carcinoma cell lines. *Cancer Res* 1990; **50**: 5382–6.
9. Fowler JE, Lau JLT, Ghosh L, Mills SE, Mounzer A. Epidermal growth factor and prostatic carcinoma: an immunohistochemical study. *J Urol* 1988; **139**: 857–61.
10. Morris GL, Green Dodd J. Epidermal growth factor receptor mRNA levels in human prostatic tumors and cell lines. *J Urol* 1990; **143**: 1272–4.
11. Qayum A, Gullick W, Clayton RC, Sikora K, Waxman J. The effects of gonadotrophin releasing hormone analogues in prostate cancer are mediated through specific tumour receptors. *Br J Cancer* 1990; **62**: 96–9.
12. Viola VM, Fromowitz F, Oravez S, *et al*. Expression of ras oncogene p21 in prostate cancer. *N Engl J Med* 1986; **314**: 133–7.
13. Carter BS, Epstein JI, Isaacs WB. ras gene mutations in human prostate cancer. *Cancer Res* 1990; **50**: 6830–32.
14. Fleming WH, Hamel A, MacDonald R, *et al*. Expression of the c-myc protooncogene in human prostatic carcinoma and benign prostatic hyperplasia. *Cancer Res* 1986; **46**: 1535–8.
15. Rijinders AWM, Van der Korput JAGM, Van Steenbrugge GJ, Romijn JC, Trapman J. Expression of cellular oncogenes in human prostatic carcinoma cell lines. *Biochem Biophys Res Comm* 1985; **132**: 548–54.
16. Bookstein R, Shew JY, Chen PL, Scully P, Lee WH. Suppression of tumorigenicity of human prostate carcinoma cells by replacing a mutated RB gene. *Science* 1990; **247**: 712–15.
17. White JW. The present position of the surgery of the hypertrophied prostate. *Ann Surg* 1893; **18**: 152–7.
18. Huggins C, Hodges CV. The effect of castration, of estrogen, and of androgen injection on serum phosphatase in metastatic carcinoma of the prostate. *Cancer Res* 1941; **1**: 292–8.

19. Nesbitt RM, Baum WC. Endocrine control of prostatic carcinoma: clinical and statistical survey of 1818 cases. *JAMA* 1950; **143**: 1317–20.
20. Veterans Administration Cooperative Urological Research Group. Treatment and survival of patients with cancer of the prostate. *Surg Gynec Obstet* 1967; **124**: 1011–19.
21. Varenhorst E, Wallentin L, Risberg B. The effects of orchidectomy, oestrogens and cyproterone acetate on the antithrombin-III concentration in carcinoma of the prostate. *Urol Res* 1981; **9**: 25–8.
22. Jacobi GH. Intramuscular cyproterone acetate treatment for advanced prostatic carcinoma: results of the first multicentre randomized trial. In: *Androgens and Antiandrogens*. Schering, Netherlands, 1983: 161–70.
23. Pavone-Macaluso M, De Voogt HJ, Viggiano G, *et al*. Comparison of diethylstilboestrol, cyproterone acetate and medroxyprogesterone acetate in the treatment of advanced prostatic cancer: final analysis of a randomized phase III trial of the European Organization for Research on Treatment of Cancer, Urological Group. *J Urol* 1986; **136**: 624–31.
24. Sogani PC, Ray B, Whitmore WF. Advanced prostatic carcinoma. *Urology* 1975; **6**: 164–6.
25. Neri R, Kassem N. Biological and clinical properties of antiandrogens. In: Bresciani F, King RJB, Lippman ME, Namer M, Raynaud JP (eds), *Hormones and Cancer 2: Proceedings of the Second International Congress on Hormones and Cancer*. Raven Press, New York 1984: 507–22.
26. Lunglmayr G. Casodex (ICI 176, 334), a new non-steroidal antiandrogen: early clinical results. *Horm Res* 1989; **32** (suppl): 77–81.
27. Waxman J. Gonadotrophin hormone releasing analogues open new doors in cancer treatment. *Br Med J* 1987; **295**: 1084–5.
28. Waxman J, Man A, Hendry WF, *et al*. Importance of early tumour exacerbation in patients treated with long-acting analogues of gonadotrophin-releasing hormone for advanced prostatic cancer. *Br Med J* 1985; **291**: 1387–8.
29. Waxman J, Williams G, Sandow J, *et al*. The clinical and endocrine assessment of three different antiandrogen regimens combined with a very long-acting gonadotrophin-releasing hormone analog. *Am J Clin Oncol* 1988; **2** (suppl 2): 152–5.
30. Waxman J, Sandow J, Abel P, Barton C, Keane P, Williams G. Three-monthly GnRH agonist (buserelin) for prostatic cancer. *Br J Urology* 1990; **65**: 43–5.
31. Labrie F, Dupont A, Giguere M, *et al*. Combination therapy with flutamide and castration (orchiectomy or LHRH agonist): the minimal endocrine therapy in both untreated and previously treated patients. *J Steroid Biochem* 1987; **27**: 525–32.
32. Crawford ED, Bertagna C, Smith JA, *et al*. A randomized controlled clinical trial of leuprolide and anandron versus leuprolide and placebo for advanced prostate cancer. *Gynecol Endocrin* 1990; **4** (suppl 2): 85.

Section IV

Urothelial Cancer

12 Oncogenes and growth factors in genitourinary tract tumours

David E Neal and Kilian Mellon

Whilst no two patients with cancer respond in exactly the same way to treatment, the oncologist is aware that characteristics of the tumour such as stage and histological grade are broad determinants of prognosis. In recent times it is the molecular biologists who have made the greatest progress, unswerving in their allegiance to the concept that discrete alterations in the molecular genetic structure of the cancer cell hold the key to carcinogenesis. In the 1980s one theory held the high ground of research into the genetics of cancer: this is the hypothesis that mutated or activated genes called oncogenes, acting in a dominant manner, might mediate the transformation of the normal to the malignant cell.

Oncogenes

The starting point for this research was the study of small oncogenic retroviruses which caused animal tumours. It was found that their single-stranded RNA was transcribed by reverse transcriptase into DNA, and these genes, after integration in the host genome, drove the cell to produce viral protein. Because a single copy of a transfected gene could transform cells, the idea gained credence that a single abnormal gene (an oncogene) could be transforming.[1] In the mid 1970s, many scientists agreed with Huebner and Todaro[2] that retroviral-like genes which were found in many mammalian cells were parasitic and inactive, but could be switched on by carcinogens. This finding was challenged by Stehlin and colleagues (the work recently winning a Nobel Prize for coauthors Bishop and Varmus) who found that normal chicken cells had a functioning gene similar to the avian Rous sarcoma virus *src* oncogene.[3] Their view—since amply supported—was that most RNA viral oncogenes have normal cellular homologues which are important in day-to-day cellular metabolism, but which can be mutated or activated by carcinogens. Indeed, it is now thought that the oncogenes of RNA viruses were captured originally from normal cellular genes.

The third strand in this web was the finding that under certain well-defined conditions, some cells grown in tissue culture—the best known of which are NIH 3T3 cells (mouse embryonic fibroblasts)—could be induced to incorporate high-molecular-weight fragments of foreign DNA into their own genome. When the DNA was taken from cells which had already been chemically transformed, many of the cells took on the appearance of transformed cells.[4] When, on the other hand, normal high-molecular-weight DNA was used the NIH 3T3 cells were not transformed. It was suggested that the transfer of oncogenes from the malignant cell lines to the NIH 3T3 cells was responsible, although one immediate objection to this view came from the observation that low-molecular-weight normal DNA could be transforming in this assay, albeit with low levels of efficiency. Shortly afterwards, it was found that DNA from the human bladder cancer cell line EJ was effective in this assay.[5] By this time, molecular biological techniques had advanced and the responsible gene was found to be identical to the oncogene of the Harvey murine sarcoma virus (termed Ha-*ras*). More surprisingly, when normal cellular DNA was examined with *ras* probes it was apparent that *ras*-like genes which produced a guanine nucleotide protein (p21) were present even in simple organisms such as yeasts.

Theoretically, oncogenes might transform cells by several distinct mechanisms, and in practice many of them have been found in tumours of different types. Firstly, the gene may be present in abnormal quantities, which is termed 'amplification'. Secondly, the gene may be activated by genetic rearrangements leading to translocation—a feature found in Burkitt's lymphoma where there is translocation of *myc* (normally found on chromosome 8) to immunoglobulin loci on chromosome 14 or 22. Thirdly, certain slow-acting oncogenic viruses such as the animal leukaemia or mammary tumour viruses contain enhancer or promoter sequences which are inserted close to the oncogene sequences leading to their inappropriate transcription. Fourthly, the oncogene may be mutated and consequently its product metabolically more active.

When the *ras* gene was cloned from normal urothelial and bladder cancer cells and used in transfection experiments, only the bladder cancer gene transformed NIH 3T3 cells, despite both cell lines producing roughly the same amount of messenger RNA encoding *ras* and the same amount of *ras* p21 protein. However, it was found that the two p21 proteins had slightly different mobilities on electrophoresis and a single base substitution at codon 12 resulting in the replacement of glycine with another amino acid was responsible.[6-8] Thus, it was found that a single point mutation in a gene could produce a strongly mutagenic protein. Another link in this complex story was forged by Barbacid and his colleagues[9] who found that chemical carcinogens such as nitroso-methylurea resulted in a similar mutation at codon 12 in the *ras* gene.

Many different oncogenes have now been identified (Table 12.1). Some were found first in viruses, whereas others such as *neu* and N-*ras* were identified first in tumours. These genes have been grouped into families on the basis of their function and evolution; some are homologous to peptide growth factors (*sis* and platelet-

Table 12.1   Oncogenes and their viral homologues

abl	TK	Abelson murine leukaemia virus
erb-A		Avian erythroblastosis virus
erb-B1	TK+GFr	Avian erythroblastosis virus
erb-B2 (*neu*)	TK+GFr	
ets		E26 virus
fes/fps	TK	Feline/avian sarcoma virus
fgr		Gardner feline sarcoma virus
fms	TK+GFr	McDonough feline sarcoma virus
fos	DNAb	FBJ osteosarcoma virus
jun	TF	
mos	TK	Moloney murine sarcoma virus
myb	DNAb	Myeloblastosis virus
myc	DNAb	Myelocytomatosis virus
p53	DNAb	
raf/mil	RNAb	Murine/avian sarcoma virus
Ha-*ras*	G	Harvey murine sarcoma virus
Ki-*ras*	G	Kirsten murine sarcoma virus
N-*ras*	G	
rel		Reticuloendotheliosis virus
ros	TK	Avian sarcoma virus
sis	GF	Simian sarcoma virus
ski		Avian SKV770 virus
src	TK	Rous sarcoma virus
yes	TK	Avian Y73 sarcoma virus

Abbreviations referring to protein product:
DNAb: DNA and nuclear binding activity.
G: guanine nucleotide binding protein.
GF: peptide growth factor
GFr: growth factor receptor.
RNAb: RNA binding activity.
TK: tyrosine kinase activity.
TF: transcription factor.

derived growth factor[10, 11]) or growth factor receptors (c-*erb*-B1 and the epidermal growth factor receptor[12]).

DNA viruses

The first oncogenes to be described in viruses and in human tumours were those isolated from RNA viruses. However, some oncogenic viruses such as the herpes virus, papillomavirus and adenovirus contain DNA; the best studied is the SV40 papillomavirus. This contains a gene (the A gene) which encodes a protein (T antigen). By means of RNA splicing different-sized T antigens are produced—a large T, a middle T and a small T. On its own, SV40 T is not strongly oncogenic, but when associated with SV40 enhancer regions it can produce tumours. For example, when recombinant genes consisting of insulin regulating sequences, SV40 enhancer and T antigen genes were inserted into mouse ova, increased transcription of large

T antigen occurred in pancreatic islet cells followed by the appearance of B cell tumours.[13] Moreover, in humans, DNA viruses such as herpes and papilloma types 16 and 18 appear to play a part in the aetiology of cervical carcinoma.[14,15] Recently, it has been shown that the adenovirus E1A protein binds to the retinoblastoma gene product,[16] decreasing its ability to function as a tumour suppressor. Such findings appear to bridge the gap between DNA oncogenes, tumour suppressor genes and proto-oncogenes.

Multistage carcinogenesis and oncogene activation

Before dealing with the different types of oncogenes which have been identified in human genitourinary tract tumours, it is worth considering some important discrepancies between the concept that single activated oncogenes can cause cancer and the realities of oncogenesis in intact animals.

It is thought, for example, that most human tumours arise, not by a single dominant mutation, but by a complex multistage process involving at least five or six different steps.[17] One important feature of these studies of oncogenes in tissue culture is the nature of the NIH 3T3 fibroblasts. Unlike most truly normal cells in tissue culture these cells are immortal—in other words they will keep on growing if they are supplied with the appropriate nutrients and sub-cultured. The fact that certain gene sequences transform this cell does not mean that they would transform a normal cell. Indeed, it is clear that in many circumstances several oncogenes acting in concert are necessary for high-efficiency transformation. Thus, both the large and middle T genes of polyomavirus are needed to complete the transformation of rat embryo fibroblasts,[18] a combination of a nuclear oncogene (*myc*) with a cytoplasmic oncogene (*ras*) enables rapid transformation of rat embryo fibroblasts[19] as does the combination of *ras* oncogenes and the adenovirus E1A oncogene.[20] In addition, the mere presence of a mutated *ras* oncogene in a cell line is insufficient to guarantee tumour formation.[21] An important concept has arisen that oncogenes of various types can cooperate in oncogenesis: this is the molecular biological equivalent of multistage carcinogenesis, though it is apparent that under certain circumstances single oncogenes can transform normal cells.

It has also become clear that other important mechanisms of genetic control are at work in the cancer cell. Firstly, recessive mechanisms may underlie some rare hereditary human tumours such as retinoblastomas and von Hippel Lindau disease;[22] and secondly, cell fusion experiments showed some years ago that the fusion of normal and tumour cells can result in the suppression of the tumour cell phenotype.[23]

Recessive mechanisms and tumour suppressor genes

In some tumours, loss of recessive genes whose protein products are concerned with suppression of tumour formation or the loss of genes inhibiting the expression of dominantly acting oncogenes may be as important as gains of dominantly acting oncogenes. It has been known for some time that losses of genetic material occur in tumours and, what is more, particular chromosome losses are associated with certain tumours.

For example, patients with retinoblastoma inherit a defective allele at the Rbl locus on the long arm of chromosome 13; a second sporadic mutation resulting in the loss of the remaining normal allele will lead to tumour formation in retina or bone.[24] Though the abnormal gene is inherited recessively, the disease appears to be inherited in a dominant way because the second sporadic mutation is very likely to occur. It is thought that the Rbl gene product is a nucleo-phosphoprotein which normally inhibits growth: its absence presumably permits tumour formation. Recent studies have also shown that the Rbl gene product binds to E1A proteins and this may be the means by which the DNA virus stimulates its own replication.[16] Other studies have shown that additional recessive mechanisms may be important in tumour formation. P53 is a nucleo-phosphoprotein, first identified through binding to the T antigen of SV40; it also competes with DNA polymerase for SV40 large T.[25] Mutated copies of p53 are very common in lung, colon and breast cancer,[26] and it now appears that normal p53 may function as a tumour suppressor gene.

It has also been shown by Harris that fusion of normal fibroblasts with a variety of tumour cells will result in suppression of malignant behaviour.[23] This is thought to be mediated by the temporary replacement by normal fibroblast genes of gene losses in the malignant cell. Genes on chromosome 4 and 11 are strongly implicated in this process and, presumably, under normal circumstances they have tumour suppressing activity.

Chromosome losses in human genitourinary tract tumours

Specific chromosomal deletions have been reported in certain genitourinary tract tumours. Deletions of parts of the short arm of chromosome 11 were reported in 5 of 12 bladder tumours,[27] although an earlier paper suggested that the loss of genetic material from the short arm of chromosome 11 was a secondary event associated with the acquisition of invasive behaviour.[28] In up to 55% of patients with familial Wilms' tumours (a combination of aniridia, mental retardation, genitourinary tract abnormalities and Wilms' tumours) deletions of the short arm of chromosome 11 have been found,[29,30] though others have failed to confirm this finding in different families, suggesting that other mechanisms may be at work.[31] Chromosome 3 has been reported to be affected in both von Hippel Lindau disease (a combination of cerebellar haemangioblastomas, retinal angiomas, phaeochromocytomas, renal cysts and renal carcinomas) and in sporadic renal carcinomas.[32,33]

Specific changes in human bladder tumours

ras *oncogenes*

The three main members of the *ras* gene family—N-*ras*, Ki-*ras* and Ha-*ras*—each encode a protein with a molecular mass of about 21 kDa. Mutated *ras* genes were the first to be identified in human tumours and in fact were first found in a human bladder cancer cell line (EJ). The p21 proteins bind guanine nucleotides (mainly GTP) and are similar to a wider class of G proteins which control adenylate cyclase and have been implicated in signal transduction across the cell membrane.[9] It appears that the p21 protein is activated when bound to GTP. However, GTP-ase activity (inherent in normal *ras* p21) results in the formation of GDP which by a negative-feedback mechanism switches off the growth signal. A GTP-ase regulating protein (GAP), present in normal cells, increases the p21 GTP-ase activity and thereby decreases the growth signal. Peptide growth factor receptors such as EGF receptors also interact with p21 proteins. Increased phosphorylation of GAP, mediated by an activated growth factor receptor, decreases its ability to diminish the p21 GTP-ase activity and thereby results in increased amounts of p21–GTP with a subsequently increased growth signal. The oncogenic mutated p21 does not bind GAP and therefore has decreased GTP-ase activity, increased GTP binding and, as a result, an increased growth promotion activity.[34]

However, over-expression of a normal *ras* protein can also cause transformation, and a mutation in the intron (that part of the gene which encodes the portion of RNA which is excised from the final processed form of mRNA leaving the cell nucleus) of the gene controlling *ras* expression has recently been shown to increase expression of the normal c-Ha-*ras* oncogene in the T24/EJ cell line.[35]

ras oncogenes have been found in a wide variety of human tumours.[9,36] They were identified by several methods ranging from the original NIH-3T3 assay, restriction length polymorphisms and more recently the RNA-ase mismatch cleavage assay[37] or the polymerase chain reaction.[38] The more recently used methods have a greater sensitivity leading to a greater reported frequency of *ras* gene involvement in some human tumours.

In bladder cancer, mutated *ras* genes have been found in about 10% of primary tumours.[39–42] Other findings, however, suggest that *ras* gene expression may be more important in bladder cancer than is suggested by this figure. For example, increased expression of *ras* p21 protein was found in many invasive bladder cancers and high-grade dysplasia both by immunohistochemistry and by immunoassay.[43] The antibody used in this study reacted with N-*ras*, Ki-*ras*, Ha-*ras* and certain types of mutated Ha-*ras* gene products: normal urothelium and grade 1 tumours stained negatively for *ras*. The same authors have also found a similar pattern of staining in prostate cancer.[44] It has been pointed out, however, that the antibody used in this study (RAP-5) may recognize cellular components distinct from p21, and others have noted that some of these antibodies stain formalin-fixed specimens in a non-specific way.[33]

A protein of 55 kDa which is antigenically related to p21 has also been found in the urine of patients with bladder cancer and a weak correlation was reported with tumour stage and grade.[45] Other studies have also indicated how activation of *ras* might make a tumour more invasive. For example, it was shown that transfection of an activated mutated *ras* gene into a low metastatic mouse bladder cancer cell line resulted in increased metastatic potential[46] and increased secretion of urokinase[47] which might increase the invasive potential of the cells.

Other oncogenes

The presence of oncogenes other than *ras* has been reported less frequently in bladder cancer. Occasional reports have suggested that increases in the protein products of *myc* and *fos* occur in bladder and prostate tumours of high grade. These reports are difficult to interpret because many were performed on paraffin-embedded archival material and both these proteins have a half-life of a few minutes. However, one recent study has shown that decreased methylation of the 3′ end of the c-*myc* gene occurs in bladder cancer and that this is more common in invasive tumours.[48] Increased methylation may impair transcription of genes and therefore the findings of decreased methylation might explain increased *myc* protein levels in tumours with a fast cell turnover. The relationship between oncogenes and growth factors has also been explored in one study of kidney cancer using a panel of 12 oncogene probes. This showed increased amounts of RNA encoding c-*erb*-B1 (EGF receptor) in 47% of cases and increased c-*myc* in 73%: an association was also found between the two.[49] Increased amounts of RNA encoding c-Ha-*ras* and c-*fms* was found in one out of 16 cases, but no increased expression of c-Ki-*ras*, N-*myc*, c-*fes*, c-*abl* or c-*erb*-B2 (*neu*) was found.

It is also uncertain whether increased *fos* or *myc* expression reflects anything other than increased cell turnover. For example, one study of renal cancer found increased *myc* protein levels correlated with grade, but also correlated with cell turnover as measured by the monoclonal antibody Ki67:[50] a finding recently supported by a study of the relationship between EGF receptors and cell turnover in bladder cancer (see later).

Oncogenes and growth factors

The continued growth of most cells in tissue culture is dependent on depletable factors in the medium, present in serum, but absent from plasma. These initial observations led to the discovery of a peptide growth factor present in platelets known as platelet-derived growth factor (PDGF). Subsequently many other peptides have been identified including epidermal growth factor (EGF) and transforming growth factors. Neoplastic cells require less serum for growth in tissue culture than normal diploid cells. This observation in conjunction with studies which identified the secretion of mitogenic growth factors in tissue cultures of neoplastic cells led to the suggestion that neoplastic cells might produce their own growth factors: this was the theory of 'autocrine production' of growth factors.

Evidence of a link between oncogenes and growth factors, supporting the autocrine theory of growth, was established following studies of the structure of the PDGF. The activated v-*sis* oncogene of the simian sarcoma virus, originally isolated from a primate fibrosarcoma, encodes a 28 kDa transforming protein, p28^{sis}, which is processed to a 24 kDa homodimer, p24^{sis}. It has been shown that the N-terminal 109 amino acids of the beta-chain of PDGF are virtually identical with p28^{sis} and that p24^{sis} is homologous with a homodimer comprised of the beta-chain of PDGF.[10,12,51] It is assumed that the viral gene product stimulates cell replication by interacting with the receptor for PDGF.

Similarly, gp65^{erbB}, the protein product of the avian erythroblastosis virus, shows considerable sequence homology with a truncated and mutated receptor for epidermal growth factor.[12]

Binding of several growth factors, including epidermal growth factor, to their receptors results in activation of tyrosine kinase which catalyses the transfer of phosphate to the tyrosine residues of protein substrates. Tyrosine kinase activity is an uncommon event in the normal cell, although common in the transformed cell. The fact that several viral transforming proteins and growth factor receptors share tyrosine kinase activity is further evidence suggesting an association between oncogenes and growth factors. The relationships between oncogenes and growth factors have previously been discussed.[52]

Conversely, certain growth factors can induce proto-oncogene expression. Within 2 hours of the addition of PDGF to stationary BALB/c 3T3 cells there is a several-fold increase in the expression of c-*myc* mRNA.[53]

Epidermal growth factor

EGF is a 53 amino acid peptide of 6 kDa, originally isolated by Cohen during the purification of nerve growth factor from mouse submaxillary gland extracts.[54] High levels of EGF in urine, in the presence of low plasma levels, favour the suggestion that renal tubules actively secrete human urinary EGF. EGF is widespread in human tissues with high levels found in milk and prostatic fluid.[55]

EGF induces cellular proliferation in certain cell lines including certain bladder tumour cell lines, but this effect has not been shown *in vivo*. EGF has been used clinically to accelerate corneal re-epithelialization following injury,[56] and has been reported to increase crypt cell proliferation in an infant with microvillous atrophy.[57] The way in which EGF stimulates cell growth and the means by which it may stimulate local invasion of tumours *in vivo* remain uncertain. EGF, however, has been found to increase transcription of the nuclear proto-oncogene c-*jun*:[58] a gene sequence which is activated during cell division.

The EGF receptor (EGFr)

The action of EGF is mediated by binding to a membrane-bound receptor which is the product of the c-*erb*-B1 gene. The EGF receptor is a 175 kDa protein consisting of an extracellular EGF-binding part, including two cysteine-rich domains, a small transmembrane segment and an intracellular domain containing the protein tyrosine kinase and three major autophosphorylation sites located on tyrosine residues. The transforming growth factor, TGF-alpha, also acts as a ligand for the EGF receptor. The EGF receptor is down-regulated from the cell membrane by ligand binding, either by EGF or TGF-alpha. Other proteins and peptides can cause down-regulation of the receptor—including a peptide encoded by the E3 region of adenovirus.[59] Down-regulation of EGF receptors by these ligands is associated with cellular activation, but the means by which this is produced by various second messengers remains obscure. Other metabolically active proteins are produced when EGF receptors are down-regulated. One study found increased secretion of plasminogen activator:[60] this is of great interest as it may be associated with increased local invasiveness of tumour cells.

EGF receptors can be detected by immunohistochemical means or by biochemical methods using radiolabelled EGF. The role of epidermal growth factor and its receptor in human cancer has been reviewed previously.[61] EGF receptors have been identified on various cell types including fibroblasts, corneal cells, kidney cells and normal basal urothelial cells.[62,63] Tumours expressing high levels of receptors for EGF include squamous cell carcinomas,[64] breast carcinomas,[65,66] gliomas,[67] lung tumours,[68] sarcomas,[69] gynaecological tumours[70] and bladder tumours.[62,63,71,72] Placenta and the A431 cell line, originally derived from a vulval squamous cell carcinoma, have especially high EGF receptor concentrations. Some authors have found low EGF receptor concentrations in high-grade carcinomas of the prostate, but other groups have shown that levels of EGF receptors in some tumours are equivalent to those in benign hyperplasia.[73] High EGF receptor concentrations have been reported in association with amplification of the EGF receptor gene in gliomas[74] and squamous cell carcinomas,[75] as well as in the A431 cell line; but in a study of 31 bladder tumours analysed by Southern blot analysis, only one tumour with high EGF receptor content had amplification of the EGF receptor gene.[71]

EGF receptors in bladder cancer

The prognosis for patients with transitional cell carcinoma of the bladder is largely dependent on the stage of the tumour (T category) and grade. Long-term survival is greatly reduced once a tumour has invaded the muscle of the bladder wall (T2–T4). About 20% of patients with initially superficial bladder tumours will develop more menacing invasive tumours. Local progression of recurrent tumours is related to T category and grade; patients with pT1 (tumour invading lamina propria) and poorly differentiated grade 3 tumours fare the worst,[76] about 30–40% developing muscle invasive disease. Patients with well-differentiated pTa tumours, on the other hand, have a very low rate of tumour progression (less than 5%). At present, there is no reliable method of predicting which individual patients with superficial tumours (pTa/pT1) will undergo stage progression.

Various factors have been suggested as being useful in this regard, including

Table 12.2   Associations among tumour category, grade and EGF receptor staining

	pTa (n=34)		pT1 (n=18)		T2 (n=16)		T3 (n=21)		T4 (n=12)	
EGFr status	+	−	+	−	+	−	+	−	+	−
Grade 1	0	2	0	0	0	0	0	0	0	0
Grade 2	5	27	5	5	5	2	1	0	2	0
Grade 3	0	0	3	5	4	5	16	4	7	3
Totals	5	29	8	10	9	7	17	4	9	3
Percentage positive	15%		44%		56%		81%		75%	

Chi squared on 4 d.o.f. for relationship among EGFr positivity and tumour category = 28; $P < 0.0001$.

staining to detect deletion of blood group substances and the presence of morphological abnormalities in the urothelium distant from the primary tumour. None has stood the test of time in predicting tumour behaviour.

Recent studies of EGF receptor status in bladder cancer have suggested that high levels of expression of this growth factor receptor may be associated with a poor outcome. Several immunohistochemical studies,[62,63,71,72] using a murine monoclonal antibody to the EGFr (EGFR1), have shown a strong correlation between EGFr positivity and tumour stage and grade (Table 12.2). However, the degree of correlation between immunohistochemical staining for EGF receptors and their detection by ligand binding in bladder cancer remains uncertain. One study found that most EGF-receptor-positive, muscle-invasive tumours had higher levels of receptors on ligand binding than superficial tumours which were EGF-receptor-positive.[77] In the superficial tumours, significantly more tumours were positive on ligand binding, suggesting that this technique may be more sensitive in detecting low levels of receptors.

Finally, a prospective study of 100 patients with bladder cancer was performed. This found that strong staining for the EGF receptor was associated with death from bladder cancer, and in superficial tumours was related to tumour recurrence and local progression. The question with studies such as this is whether this statistical association is a non-specific phenomenon. For example, strong staining for the EGF receptor was associated with grade and stage and tumour multiplicity. A multivariate analysis was, therefore, carried out to determine whether EGF receptor status was independently associated with poor outcome, and the previously noted associations were confirmed suggesting that EGF receptor status may function as an independent variable.[72]

EGFr status and cell division in bladder cancer

Recently, we have performed a combined study of EGF receptor status and cell cycling in a further 55 bladder tumours using staining with EGFR1 to assess receptor status and the monoclonal antibody Ki67 to determine cell turnover. The Ki67 antibody recognizes an unknown nuclear antigen expressed by actively dividing cells; i.e. S, G2 and M phase cells and G1 cells after mitosis. This study has confirmed the previously noted association of EGFr positivity with T category and histopathological grade. Significantly more cells were actively dividing in muscle-invasive tumours (mean ± SD: 11.3 ± 6.3%) compared with superficial tumours (3.9 ± 2.8%), as they were in grade 3 tumours (10 ± 7.1%) compared with grade 1 and 2 tumours (4.6 ± 3.0%). A further finding of this study was of a significant positive association between EGF receptor positivity and Ki67 reactivity, indicating that tumours with high EGFr content tended to have increased growth fractions. In addition, a significant area of overlap in Ki67 counts was found when grade 3 tumours were compared with grade 1 and 2 tumours, suggesting that some low-grade tumours had high cell turnovers. Further studies will determine whether such tumours have a worse clinical outcome.

Expression of the c-*erb*-B2 (*neu*) oncoprotein

The proto-oncogene c-*erb*-B2 (*neu*) encodes a transmembrane glycoprotein which is similar to the EGF receptor. Amplification of the c-*erb*-B2 gene and over-expression of its protein product have been reported mainly in adenocarcinomas arising in various sites, and in breast cancer is associated with a poor prognosis.[78] A previous study of over 40 paraffin-embedded bladder tumours had failed to demonstrate any increased expression of this oncoprotein (unpublished data). However, a more recent study using frozen sections stained immuno-histochemically with a monoclonal antibody (CB-11) against a synthetic peptide representing residues close to the C-terminus of the predicted oncoprotein sequence, has shown that 17 out of 45 (38%) tumours showed positive staining. Five tumours showed areas of strong positive staining (four muscle-invasive tumours and one pTaG2 tumour which rapidly progressed). Weak positive staining was noted in a further four muscle-invasive tumours and in eight superficial tumours. The prognostic significance of c-*erb*-B2 oncoprotein in bladder tumours must now be evaluated.

Other growth factors and other genitourinary tract tumours

EGF receptors have been found in prostate cancer and in benign hyperplasia.[73] Its activity is decreased by certain kinases; one of these is the prostatic-specific acid phosphatase.[79] Androgens have also been found to modulate EGF receptor activity,[80] mainly resulting in decreased EGF receptor levels in the prostate. Another family of peptide growth factors are the fibroblast growth factors. Acidic fibroblast growth factor is limited in its distribution to the brain and retina.[81] Basic fibroblast growth factor is a peptide of 146 amino acids and has been given a number of names including prostatic growth factor and endothelial growth factor.[81] It has a ubiquitous distribution in many mesodermal and neuroectodermal tissues, but is characteristically found in the vascular system. The main fraction of prostatic extracts which promotes growth in cells in tissue culture is found bound to heparin in Sephadex columns: this is basic fibroblast growth factor.[82] Messenger RNA encoding basic FGF has been isolated from human benign prostatic hyperplasia and carcinoma,[83] and it has also been found in the testis[84] and in kidney and renal cell carcinomas.[85] Increased levels have also been found in the urine of patients with bladder or renal cancer.[86]

Other peptide growth factors have not yet been explored in depth. Insulin-like growth factor I (Somatomedin C), insulin-like growth factor II and their receptors may be found on certain tumour cells. There is some evidence that their levels may be mediated by steroid hormones, at least in breast cells, and it is likely that their function in the prostate will be studied in the near future. Increased amounts of insulin-like growth factor II have been found in Wilms' tumours.[87]

One family of growth factors of major importance in tumours are the transforming growth factors, alpha and beta.[61] They are secreted by many tumour cell types and are found in high levels in pleural effusions and in the urine of patients with metastatic disease.[88-90] TGF-alpha also activates the EGF receptor. Increased levels of TGF-alpha have been found in renal tumours[89] and are frequently associated with increased levels of EGF receptor expression.[91] In addition, increased amounts of TGF-alpha activity have been reported in tumour ascitic fluid and in the urine of patients with metastatic disease. This suggests that tumours elaborate these peptide growth factors which may be important in local growth and invasion.

Conclusions

Studies of oncogenes and peptide growth factors in urological cancer are beginning to provide information about the genetic changes which underpin the malignant phenotype. For the future, it is to be hoped that measurement of these changes will yield clinically useful prognostic information. The use of immuno-modulators has already shown potential benefit in patients with otherwise untreatable renal cancer. It may be that other modulators of growth factor receptor function, such as peptide antagonists, will find a place in the overall management of patients with malignant disease.

References

1. Andersson P, Goldfarb MP, Weinberg RA. A defined subgenomic fragment of *in vitro* synthesized Moloney sarcoma virus DNA can induce cell transformation upon transfection. *Cell* 1975; **16**: 63–75.

2. Huebner RJ, Todaro GJ. Oncogenes of RNA tumour viruses as determinants of cancer. *Proc Natl Acad Sci (USA)* 1969; **64**: 1087–94.

3. Stehlin D, Varmus HE, Bishop JM, Vogt PA. DNA related to the transforming gene(s) of avian sarcoma viruses is present in normal avian DNA. *Nature (Lond)* 1976; **260**: 170–3.

4. Shih C, Shilo BZ, Goldfarb MP, Danneberg A, Weinberg RA. Passage of phenotypes of chemically transformed cells via transfection of DNA and chromatin. *Proc Natl Acad Sci (USA)* 1979; **76**: 5714–18.

5. Krontiris TG, Cooper GM. Transforming activities of human tumour DNAs. *Proc Natl Acad Sci (USA)* 1981; **78**: 1181–4.

6. Reddy EP, Reynolds RK, Santos E, Barbacid M. A point mutation is responsible for the acquisition of transforming properties by the T24 human bladder carcinoma oncogene. *Nature (Lond)* 1982; **300**: 149–52.

7. Capon DJ, Chen EY, Levinson AD, Seeburg PH, Goeddel DV. Complete nucleotide sequences of the T24 human bladder carcinoma oncogene and its normal homologue. *Nature (Lond)* 1983; **302**: 33–7.

8. Weinberg RA. The genetic origins of human cancer. *Cancer* 1988; **61**: 1963–8.

9. Barbacid M. *ras* genes. *Ann Rev Biochem* 1987; **56**: 779–827.

10. Doolittle RF, Hunkapillar MW, Hood LE, *et al*. Simian sarcoma virus oncogene v-sis is derived from the gene (or genes) encoding a platelet derived growth factor. *Science (Wash DC)* 1983; **221**: 275–7.

11. Waterfield MD, Scrace T, Whittle N, *et al*. Platelet derived growth factor is structurally related to the putative transforming protein p28sis of simian sarcoma virus. *Nature (Lond)* 1983; **304**: 35–9.

12. Downward J, Yarden Y, Mayes E, *et al*. Close similarity of epidermal growth factor receptor and v-erb-B oncogene protein sequences. *Nature (Lond)* 1984; **307**: 521–7.

13. Hanahan D. Heritable formation of pancreatic B-cell tumours in transgenic mice expressing recombinant insulin/simian virus 40 oncogenes. *Nature (Lond)* 1985; **315**: 115–22.

14. Dreesman GR, Burek J, Adam E, *et al*. Expression of herpes virus induced antigens in human cervical cancer. *Nature (Lond)* 1980; **283**: 591–3.

15. Schwarz E, Freese UK, Gissman L, *et al*. Structure and transcription of human papillomavirus sequences in cervical carcinoma cells. *Nature (Lond)* 1985; **314**: 111–14.

16. Whyte P, Buchkovich KJ, Horowitz JM, Friend SH, Raybuck M, Weinberg RA, Harlow E. Association between an oncogene and an anti-oncogene: the adenovirus E1A proteins bind to the retinoblastoma gene product. *Nature (Lond)* 1988; **334**: 124–9.

17. Nowell P. The clonal evolution of tumour cell populations. *Science (Wash DC)* 1976; **194**: 23–8.

18. Rassoulzadegan M, Cowie A, Carr A, Glaichenhaus N, Kamen R, Cuzin F. The role of individual polyoma virus early proteins in oncogenic transformation. *Nature (Lond)* 1982; **300**: 713–18.

19. Land H, Parada LF, Weinberg RA. Tumorogenic conversion of primary embryo

fibroblasts requires at least two cooperating oncogenes. *Nature (Lond)* 1983; **304**: 596–602.

20.   Ruley HE. Adenovirus early region 1A enables viral and cellular transforming genes to transform primary cells in culture. *Nature (Lond)* 1983; **304**: 602–6.

21.   Senger DR, Perruzi CA, Unnisa Ali I. T24 human bladder carcinoma cells with activated Ha-*ras* protooncogene: nontumorogenic cells susceptible to malignant transformation with carcinogen. *Proc Natl Acad Sci (USA)* 1988; **85**: 5107–11.

22.   Klein G. The approaching era of the tumor suppressing genes. *Science (Wash DC)* 1987; **238**: 1539–45.

23.   Harris H. The analysis of malignancy by cell fusion: the position in 1988. *Cancer Res* 1988; **48**: 3302–6.

24.   Knudsen AG. Hereditary cancer, oncogenes and anti-oncogenes. *Cancer Res* 1985; **45**: 1437–43.

25.   Gannon JV, Lane DP. p53 and DNA polymerase compete for binding to SV40 antigen. *Nature (Lond)* 1987; **329**: 454–8.

26.   Nigro JM, Baker SJ, Preisinger AC. Mutations in the p53 gene occur in diverse tumour types. *Nature (Lond)* 1989; **342**: 705–8.

27.   Fearon ER, Feinberg AP, Hamilton SH, Vogelstein B. Loss of genes on the short arm of chromosome 11 in bladder cancer. *Nature (Lond)* 1985; **318**: 377–80.

28.   Gibas Z, Prout GR, Connolly JG, Edson-Pontes J, Sandberg AV. Nonrandom changes in transitional cell carcinoma of the bladder. *Cancer Res* 1984; **44**: 1257–64.

29.   Fearon ER, Vogelstein B, Feinberg AP. Somatic deletion and duplication of genes on chromosome 11 in Wilms' tumour. *Nature (Lond)* 1984; **309**: 176–8.

30.   Koufos A, Hansen MF, Lampkin BC, *et al.* Loss of alleles at loci on chromosome 11 during genesis of Wilms' tumour. *Nature (Lond)* 1984; **309**: 170–2.

31.   Grundy P, Koufos A, Morgan K, Li FP, Meadows AT, Cavanee WK. Familial predisposition to Wilms' tumour does not map to the short arm of chromosome 11. *Nature (Lond)* 1988; **336**: 374–6.

32.   Kovacs G, Erlandsson R, Boldog F, *et al.* Consistent chromosome 3p deletion and loss of heterozygosity in renal cell carcinoma. *Proc Natl Acad Sci (USA)* 1988; **85**: 1571–5.

33.   Green AR. Recessive mechanisms of malignancy. *Br J Cancer* 1988; **58**: 115–21.

34.   Sigal IS. The ras oncogene: a structure and some function. *Nature (Lond)* 1988; **332**: 485–6.

35.   Cohen JB, Levinson AD. A point mutation in the last intron responsible for increased expression and transforming activity of the c-Ha-*ras* oncogene. *Nature (Lond)* 1988; **334**: 119–24.

36.   Bos JL. *ras* oncogenes in human cancer: a review. *Cancer Res* 1989; **49**: 4682–9.

37.   Forrester K, Almoguera C, Han K, Grizzle WE, Perucho M. Detection of high incidence of Ki-*ras* oncogenes during human colon tumorigenesis. *Nature (Lond)* 1987; **327**: 298–303.

38.   Burmer GC, Rabinovitch PS, Loeb LA. Analysis of c-Ki-*ras* mutations in human colon carcinoma by cell sorting, polymerase chain reaction and DNA sequencing. *Cancer Res* 1989; **49**: 2141–6.

39.   Fujita J, Yoshida O, Yasohito Y, Rhim JS, Hatanaka M, Aaronson SA. Ha-*ras* oncogenes are activated by somatic alterations in human urinary tract tumours. *Nature (Lond)* 1984; **309**: 464–6.

40.   Fujita J, Srivastava SK, Kraus MH, Rhim JS, Tronick SR, Aaronson SA. Frequency of molecular alterations affecting *ras* protooncogenes in human urinary tract tumors. *Proc Natl Acad Sci (USA)* 1985; **82**: 3849–53.

41. Malone PR, Visvanathan KV, Ponder BA, Shearer RJ, Summerhayes IC. Oncogenes and bladder cancer. *Br J Urol* 1985; **57**: 664–7.

42. Visvanathan KV, Pocock RD, Summerhayes IC. Preferential and novel activation of H-*ras* in bladder cancer. *Oncogene Res* 1988; **3**: 77–86.

43. Viola MV, Fromowitz F, Oravez S, Deb S, Schlom J. *ras* oncogene p21 expression is increased in premalignant lesions and high grade bladder carcinoma. *J Exp Med* 1985; **161**: 1213–18.

44. Viola MV, Fromowitz F, Oravez S, *et al.* Expression of ras oncogene p21 in prostate cancer. *N Engl J Med* 1986; **314**: 133–7.

45. Stock LM, Brosman SA, Fahey JL, Liu BC-S. *ras* related oncogene protein as a tumor marker in transitional cell carcinoma of the bladder. *J Urol* 1987; **137**: 789–92.

46. Pohl J, Radler-Pohl A, Franks LM, Schirrmacher V. Analysis of metastatic competence of mouse bladder carcinoma cells after transfection with activated Ha-*ras* or N-*ras* oncogenes. *J Cancer Res Clin Onc* 1988; **114**: 373–9.

47. Brunner G, Pohl J, Erkell LJ, Radler-Pohl A, Schirrmacher V. Induction of urokinase activity and malignant phenotype in bladder carcinoma cells after transfection of the activated Ha-*ras* oncogene. *J Cancer Res Clin Onc* 1989; **115**: 139–44.

48. Senno L, Maestri I, Piva R, *et al.* Differential hypomethylation of the c-*myc* proto-oncogene in bladder cancers at different stages and grade. *J Urol* 1989; **142**: 146–9.

49. Yao M, Shuin T, Misaki H, Kubota Y. Enhanced expression of c-*myc* and epidermal growth factor receptor (c-*erb*-B1) genes in primary human renal cancer. *Cancer Res* 1988; **48**: 6753–7.

50. Kinouchi T, Saiki S, Naoe T, *et al.* Correlation of c-*myc* expression with nuclear polymorphism in renal cell carcinoma. *Cancer Res* 1989; **49**: 3627–30.

51. Johnsson A, Heldin C-H, Wasteson A, Westermark B, Deuel TF, Huang JS, Seeburg DH, Gray A, Ullrich A, Scrace G, Stroobant P, Waterfield MD. The c-*sis* gene encodes a precursor of the B chain of platelet-derived growth factor. *EMBO J* 1984; **3**: 921–8.

52. Neal DE. Growth factors in tumour biology. In: Waxman J, Coombes RC (eds), *The New Endocrinology of Cancer*. London: Edward Arnold, 1987: 19–37.

53. Kelly K, Cochran BH, Stiles CD, Leder P. Cell-specific regulation of the c-*myc* gene by lymphocyte mitogens and platelet-derived growth factor. *Cell* 1983; **35**: 603–10.

54. Cohen S. Isolation of a mouse submaxillary gland protein accelerating incisor eruption and eyelid opening in the newborn animal. *J Biol Chem* 1962; **237**: 1555–62.

55. Gregory H, Willshire IR, Kavanagh JP, *et al.* Urogastrone-epidermal growth factor concentration in prostatic fluid of normal individuals and patients with benign prostatic hypertrophy. *Clin Sci* 1986; **70**: 359–63.

56. Reim M, Kehrer T, Lund M. Clinical application of epidermal growth factor in patients with most severe eye burns. *Ophthalmologica* 1988; **197**: 179–84.

57. Walker-Smith JA, Phillips AD, Walford N, *et al.* Intravenous epidermal growth factor/urogastrone increases small intestinal cell proliferation in congenital microvillous atrophy. *Lancet* 1985; **ii**: 1239–40.

58. Quantin B, Breathnach R. Epidermal growth factor stimulates transcription of the c-jun proto-oncogene in rat fibroblasts. *Nature (Lond)* 1988; **334**: 538–9.

59. Carlin C, Tollefson AE, Brady HA, Hoffman BL, Wold WSM. Epidermal growth factor receptor is down regulated by a 10,400 MW protein encoded by the E3 region of adenovirus. *Cell* 1989; **57**: 135–44.

60. Gross JL, Krupp MN, Rifkin DB, Lane MD. Down regulation of epidermal growth factor receptor correlates with plasminogen activator activity in human A431 epidermoid carcinoma cells. *Proc Natl Acad Sci (USA)* 1983; **80**: 2276–80.

61. Harris, AL, Neal DE. Epidermal growth factor and its receptor in human cancer. In: Sluyser M (ed), *Growth Factors and Oncogenes in Breast Cancer*. Chichester: Ellis Horwood, 1987: 60–90.

62. Neal DE, Marsh C, Bennett MK, Abel PD, Hall RR, Sainsbury JRC, Harris AL. Epidermal growth factor receptors in human bladder cancer: comparison of invasive and superficial tumours. *Lancet* 1985; **i**: 366–8.

63. Messing EM, Hanson P, Ulrich P, Erturk E. Epidermal growth factor—interactions with normal and malignant urothelium: *in vivo* and *in situ* studies. *J Urol* 1987; **138**: 1329–35.

64. Yamamoto T, Kamata N, Kawano H, *et al.* High incidence of amplification of the epidermal growth factor receptor gene in human squamous carcinoma cell lines. *Cancer Res* 1986; **46**: 414–16.

65. Fitzpatrick SL, Brightwell J, Wittliff JL, Barrows GH, Schultz GS. Epidermal growth factor binding by breast tumor biopsies and relationship to estrogen receptor and progestin receptor levels. *Cancer Res* 1984; **44**: 3448–53.

66. Sainsbury JRC, Farndon JR, Sherbet GV, Harris AL. Epidermal growth factor receptors and oestrogen receptors in human breast cancer. *Lancet* 1985; **i**: 364–6.

67. Libermann TA, Razon N, Bartal AD, Yardin Y, Schlessinger J, Soreq H. Expression of epidermal growth factor receptors in human brain tumours. *Cancer Res* 1984; **44**: 753–60.

68. Dazzi H, Haseleton PS, Thatcher N, *et al.* Expression of epidermal growth factor receptor (EGFr) in non-small cell lung cancer: use of archival material and correlation of EGFr with histology, tumour size, nodal status and survival. *Br J Cancer* 1989; **59**: 746–9.

69. Gusterson B, Cowley G, McIlhinney J, Ozanne B, Fisher C, Reeves B. Evidence for increased epidermal growth factor receptors in human sarcomas. *Int J Cancer* 1985; **36**: 689–93.

70. Gullick WJ, Marsden JJ, Whittle N, Ward B, Bobrow L, Waterfield MD. Expression of epidermal growth factor receptors on human cervical, ovarian and vulval carcinomas. *Cancer Res* 1986; **46**: 285–92.

71. Berger MS, Greenfield C, Gullick WJ, Haley J, Downward J, Neal DE, Harris AL, Waterfield MD. Evaluation of epidermal growth factor receptors in bladder tumours. *Br J Cancer* 1987; **56**: 533–7.

72. Neal DE, Sharples L, Smith K, Fennelly J, Hall RR. The epidermal growth factor receptor and the prognosis of bladder cancer. *Cancer* 1990; **65**: 1619–25.

73. Davies P, Eaton C. Binding of epidermal growth factor by human normal, hypertrophic and carcinomatous prostate. *Prostate* 1989; **41**: 123–32.

74. Livermann TA, Nusbaum HR, Razon N, Kris R, Lax I, Soreq H, Whittle N, Waterfield MD, Ullrich A, Schlessinger J. Amplification, enhanced expression and possible rearrangement of EGF receptor gene in primary brain tumours of glial origin. *Nature* 1985; **313**: 144–7.

75. Merlino GT, Young-hua X, Richert N, *et al.* Elevated epidermal growth factor receptor gene copy number and expression in a squamous carcinoma cell line. *J Clin Invest* 1985; **75**: 1077–9.

76. Anderstrom C, Johansson S, Nilsson S. The significance of lamina propria invasion on the prognosis of patients with bladder cancer. *J Urol* 1980; **124**: 23–6.

77. Smith K, Fennelly JA, Neal DE, Hall RR, Harris AL. Characterization and quantitation of the epidermal growth factor receptor in invasive and superficial bladder cancer. *Cancer Res* 1989; **49**: 5810–15.

78. Barnes DM. Breast cancer and a proto-oncogene. *Br Med J* 1989; **299**: 1061.
79. Lin ML, Clinton GM. The epidermal growth factor receptor from prostatic cells is dephosphorylated by a prostate specific phospho tyrosyl phosphatase. *Mol Cell Biol* 1988; **8**: 5477–85.
80. Traish AM, Wotiz HH. Prostatic epidermal growth factor receptors and their regulation by androgens. *Endocrinol* 1987; **121**: 1461–7.
81. Gospodorowicz D, Ferrara N, Schweigere L, Neufeld G. Structural characterisation and biological functions of fibroblast growth factor. *Endocrine Rev* 1987; **8**: 95–114.
82. Jacobs SC, Story MT, Sasse J, Lawson RK. Characterisation of growth factors derived from the rat ventral prostate. *J Urol* 1988; **139**: 1106–10.
83. Mydlo JH, Michaeli J, Heston WDW, Fair WR. Expression of fibroblast growth factor mRNA in benign prostatic hyperplasia and prostate carcinoma. *Prostate* 1988; **13**: 241–7.
84. Story MT, Sasse J, Kakusa D, Jacobs SC, Lawson RK. A growth factor in bovine and human testis structurally related to basic fibroblast growth factor. *J Urol* 1988; **140**: 422–77.
85. Mydlo JH, Heston WDW, Fair WR. Characterization of a heparin binding growth factor from adenocarcinoma of the kidney. *J Urol* 1988; **140**: 1575–9.
86. Chodak GW, Hospellorn V, Judge SM, Mayforth R, Koeppen H, Sasse J. Increased levels of fibroblast growth factor-like activity in urine from patients with bladder or kidney cancer. *Cancer Res* 1988; **48**: 2083–8.
87. Reeve AE, Eccles MR, Wilkins RJ, Bell GI, Millow LJ. Expression of insulin-like growth factor-II transcripts in Wilms' tumour. *Nature (Lond)* 1985; **317**: 258–60.
88. Gregory H, Thomas CE, Willshire IR, *et al.* Epidermal and transforming growth factor alpha in patients with breast tumours. *Br J Cancer* 1989; **59**: 605–9.
89. Derynck R. Transforming growth factor alpha. *Cell* 1988; **54**: 593–5.
90. Arteaga CL, Hanauske AR, Clark GM, *et al.* Immunoreactive alpha transforming growth factor activity in effusions from cancer patients as a marker of tumor burden and prognosis. *Cancer Res* 1988; **48**: 5023–8.
91. Sargent ER, Gomella LG, Belldegrun A, Linehan WM, Kasid A. Epidermal growth factor gene expression in normal human kidney and renal cell carcinoma. *J Urol* 1989; **142**: 1364–8.

13 Prognostic indices for superficial bladder cancers

Paul D Abel

Bladder cancer is a heterogeneous disease and its clinical course is unpredictable. There have been many attempts to classify the disease by studying a whole variety of prognostic parameters. However, none gives information of specific value to an individual patient. The commonly used prognostic indices give useful information of a general nature, and this chapter will consider these in detail as well as some of the newer techniques for assessing tumour behaviour. It is only when the future clinical behaviour of an individual tumour can be predicted that the most appropriate treatment will be possible.

Depth of bladder wall infiltration by tumour

Geraghty[1] was the first individual to record an association between increasing depth of bladder wall infiltration by tumour and impaired prognosis with the development of metastases. However, depth of invasion was not used within a clinical staging system until 1946 by Jewett and Strong.[2] This system has since been adapted by the UICC[3] and is now the most commonly used guide to predicting prognosis in bladder cancer. There are clinical pre-treatment (T) and pathological post-resection (pT) categories. There are also nodal (N) and metastatic (M) categories. The criteria for each category were laid down both to fulfil the TNM requirements and to set a standard which should enable valid comparisons to be made between different centres and different treatments.[3,4]

These T and pT categories are limited in value because of errors in clinical and pathological assessment of depth of tumour infiltration. Skinner[5] compared the clinical assessment of depth of invasion (the T category) at bimanual examination prior to cystectomy with the pT category of the corresponding cystectomy specimen and found clinical staging errors of more than 50%. Similar discrepancies were reported from Baker[6] when he compared the pT category assigned after transurethral resection biopsies with those of the corresponding complete surgical cystectomy specimen. An additional problem is that the presence of full-thickness bladder wall is an essential requirement for the assignation of pT category. Chisholm *et al.*[7] found that this resulted in the categorization of many T3 tumours as pTx because full-thickness bladder wall was not always available in biopsy material from transurethral resection. They also reported that it was impossible to distinguish Ta from T1 tumours clinically. The biggest problem identified by all authors, however, appears to be reconciling pre- and post-treatment categories T2 to T3b.

Some of the difficulties in comparing results of treatments and prognoses between centres and populations may be due to differences in interpretation of tumour grade and pT category by pathologists. Ooms *et al.*[8] compared the consistency of grading of 57 bladder tumours assessed in one session by seven pathologists sitting apart. All the pathologists showed virtually the same degree of intra-individual inconsistency of about 50%. Some of these pathologists reviewed the slides in a second session seven months later and, in almost 50% of tumours, a different grade was assigned by the same individual. Pathologists may also disagree in allocating pT category. One report found that 15% of cases were assigned a different pT category from that of the original when all the tumours were reviewed by one pathologist sitting in continuous session.[9] These studies are important because they suggest that interpretation of pT category and grade is subjective and dependent on observer bias. Comparison of results of treatment and/or prognosis between different centres can therefore be difficult, especially when only small numbers of patients are involved, because of the uncertainty that like has been compared with like. It would appear essential that both clinical and pathological characteristics of each patient's tumour should be reviewed by all clinicians concerned with management so that a consensus on an appropriate classification (of grade and pT category) can be made for each individual. This should improve the accuracy of clinical staging and of pathology reporting, make treatment decisions more rational and make data on prognosis more reliable. Further, comparison of results between centres may become more useful. Ultimately, reliable distinction between characteristics of prognostic significance that may be of value to the individual patient might be distinguished from those that may have no significance.

Having said that, large series have confirmed depth of invasion to be a generally useful prognostic indicator. Skinner[5] reviewed more than 1500 cases: the five-year survival rate for patients with tumours of pTa/pT1 category was 67%, pT2 was 40%, pT3a was 36% and pT3b was 18%. Cifuentes Delatte *et al.*[10] studied over 1700 patients and reported 55% with pT/pT1 tumours, but only 15% with muscle infiltrating tumours, survived 10 years. Although prognosis was significantly worsened by any degree of muscle infiltration, some of the tumours that had penetrated no deeper than the lamina propria had already produced occult metastatic disease. However, whilst it may be thought for example that early diagnosis may influence prognosis in bladder cancer, Bishop[11] has concluded, from a survey of data on both haematuria screening clinics and the use of urine cytology in 'at-risk' groups, that early diagnosis has at best only marginal influence on survival times.

Routine clinical practice has generally involved the classification of depth of invasion into two broad categories for treatment purposes. These are *superficial* and *muscle infiltrating or deeper*. The superficial group are generally perceived to have a better prognosis than those which infiltrate muscle. Between 70% and 80% of patients with bladder cancer have superficial disease (pTa/pT1) on initial presentation and the remainder have tumours that infiltrate at least into muscle. [12,13] Animal models and observations of the histological spectrum of bladder cancer in man suggest a disease progressing through an orderly sequence of events from initially non-invasive tumours to, progressively, invasion of lamina propria, detrusor muscle, perivesical fat and finally metastases. [14] Clinical practice, however, reveals that bladder cancer may evolve through a wide variety of developmental pathways which put this thesis in doubt, [15] and it is frequently overlooked that over 80% of transitional cell cancers (TCC) that infiltrate muscle are invasive at the time of presentation and have no previous history of superficial disease. [16]

'Superficial' bladder cancer

Prior to 1978, 'superficial bladder cancer' included together all TCC that had not invaded muscle. These were designated pT1. Since 1978, superficial bladder tumours have been divided into pTa (extending up to but no deeper than basement membrane) and pT1 (extending into lamina propria but no deeper). [3] pTa tumours comprise approximately 60–70% of all superficial tumours (that is more than 50% of all bladder tumours) and it is imperative to note that they are rarely invasive. [13] It has been shown that between 50% and 70% of patients with superficial tumours will develop new superficial tumours, often within 12 months of diagnosis, and about 10–20% of these progress to muscle infiltration. [12,13,17,18] Present follow-up policies aim to identify new tumour development at a stage before progression occurs. This, however, assumes that all new tumours have the potential to progress, an assumption that is unproven. The clinical difficulty in superficial bladder cancer is to identify the patients who will develop new tumours which will invade and metastasize from those who may either develop no further tumours at all or new tumours without life-threatening potential.

The subdivision of superficial TCC into pTa and pT1 has been extremely useful, resulting in the identification of significant differences in behaviour between the two groups. Heney *et al.* [18] in a prospective study of 249 patients with a median follow-up of 39 months, found 4% of non-invasive (pTa) but 30% of pT1 tumours progressed (progression is defined here as the development of muscle invasion and metastases). Cutler *et al.* [13] reported that, of the pT1 patients who progressed to muscle infiltration, two-thirds did so within 12 months of initial diagnosis. Both these studies involved multi-centre collaboration so that it is possible that patients from individual centres were not entered consecutively. Pauwels *et al.* [19] studied prospectively a group of 91 patients followed for a mean of 24 months, and reported progression rates of 6% (pTa) and 30% (pT1). One prospective study of a consecutively presenting group of patients from a single centre showed 46% of pT1 but no pTa TCC progressing to muscle infiltration within three years of diagnosis; all of the patients who progressed died of bladder cancer.[20] In this latter series, pT category and grade were reassigned by a single pathologist sitting in continuous session. Lutzeyer *et al.*[21] assessed the risk of progression to be 20% (pTa) and 24% (pT1); but this study was retrospective and progression was not defined, so that patients with pTa tumours who developed pT1 tumours may have been included. Smith *et al.*[22] reported that initial pT category of superficial tumour bore no significant relationship to the subsequent recurrence rate but patients in this study had a short follow-up of only 1.6 years.

At last, attitudes to follow-up are changing as a result of these behavioural differences. For example, one group has based rationalization of its follow-up policy on the basis of a retrospective study of the behaviour of 170 patients with pTa TCC.[23] In a period of one to 15 years, only five patients progressed (to muscle infiltration), whereas 61% developed new non-invasive tumours. The highest rate of new tumour occurrence was in the first year after diagnosis and was especially prominent in patients with multiple tumours at presentation. It is progression that may prove fatal to the patient and it is important not to assume new tumour occurrence will invariably lead to muscle infiltration.

It seems clear from these studies that pT1 TCC have a significantly worse prognosis than pTa TCC. Studies that include these two subgroups together as one 'superficial' group can no longer be considered satisfactory. An additional possible complicating factor in interpreting results is that many patients within these studies received different treatments.

Basement membrane

Clear identification of the basement membrane (BM) is essential for accurate assessment of lamina propria invasion.[24] This may be difficult with conventional haematoxylin and eosin sections. The use of antibodies to BM components may help to define this structure and could increase the accuracy of assigning pTa/pT1 category. Barsky *et al.*[25] suggested that the ability of a tumour to produce its own BM may provide prognostic information. In invasive bladder cancer, a correlation between short-term behaviour (three years) and BM staining has recently been reported. All patients with invasive TCC who had widely fragmented BM or BM absent in more than 5% of the tumour area had a significantly poorer prognosis.[26]

Differentiation grade

Broders[27] was the first to establish the importance of tumour grade—'malignant tumours of the bladder vary in behaviour according to the proportion of undifferentiated cells they contain'. Marshall[28] showed that grade acted independently of stage to indicate potential curability; high-grade superficial tumours killed their patients twice as often as low-grade tumours (37% against 71%) within five years.

In Skinner's series,[5] over 50% of those with high-grade invasive tumours died of metastases. Cifuentes Delatte *et al.*[10] found that 55% of patients with low-grade but only 16% with high-grade tumours survived 10 years. In a group of 365 patients treated conservatively, 5% of patients with grade 1 and 16% with grade 2 tumours died of their disease at five years, in contrast to 60% with grade 3 disease.[29] Other reports are in agreement with these findings.[13,17]

Particular problems with grading occur in the definition of WHO grade 2 lesions. Recently, characteristics of two new subgroups of grade 2 tumour have been defined. The grade 2a tumour demonstrates normal polarity and has been shown to have markedly different recurrence and progression rates from grade 2b tumours (5% and 31% respectively for category Ta tumours after 12 months' follow-up).[19] Morphometry is a newer method of tumour grading and, following comparison with grading by pathologists, Ooms *et al.*[30] concluded that it was valuable because it was more objective.

The relationship between pT category and grade

There is an association between low-grade tumours and both low-stage disease and a good prognosis. In comparison, high-grade tumours also tend to be high-stage and are associated with a worse prognosis.[13,31,32] Friedell *et al.*[33,34] found only 6% of grade 1 lesions to be invasive and almost never to metastasize, whereas 52% of grade 2 and 82% of grade 3 tumours were invasive and more frequently metastatic than grade 1. Worsening of grade in recurrent tumours has prognostic significance, both when considered alone[35] and in combination with stage.[36] In general, multiple, large and high-grade tumours are more likely to be associated with recurrence.[34,37]

Dysplasia and carcinoma-in-situ

If superficial TCC have been completely resected, the term 'recurrences' for tumours found at subsequent check cystoscopies is inappropriate; these are new occurrences, developing from the malignant potential of the residual, apparently normal urothelium. Melicow[38] was the first to study macroscopically apparently normal urothelium in between areas of gross bladder cancers. In 10 total-cystectomy specimens, cellular abnormalities ranging from hyperplasia and dysplasia to carcinoma-in-situ (CIS) were identified. These changes were absent in five control bladders from patients without bladder disease. Melicow and Hollowell[39] subsequently showed that similar abnormalities could occur in any part of the urothelium and it was inferred that focal areas of cancerous change, unseen by the naked eye, could be present during removal of an obvious tumour. Later, these abnormal areas would form new tumours (new occurrences).

In 1960 Eisenberg *et al.*[40] documented similar changes but, more importantly, they showed (in a small group of patients with superficial tumours followed for five years) that these changes were of prognostic significance and hence clinically relevant. All patients with cellular atypia in normal-looking mucosa had a bad prognosis. In contrast, patients with no mucosal atypia had controllable disease.

Schade and Swinney[41,42] extended this research prospectively, taking multiple biopsies of normal-looking mucosa in bladder cancer patients. They found pre-cancerous abnormalities in over 80% of cases. When the long-term follow-up data were presented,[43] it was clear that the fate of patients was related to the presence or absence of associated mucosal abnormalities. CIS in particular gave a significantly worse prognosis. In categories T1/T2, half of the patients with coexistent CIS had bladder cancers uncontrollable by endoscopic means alone, in contrast to none of 41 patients without CIS. This was regardless of the characteristics of the primary tumour or its grade or category. Althausen *et al.*[44] reviewed the histology slides from a group of patients with grade 1 or 2 papillary bladder tumours treated endoscopically. Seven per cent of patients with normal, 36% with atypia but 83% with CIS in the intervening mucosa, developed invasive disease within four years. Interestingly, not one of the original pathology reports mentioned the presence of any atypia in mucosa close to the tumours. Recent workers have consistently confirmed these findings,[13,22,45] and clearly the presence and extent of microscopic mucosal dysplasia is an important consideration in assessing the ultimate clinical course of bladder cancer. No relationship between other mucosal abnormalities, such as cystitis cystica and squamous metaplasia, has been found to be associated with the prognosis of bladder cancer.[46]

This field would appear to be one of the most fruitful areas for future research on prognostic indices. After frank TCC have been completely removed, only the remaining urothelium can have the potential to develop new cancers. More sophisticated techniques than morphological appearance by light microscopy may offer increased sensitivity in the detection of abnormalities in what is apparently 'normal' urothelium—for example, early reports of DNA cytophotometry to study endoscopically normal urothelium revealed 45% of histologically 'normal' biopsies to have abnormal changes.[47]

Tumour multiplicity

This is associated with increased risk of recurrent disease. Lutzeyer *et al.*[21] reported progression rates in solitary pTa and pT1 tumours of 18% and 33%. For multiple tumours, the figures were 43% and 46% respectively. Cutler *et al.*[13] showed that patients with single tumours had a 67% chance of recurrence, in contrast to a 90% chance if their growths were initially multiple. The disease-free interval for patients with multiple tumours was also shorter. Dalesio *et al.*[48] found the number of tumours at diagnosis to be the single most important factor (among tumour size, grade, treatment and patient's age) to influence the new tumour rate. A poor prognosis was also associated with a tumour size greater than 3 cm and a recurrence rate of more than once a year. The presence of more than one TCC suggests that multifocal disease is present and may simply reflect part of the spectrum of dysplasia and CIS.

Tumour vessel invasion

McDonald and Thompson,[49] in a series of 274 patients, described the effect of vascular invasion in bladder tumours, either perineural lymphatics (64 cases), venules (23 cases) or both (15 cases). This was observed more frequently in association with increasing bladder wall infiltration by tumour. It also conferred prognostic significance: only 12% with vascular invasion survived five years, compared with 38% without invasion. Others have confirmed these results. Jewett and Eversole[50] reported lymphatic permeation in 40% of deeply infiltrating tumours, compared with only 2.5% of superficial tumours. Slack and Prout[51] found lymphatic vessel invasion in 74% of solid invasive tumours but in only 25% of papillary invasive tumours, and noted that the presence of lymph vessel invasion conferred a poorer prognosis. Heney *et al.*[52] reported a relationship between vessel invasion and the presence of lymph node metastases in 86 patients undergoing radical cystectomy for invasive cancer. Lymph node metastases were present in 24 cases, of which 18 also had small vessel invasion in the primary tumour. Bell *et al.*[53] used special elastic stains to improve identification of vessels in tissue sections. Invasion was seen in 42% of patients, of whom 29% survived for five years, compared with 51% survival if there was no vessel involvement. Further advances in the detection of vascular invasion, for example by using the lectin Ulex europeus 1 to identify endothelium,[54] may increase the sensitivity of identifying vascular invasion as a prognostic indicator.

Lymph node metastases

The presence of lymph node metastases correlates with a poor prognosis. Following radical cystectomy, 24 of 86 patients (28%) were found to have nodal metastases; of these, 4% with involved nodes, but 41% without, survived for five years.[52] Bloom *et al.*[55] reported corresponding figures of 16% and 53% respectively. Prout *et al.*[15] found the extent of local tumour to be directly related to the incidence of positive pelvic nodes, and that nodal involvement suggested the presence of occult metastases elsewhere.

Marker chromosomes

Marker chromosomes are defined as abnormal chromosomes appearing in the metaphase of the cell cycle which defy systematic arrangement because of abnormal morphology. They may be seen as giant forms, ring forms or abnormalities in centromere location and arm length. Falor and Ward[56,57] examined 53 bladder cancers. Diploid tumours of both pTa and pT1 categories without marker chromosomes had a 10% recurrence rate and 95% survival. In contrast, the presence of marker chromosomes was associated with an increase in aneuploidy; this group of patients all had recurrences, and five-year survival rates were 55%

(pTa) and 40% (pT1). In a follow-up series, including over 600 cases, only three tumours infiltrating muscle or deeper did not have a marker chromosome.[58] Sandberg[59] reported similar relationships between aneuploidy, marker chromosomes and malignant potential. It seems surprising that this technique has not received more attention.

ABO(H) blood group antigens (BGA)

BGA are terminal carbohydrate residues on the cell surfaces of erythrocytes and normal epithelium, including urothelium.[60] Reduction or loss of BGA in presenting tumours has been reported to be associated with a poor prognosis, whereas retention of BGA indicates a good prognosis. Although this relationship largely holds true for BGA positive tumours, significant numbers of BGA negative tumours, expected to do badly, in fact have a good prognosis, limiting the usefulness of the test in clinical practice. Recent work[61–63] has suggested that methods for detecting BGA on tissue sections of normal urothelium may be responsible for the conflicting results between different centres: BGA are probably carried predominantly on glycolipid backbones in the urothelium, resulting in their extraction by the lipid solvents necessarily required for the processing of formalin-fixed, paraffin-embedded material. A prospective study of BGA expression in TCC using cryostat material showed a poor correlation between the presence or absence of BGA and prognosis.[64] The test requires considerable refinement before it may be of use in routine clinical practice.

The 'T' antigen

This is also a cell-surface carbohydrate, present on the surface of normal erythrocytes and urothelium where it is 'masked' by sialic acid and usually detectable only after desialyation using the enzyme neuraminidase.[65] Coon *et al.*[66] related T antigen expression to subsequent bladder cancer prognosis. Tumour cells expressing T antigen only after neuraminidase treatment (like normal cells) had a good prognosis. Those expressing T antigen without neuraminidase had an intermediate prognosis (cells had not synthesized sialic acid). Those in which T antigen was not detected with or without neuraminidase had the worst prognosis (the cells had synthesized neither sialic acid nor T antigen). In a follow-up report, Summers *et al.*[67] showed that BGA negative tumours could be further sub-classified by T antigen expression, giving a better prediction of future behaviour than when BGA were used alone. Further studies on changes in carbohydrate structures during malignant transformation of urothelium are warranted.

Tumour markers

Tumour markers of high sensitivity and specificity would help considerably in the management of patients with bladder cancer, but none has yet been identified. Ackermann[68] reviewed the role of carcinoembryonic antigen and reported that elevated levels have been found in the blood of 41–85% of patients. These wide differences are probably related both to tumour heterogeneity and the poor standardization of techniques for its detection between centres. Some newer serum markers, such as tissue polypeptide antigen, are reported to be sensitive predictors of metastatic urinary cancers and to be useful in monitoring response to treatment, but are unlikely to be helpful in primary diagnosis.[69] CA 19.9 may have value in monitoring the natural history of bladder cancer in patients with raised levels at diagnosis.[70]

The biological and clinical potential of human chorionic gonadotrophin (HCG) in bladder cancers has been extensively reviewed by Iles and Chard.[71] They concluded that HCG expression, particularly beta-HCG, was a common phenomenon in bladder cancer and this may reflect the ability of some mucosal cells to secrete it. Clinically, beta-HCG has been associated with advanced disease and radioresistance and may indicate chemosensitivity in some tumours. Immunohistochemical or quantitative assays in serum and urine may be of value in the identification of aggressive forms of the disease and the monitoring of treatment.

Conclusions

It is clear from the above survey that no single characteristic of a bladder tumour reliably correlates with future behaviour. In fact, many tumours with similar features may behave clinically in a wide variety of ways. The paucity of specific relationships between structure and function in bladder cancer results in the tendency to direct treatment regimens toward the behaviour of the broad group of patients rather than toward that which may be most appropriate in any individual patient. Only after the identification of those cellular changes attributed to cancers which contribute to their biological behaviour (and the discarding of those which are irrelevant to the process of invasion and metastases) can treatment be directed towards the individual, and appropriate comparisons of prognosis and clinical treatment between centres be made possible.[72]

The most useful recent advance in the management of TCC has been recognition of the importance of any invasion by tumour through the basement membrane. The present grouping of superficial cancer into categories pTa and pT1 identifies two broadly different behavioural phenotypes. Patients now need to be subcharacterized in clinical practice, perhaps with the introduction of new terminology such as 'superficial non-invasive' for pTa and 'superficial invasive' for pT1. It can no longer be acceptable for reports of prognostic indices and/or treatment to include these two groups together.

Acknowledgement

The Editor of the *British Journal of Urology* has kindly allowed the use of previously published material in this report (*British Journal of Urology* 1988; **62**: 103–9).

References

1. Geraghty JT. Treatment of malignant disease of the prostate and bladder. *J Urol* 1922; **7**: 33–65.
2. Jewett HJ, Strong GH. Infiltrating carcinoma of the bladder: relation of depth of penetration of the bladder wall to incidence of local extension and metastases. *J Urol* 1946; **55**: 366–72.
3. UICC (Union Internationale Contre le Cancer) *TNM Classification of Malignant Tumours*, 3rd edn. Geneva: UICC, 1978.
4. Jacobi GH, Engelmann U, Hohenfellner R. Classification of bladder tumours. In: Zingg EJ, Wallace DM (eds), *Bladder Cancer*. Berlin: Springer, 1985: 117–40.
5. Skinner DG. Current perspectives in the management of high grade invasive bladder cancer. *Cancer* 1980; **45**: 1866–74.
6. Baker R. The accuracy of clinical *vs* surgical staging. *JAMA* 1968; **206**: 1770–3.
7. Chisholm GD, Hindmarsh JR, Howatson AG, *et al*. TNM (1978) in bladder cancer: use and abuse. *Br J Urol* 1980; **52**: 500–5.
8. Ooms ECM, Anderson WAD, Alons CL, *et al*. Analysis of the performance of pathologists in the grading of bladder tumours. *Hum Path* 1983; **14**: 140–3.
9. Abel PD, Henderson D, Bennett MK, *et al*. Differing interpretations of the pT category and grade of transitional cell cancer of the bladder by pathologists. *Br J Urol* 1988; **62**: 339–42.
10. Cifuentes Delatte L, Garcia de la Pena E, Vela Navarrete R. Survival rates of patients with bladder tumours: an experience of 1744 cases. *Br J Urol* 1982; **54**: 267–74.
11. Bishop MC. The dangers of a long urological waiting list. *Br J Urol* 1990; **65**: 433–40.
12. Gammelgaard PA, Sorensen BL. The Copenhagen bladder cancer project. In: Pavone-Macaluso M, Smith PH, Edsmyr F (eds), *Bladder Tumours and Other Topics in Urological Oncology*. London: Plenum Press, 1978: 113–15.
13. Cutler SJ, Heney NM, Friedell GH. Longitudinal study of patients with bladder cancer: factors associated with disease recurrence and progression. In: Bonney WW, Prout GR (eds), *Bladder Cancer*. Baltimore: Williams & Wilkins, 1982: 35–46.
14. Droller MJ. Transitional cell cancer: upper tracts and bladder. In: Walsh PC, Gittes RF, Perlmutter AD, Stamey TA (eds), *Campbell's Urology*. New York: WB Saunders, 1986: 1343–440.
15. Prout GR, Griffin PP, Shipley WU. Bladder carcinoma as a systemic disease. *Cancer* 1979; **43**: 2532–9.
16. Kaye KW, Lange PH. Mode of presentation of bladder cancer: reassessment of the problem. *J Urol* 1982; **128**: 31–3.
17. Heney NM, Nocks BN, Daly JJ, *et al*. Ta and T1 bladder cancer: location, recurrence and progression. *Br J Urol* 1982; **54**: 152–7.
18. Heney NM, Ahmed S, Flanaghan MJ, *et al*. Superficial bladder cancer: progression and recurrence. *J Urol* 1983; **130**: 1083–6.

19. Pauwels RPE, Schapers RFM, Smeets AWGB, *et al.* Grading in superficial bladder cancer. 1: Morphological criteria. *Br J Urol* 1988; **61**: 129–34.
20. Abel PD, Hall RR, Williams G. Should pT1 transitional cell cancers of the bladder still be classified as superficial? *Br J Urol* 1988; **62**: 235–9.
21. Lutzeyer W, Rubben W, Dahm H. Prognostic parameters in superficial bladder cancer: an analysis of 315 cases. *J Urol* 1982; **127**: 250–2.
22. Smith G, Elton RA, Beynon LL, *et al.* Prognostic significance of biopsy results of normal looking mucosa in cases of superficial bladder cancer. *Br J Urol* 1983; **55**: 665–9.
23. Morgan JDT, Bowsher W, Griffiths DFR, Matthews PN. Rationalisation of follow-up in patients with non-invasive bladder tumours: a preliminary report. *Br J Urol* 1991; **67**: 158–61.
24. Mostofi FK. *Histological Typing of Urinary Bladder Tumours.* International Histological Classification of Tumours no. 10. Geneva: World Health Organization, 1973.
25. Barsky SH, Siegal GP, Jannotta F, *et al.* Loss of basement membrane components by invasive tumours but not by their benign counterparts. *Lab Invest* 1983; **49**: 140–7.
26. Daher N, Abourachid H, Bove N, *et al.* Collagen IV staining pattern in bladder carcinoma: relationship to prognosis. *Br J Cancer* 1987; **55**: 665–71.
27. Broders AC. Epithelioma of the genito-urinary organs. *Ann Surg* 1922; **75**: 574–604.
28. Marshall VF. Current clinical problems regarding bladder tumours. *Cancer* 1956; **9**: 543–50.
29. Gilbert HA, Logan JL, Kagan AR, *et al.* The natural history of papillary transitional cell carcinoma of the bladder and its treatment in an unselected population on the basis of histological grading. *J Urol* 1978; **119**: 488–92.
30. Ooms ECM, Kurver PHJ, Veldhuizen RW, *et al.* Morphometric grading of bladder tumours in comparison with histologic grading by pathologists. *Hum Path* 1983; **14**: 144–50.
31. Narayana AS, Loening SA, Slyman DJ, *et al.* Bladder cancer: factors affecting survival. *J Urol* 1983; **130**: 56–60.
32. Kern WH. The grade and pathologic stage of bladder cancer. *Cancer* 1984; **53**: 1185–9.
33. Friedell GH, Bell JR, Burney SE, *et al.* Histopathology and classification of urinary bladder carcinoma. *Urol Clin N Am* 1976; **3**: 53–70.
34. Friedell GH, Nagy GK, Cohen SM. Pathology of human bladder cancer and related lesions. In: Bryan GT, Cohen SM (eds), *The Pathology of Bladder Cancer.* Florida: CRC Press, 1984: 11–42.
35. England HR, Paris AMI, Blandy JP. The correlation of T1 bladder tumour histology with prognosis and follow-up requirements. *Br J Urol* 1981; **53**: 593–7.
36. Barnes R, Hadley H, Dick A, *et al.* Changes in grade and stage of recurrent bladder tumours. *J Urol* 1977; **118**: 117–8.
37. Pocock RD, Ponder BAJ, O'Sullivan JP, *et al.* Prognostic factors in non-infiltrating carcinoma of the bladder: a preliminary report. *Br J Urol* 1982; **54**: 711–15.
38. Melicow MM. Histological study of vesical urothelium intervening between gross neoplasms in total cystectomy. *J Urol* 1952; **68**: 261–79.
39. Melicow MM, Hollowell JW. Intraurothelial cancer: carcinoma-in-situ, Bowen's disease of the urinary system: discussion of thirty cases. *J Urol* 1952; **68**: 763–72.
40. Eisenberg RB, Roth RB, Schweinberg MH. Bladder tumours and associated proliferative mucosal lesions. *J Urol* 1960; **84**: 544–9.

41. Schade ROK, Swinney J. Pre-cancerous changes in bladder epithelium. *Lancet* 1968; **II**: 943–6.
42. Schade ROK, Swinney J. The association of urothelial atypism with neoplasia: its importance in treatment and prognosis. *J Urol* 1973; **109**: 619–22.
43. Schade ROK, Swinney J. The association of urothelial abnormalities with neoplasia: a 10-year follow-up. *J Urol* 1983; **129**: 1125–6.
44. Althausen AF, Prout GR, Daly JJ. Non-invasive papillary carcinoma of the bladder associated with carcinoma-in-situ. *J Urol* 1976; **116**: 575–80.
45. Wolf H, Olsen PR, Hojgaard K. Urothelial dysplasia concomitant with bladder tumours: a determinant for future new occurrences in patients treated by full course radiotherapy. *Lancet* 1985; **I**: 1005–8.
46. Weiner DP, Koss LG, Sablay B, *et al*. The prevalence and significance of Brunn's nests, cystitis cystica and squamous metaplasia in normal bladders. *J Urol* 1979; **122**: 317–21.
47. O'Brien A, Dorman A, Butler M, *et al*. A DNA cytophotometric study of neoplastic field change in the human urinary bladder (abstract). *Br J Cancer* 1987; **56**: 229.
48. Dalesio O, Schulman CC, Sylvester R, *et al*. Prognostic factors in superficial bladder tumours. *J Urol* 1983; **129**: 730–3.
49. McDonald JR, Thompson GT. Carcinoma of the urinary bladder: a pathologic study with special reference to invasiveness and vascular invasion. *J Urol* 1948; **61**: 435–45.
50. Jewett HJ, Eversole SL. Carcinoma of the bladder: characteristic modes of local invasion. *J Urol* 1960; **83**: 383–9.
51. Slack NH, Prout GR. The heterogeneity of invasive bladder carcinoma and different responses to treatment. *J Urol* 1980; **123**: 644–52.
52. Heney NM, Proppe K, Prout GR, *et al*. Invasive bladder cancer: tumour configuration, lymphatic invasion and survival. *J Urol* 1983; **130**: 895–7.
53. Bell JT, Burney SW, Friedell GH. Blood vessel invasion in human bladder cancer. *J Urol* 1971; **105**: 675–8.
54. Fujime M, Lin CW, Prout GR. Identification of vessels by lectin-immunoperoxidase staining of endothelium: possible applications in urogenital malignancies. *J Urol* 1984; **131**: 566–70.
55. Bloom HTG, Hendry WF, Wallace DM, *et al*. Treatment of T3 bladder cancer: controlled trial of pre-operative radiotherapy and radical cystectomy versus radical radiotherapy. *Br J Urol* 1982; **54**: 136–51.
56. Falor WH, Ward RM. Cytogenic analysis: a potential index for recurrence of early carcinoma of the bladder. *J Urol* 1976; **115**: 49–52.
57. Falor WH, Ward RM. Prognosis in early carcinoma of the bladder based on chromosomal analysis. *J Urol* 1978; **119**: 44–8.
58. Summers JL, Falor WH, Ward R. A 10-year analysis of chromosomes in non-invasive papillary carcinoma of the bladder. *J Urol* 1981; **125**: 177–8.
59. Sandberg AA. Chromosome markers and progression in bladder cancer. *Cancer Res* 1977; **37**: 2950–6.
60. Watkins WM. Biochemistry and genetics of the ABO, Lewis and P blood-group systems. In: Harris H, Hirschorn K (ed.), *Advances in Human Genetics*. New York: Plenum Press, 1980: 1–136.
61. Limas C, Lange P. Altered reactivity for ABH antigens in transitional cell carcinomas of the urinary bladder: a study of the mechanisms involved. *Cancer* 1980; **46**: 1366–73.

62.   Limas C, Lange P. ABH antigen detectability in normal and neoplastic urothelium: influence of methodologic factors. *Cancer* 1982; **49**: 2476–84.
63.   Thorpe SJ, Abel PD, Slavin G, *et al.* Blood group antigens in the normal and neoplastic bladder epithelium. *J Clin Pathol* 1983; **36**: 873–82.
64.   Abel PD, Thorpe SJ, Williams G. Blood-group antigen expression in frozen sections of presenting bladder cancer: 3-year prospective follow-up of prognostic value. *Br J Urol* 1989; **63**: 171–5.
65.   Springer GF, Desai PR, Murthy MS, *et al.* Precursors of the blood-group MN antigens as human carcinoma associated antigens. *Transfusion* 1979; **19**: 233–49.
66.   Coon JS, Weinstein RS, Summers JL. Blood-group precursor T-antigen expression in human bladder carcinoma. *Am J Clin Pathol* 1982; **77**: 692–9.
67.   Summers JL, Coon JS, Ward RM, *et al.* Prognosis in carcinoma of the urinary bladder based upon tissue blood-group ABH and Thomsen–Freidenreich antigen status and karyotype of the initial tumour. *Cancer Res* 1983; **43**: 934–9.
68.   Ackerman R. Immunological aspects of bladder cancer. In: Zingg EJ, Wallace DMA (eds), *Bladder Cancer*. Berlin: Springer, 1985: 52–76.
69.   Khanna OP, Wu B. Tissue polypeptide antigen as a predictor for genitourinary cancers and their metastases. *Urology* 1987; **30**: 106–10.
70.   Abel PD, Cornell C, Buamah PK, *et al.* Assessment of serum CA 19.9 as a tumour marker in patients with carcinoma of the bladder and prostate. *Br J Urol* 1987; **59**: 427–9.
71.   Iles RK, Chard T. Human chorionic gonadotrophin expression by bladder cancers: biology and clinical potential. *J Urol* 1991; **145**: 453–8.
72.   Pauli BU, Alroy J, Weinstein RS. The ultrastructure and pathobiology of urinary bladder cancer. In: Bryan GT, Cohen SM (eds), *The Pathology of Bladder Cancer*, vol. 2. Florida: CRC Press, 1984: 41–140.

14 Radical surgery in locally advanced bladder cancer

EJ Zingg and UE Studer

The treatment of patients with advanced bladder cancer remains controversial. Single-modality treatments such as cystectomy or radiotherapy, and multimodal therapies such as cystectomy with radiotherapy or chemotherapy, lead to cure in a proportion of patients. A comparison of the results of these different treatments is difficult because of the lack of prospective, randomized studies, differing preoperative staging criteria, and variable patient selection. The identification of patients suitable for surgery has been facilitated by the development and extensive use of diagnostic imaging tools. Bone scanning and axial computed tomography identify patients with overt dissemination.

Bladder wall infiltration, regional and distant dissemination

Eighty-two per cent of bladder tumours are confined to the bladder when initially diagnosed, 9% show regional spread, and 6% have distant metastases.[1] When first assessed, 20–36% of all bladder tumours are already at an advanced stage T2–T4.[2] However, 80–95% of patients presenting with invasive carcinoma do not have a previous history of treated superficial bladder tumours but are diagnosed *de novo* (Table 14.1).[3]

Prout and Kopp[2] distinguish two separate tumour groups: *superficial* which progress to invasive carcinomas; and *de novo* carcinomas which are invasive from the very beginning and which are likely to be accompanied by regional and/or distant metastases. The relative proportions of these two tumour groups is thought to depend on the socioeconomic situations of the patients, the availability of adequate medical care, and patient and physician awareness.[8]

Clinically, there are significant differences between two major forms of transitional epithelium carcinomas of the bladder: *superficial* tumours (Ta, T1) and *deeply invasive* tumours (T2). Additionally, a clear distinction between the non-invasive Ta

Table 14.1   Advanced bladder carcinoma at diagnosis: percentage of cases with invasion presenting *de novo*

Authors	Number of patients	Invasion at the time of first presentation
Brawn (1982)[4]	104	84 (80.8%)
Kaye and Lange (1982)[5]	166	139 (84%)
Hopkins *et al.* (1983)[6]	90	82 (91%)
Berne series (1990)[7]	97	93 (96%) (for stage T3b)

and the microinvasive T1 tumours also seems very important. Superficial tumours (Ta) confined to the mucosa and of a low or moderate grade of differentiation lead to progression in only 3–4% of patients.[9] In this group, with adequate treatment the five-year survival is 80–90%.

There are further major distinctions within the T1 subgroup, where the high-grade (G3) T1 tumours have a high probability of tumour extension into lymphatic spaces and vessel systems.[2,9,10–14]

Between 40% and 50% of the patients with T1/G3 tumours subsequently develop muscle invasion.[2,9,11,12] In these patients with progressive disease the three- and five-year survival rates fall to 50% and 20% respectively.[9,13,14] The simultaneous occurrence of carcinoma-in-situ has an adverse effect on prognosis.[9,15] In T1 tumours there is concomitant carcinoma-in-situ in the prostatic glands and the urethra in 20% of cases,[16–18] and the involvement of the distal ureters by carcinoma-in-situ in 8% to 50% of patients.[19,20]

Overt invasion of the detrusor muscle is an ominous prognostic factor: the patient has, at best, little more than a 50–60% chance of survival. Prognosis is compromised by the possibility of concomitant nodal or distant metastases. If such are present there is limited hope for curative therapy.

The relationships between the depth of tumour infiltration, lymph node involvement and distant metastases have been known since the investigations of Jewett and Strong in 1946.[21] The more invasive the tumour, the poorer the prognosis because the probability of regional lymph node and systemic disease increases. These relationships between the T, N and M stages have been described in many series of patients treated by total cystectomy and pelvic lymph node dissection (Table 14.2). It should be noted that patients who underwent cystectomy and pelvic lymphadenectomy consisted of a preselected group which excluded patients with

Table 14.2   Pelvic node metastatic disease

Tumour stage	Skinner (1982)[22]	Whitmore (1983)[23]
P1	6%	5%
P2	30%	<10%
P3a	31%	
P3b	65%	20%
P4		40%

overt distant metastases. Therefore, these figures do not necessarily provide accurate information about the overall percentage of regional and disseminated metastases in patients with advanced tumours at the time of initial diagnosis.[24]

Lymph node metastases are present in 20–35% of those patients with muscle invasion.[22,25,26] When extension into the perivesical tissue is present, the incidence of lymph node invasion may reach 60%. Between 50% and 65% of the patients with penetration of the tumour into the perivesical fat or who have metastases in the regional pelvic lymph nodes develop disseminated disease within 30 months.[27] It is very unlikely that surgery is curative in cases with lymph node dissemination.

Zincke *et al.*[28] found that only three out of 57 patients with stage pT1–4 N+ tumours were alive after 30, 53 and 73 months respectively. Patients with only one positive lymph node had a slightly longer survival time than those with more than three affected lymph nodes. Camey[25] found regional lymph node metastases in 26% of 215 patients treated by cystectomy and lymphadenectomy. Patients in stage pN1 had significantly better survival rates than those presenting with stages pN2–pN4. In 1987, Skinner[29] reported a 38% five-year survival rate in 79 patients with histologically proven lymph node metastases. In this study, disease bulk in lymph nodes correlated with a better prognosis, and the five-year survival rate was 48% in patients with fewer than three positive nodes where tumour involved less than 10% of the nodes. Unfortunately, no detailed indication was given of the location of the diseased nodes in patients with a good outcome. It is obviously important to know whether the nodes with microscopic disease were in the perivesical fat or along the major pelvic vessels. Whitmore[23] concluded that in patients with pT3 tumours lymphadenectomy in addition to radical cystectomy led to an additional cure rate of only about 2%.

An overview of the literature has shown that the absolute number of survivors after lymphadenectomy in patients with positive lymph nodes is small and that in these patients the number and location of the involved lymph nodes has often been unreported (Table 14.3).[30]

On the basis of experiences reported in the literature, it can be concluded that

Table 14.3 Pelvic node metastases in bladder cancer: survival after pelvic lymphadenectomy

Authors	*Number of patients*	*Macro-/micro-metastases*	*Five-year survival*
Leadbetter and Cooper (1950)[31]	4	Macro	0
Laplante and Brice (1973)[32]	39	Micro?	5/39 (13%)
Dretler *et al.* (1973)[33]	12	Micro	4/12 (33%)
Reid *et al.* (1976)[34]	24	?	5/24 (25%)
Clark (1978)[35]	12	Micro	3/12 (25%)
Smith and Whitmore (1981)[36]	134	? (N1–N4)	9/134 (7%)
	30	N1	5/30 (17%)
Bloom *et al.* (1982)[26]	15	?	2/15 (15%)
Skinner (1982)[22]	36	Micro?	12/36 (35%)
Skinner (1987)[29]	79	Micro+macro	38%

surgery can be curative in patients with a solitary micrometastasis. Nevertheless, there is still a possibility in such patients that general dissemination has occurred. This is underlined by the fact that, in patients with regional lymph node involvement after radical surgery, it is not so much the local recurrence as the distant metastases which influence the outcome.[22,28,36] It is debatable whether patients with pN1 disease require systemic chemotherapy.[36-39] However, since at least 50% of those who die show evidence of disseminated disease, it is generally agreed that in patients with regional tumour spread (pN2–pN4) surgery alone is suboptimal treatment as the carcinoma has extensively disseminated. Surgery in such cases is not curative but, at the very best, a means of local control of tumour. In 1989, Gervasi *et al.*[40] demonstrated an analogous situation in prostatic carcinoma: the incidence of distant metastases after 10 years was 31% in patients with negative regional lymph nodes but 83% in patients with positive lymph nodes.

The proportion of poorly differentiated tumours increases as the depth of invasion increases.[41] Similarly, the more undifferentiated the tumour, the greater the probability of deeply invasive growth. In both these cases regional and distant metastases are all the more likely. In both groups of patients, prognosis depends not so much on the extent of the invasion but on the potential biological behaviour of the tumour. Given adequate surgical treatment there are no differences between the results obtained with undifferentiated superficially muscle invading tumours and those with deep muscular infiltration, provided no regional or distant lymph node metastases are invaded and no metastatic tumour is found at surgery.[24,27]

Diagnostic procedures

The aim of diagnostic procedures in advanced bladder carcinoma is to obtain indications of the extent of the tumour and its potential biological behaviour. On the basis of such findings, therapeutic measures can be initiated and the prognosis defined. A single diagnostic examination is not enough, but when all modern diagnostic investigations are taken together we usually obtain an idea of the biological potential of the tumour and the chances of cure for each individual patient. A determination of the biological malignant potential of each tumour is therefore of the greatest importance for future research, and requires investigation in order to further define prognosis in our patients.

Bimanual examination under anaesthesia alone is inadequate as the tumour is understaged in 40–50% of cases.[42,43] Computed tomography by itself is insufficient for an assessment of any local invasion,[7,44] with up to 90% inaccuracy.

The extent of invasion often cannot be assessed because of previous irradiation and/or transurethral resection. Also, peritumoural inflammation and reactive changes cannot be distinguished from tumour. Chronic infection by itself or combined with reduced bladder capacity may simulate tumour invasion of the bladder wall. The diagnosis of regional lymph node metastases is associated with errors of a similar order of magnitude. Computed tomography can only demonstrate enlarged lymph nodes but cannot evaluate their structure. Reactive enlarged lymph nodes are wrongly interpreted as grossly affected by the tumour.[44–46] Ureteric obstruction shown by intravenous urography or ultrasound indicates a poor prognosis.[47]

Cystoscopy is often underrated as an investigative procedure and is performed only for biopsy purposes. However, a reduced bladder capacity, an asymmetric bladder wall structure, mucosal changes indicating *in situ* carcinoma, and changes in the prostatic urethra provide important information and indicate a multifocal and probably invasive tumour.

At cystoscopy, random mucosal biopsies of the bladder are always indicated for the detection of concomitant carcinoma in-situ or epithelial atypias. In transitional epithelial carcinoma of the bladder these changes may be found in the prostatic urethra in 10–42% of cases.[48] If a carcinoma-in-situ of the bladder is present, prostatic involvement may be as high as 46–68%.[48–51] Carcinoma-in-situ of the prostatic urethra or of the excretory ducts of the prostate without invasion of the basal membrane or without prostatic stromal invasion does not adversely affect the prognosis after cystoprostatectomy. The incidence of prostatic involvement seems to be increasing. This may be due to the more meticulous examination of the prostate or to a real increased prevalence of carcinoma-in-situ in bladder and prostate.[52]

Invasion of the prostatic stroma by urothelial carcinoma is an ominous prognostic sign,[18,50,53,54] such that cystoprostatectomy is indicated.

Indications for curative surgery

There are three approaches to the primary surgical management of invasive bladder cancer: transurethral resection, segmental or partial cystectomy, and radical cystectomy.

Transurethral resection

The indication for transurethral resection for invasive tumour is controversial and rare. The tumour should be solitary and should not exceed a diameter of 2 cm. Random mucosal biopsies from other quadrants should be normal. The resection must extend into the perivesical fatty tissue. The procedure is not appropriate for tumours in the posterior part of the bladder and a second transurethral resection is mandatory. Adjuvant chemotherapy after complete resection has been advocated.[55,56]

Segmental or partial cystectomy

A segmental cystectomy (partial cystectomy, segmental resection) would seem to be a logical form of treatment for a localized invasive bladder carcinoma. The patients for such a procedure will always be highly selected. There are two well-established indications: a tumour arising in a diverticulum; and an adenocarcinoma of urachal origin arising in the vault of the bladder. In other situations in which a segmental cystectomy is considered, the following criteria must be met: the tumour must be solitary; selected mucosal biopsies in bladder and prostate must exclude carcinoma-in-situ or dysplasia elsewhere; the carcinoma should be situated in the mobile posterior part or the vault of the bladder; and an adequate clearance of 3 cm from the bladder neck has to be assured. When a ureteric orifice is involved, reimplantation of the ureter is necessary. The indications for this procedure are extremely rare. A segmental resection can only be used in a bladder with adequate capacity and previous radical radiotherapy excludes segmental cystectomy. To prevent possible tumour cell implantation during the surgical procedure, a short course (5–20 Gy) of preoperative radiation has been suggested by some authors.[57]

From the published data it can be seen that the five-year survival rate following partial cystectomy for superficially invasive tumours is between 47% and 75%, the operative mortality is 1–7% and the risk of tumour implantation is 1–3%.[58–62] However, very little can be concluded from these reports as the numbers were small, the cases were highly selected, and the criteria for selection not clearly defined.

Radical cystectomy

There are two new concepts which require consideration in the context of any discussion of radical cystectomy. The first is the use of first-line chemotherapy with a complete response rate of up to 30%,[37] as this has the potential for bladder preservation in some patients. Radical cystectomy would mean, therefore, over-treatment and could be avoided. Nevertheless, complete responses are mostly seen in small tumours which had been at least partially resected by a previous TUR. Moreover, despite a complete response with negative cystoscopy, negative cytology and negative biopsy, residual cancer tissue may be found following careful histological examination of the cystectomy specimens.

Secondly, the use of continent urinary reservoirs or bladder replacement procedures after radical cystectomy improves the quality of life when compared with cutaneous diversions and reduces the impact of radical surgery on the patients.

The indications for primary radical surgical management of invasive tumours depend on the tumour and each patient's general condition, the individual urological surgeon's opinion and the technical facilities in his hospital. The surgeon must decide what is the best treatment in his hands, in his hospital and for each patient.

As a general rule the indications for radical cystectomy are:

- large, deeply invasive, undifferentiated tumours (T2–T4a)
- multifocal, undifferentiated cancer of stage T1
- multifocal, rapidly recurring Ta/T1 tumours, refractory to transurethral resection and postoperative intravesical therapy (BCG, mitamycin, etc.)

The major contraindication is known juxtaregional nodal metastases.

Surgical techniques of radical cystectomy

The optimal surgery for invasive carcinoma comprises radical cystectomy and bilateral pelvic lymphadenectomy.

Pelvic lymphadenectomy consists of the bilateral removal of the perivascular adipose tissue and of the lymph nodes along the most distal part of the common iliac vessels, around the external iliac vessels, the obturator nerve and along the hypogastric vessels and the pelvic wall. The proximal extent of the lymph node dissection is at the crossing with the ureter. The genitofemoral nerve represents the lateral limit of the dissection. The circumflex iliac vein and Cooper's ligament, respectively, are the distal limits of the dissection, including the resection of the lymph node of Rosenmüller. We prefer to ligate the distal lymphatic connections in order to avoid lymphatic fistulas or the development of a lymphocoele. The lymphatic tissue can be swept by blunt dissection out of the obturator fossa. The obturator nerve is protected; the hypogastric vein should be carefully protected.[63–65]

Whishnow *et al.*[66] recommended less extensive lymphadenectomy because 90% of the metastases are found within the bifurcation of the iliac arteries. Nevertheless, because some patients can be cured when all the lymph nodes containing micrometastases are completely removed, and because, for obvious reasons, these cannot be detected and localized at surgery, a meticulous lymph node dissection seems justified. Moreover, according to Skinner[29] and Zincke *et al.*[28] the extended dissection makes the operation easier and safer and does not increase the morbidity of the cystectomy.

A frozen section of the lymph nodes is necessary only when there are palpable, enlarged glands and if the histological result would influence the therapeutic decision. In cases of multiple lymph node metastases (N2–N4), lymph node dissection has no benefit. The further action to be taken is therefore determined by the local tumour situation and the general clinical condition of the patient.

If radical cystectomy is possible and the patient suffers from bleeding, frequency, urgency and urinary incontinence, cystectomy and urinary diversion may be necessary for local control of the tumour and the symptoms. Postoperatively, adjuvant chemotherapy can be considered. If the patient has only a few symptoms from his bladder tumour and lymph node metastases are present, bladder preservation may well be justified and systemic treatment can be started postoperatively. If the extent of the local tumour is too advanced and makes a palliative cystectomy impossible, at least two therapeutic alternatives are possible: supravesical diversion followed by radiotherapy or chemotherapy (in patients with marked subjective symptoms); or abandoning the operation and subsequent chemotherapy. With our present-day preoperative imaging using axial computer tomography and magnetic resonance imaging, it is rare to find an inoperable situation only at surgery. According to Skinner the incidence of inoperable cases in patients who are explored with curative intent is only 3.7%.

After having performed the lymphadenectomy and mobilized the bladder along the pelvic wall, thus assuring that the bladder can be removed, the ureters are transected 2–3 cm cranial to their ureterovesical junctions. A biopsy is sent for fresh-frozen section and histological analysis. In the juxtavesical section of the ureter malignant changes in the form of a carcinoma-in-situ or dysplasia are found in 16–18% of cases.[19,67] In the lower third of the pelvic ureter, at the site of the subsequent ureteroenteric anastomosis, the frequency of malignant changes is only 9%.[67] Ureteric involvement is more frequent in patients with multifocal, extensive tumour disease of the bladder or when transitional cell carcinoma is present in the prostatic gland ducts.[66] Johnson *et al.*,[68] however, considered that the fresh-frozen investigation of the distal ureter was not necessary, since in their series unsuspected malignant disease was present in only 2% and dysplasia in only 19 out of 403 patients. In none of the patients did a recurrence of the carcinoma develop later at the ureteroenteric anastomosis. This relatively low incidence of ureteric involvement may also reflect the problem of patient selection for cystectomy. At least in patients with multifocal bladder carcinoma and/or concomitant carcinoma-in-situ, we recommend resection of the ureters at a safe distance from the bladder, if possible at their crossing with the iliac arteries, together with frozen sections of the ureteric resection sites.

Exposure and subsequent ligature of the superior and inferior vesical arteries (forming the dorsolateral vesical pedicle) is the next step. The posterior gluteal artery is spared. In men, the retrovesical peritoneum is incised at its lowest point in the prerectal area, thus giving access to the prerectal space. Denonvillier's fascia is separated by blunt dissection from the anterior rectal wall and is removed together with the seminal vesicles and the prostate. In the few cases in which the location of the bladder cancer makes it possible to resect, on one or both sides, the medial pararectal vesical and prostatic pedicles in direct contact with the organ, an attempt at nerve-sparing cystectomy can be made.[69] A careful radical prostatectomy together with the cystectomy seems to be important. In 26–38% of prostates removed during radical cystectomy for bladder carcinoma, foci of prostatic cancer are found, mostly localized in the apical segment.[70,71]

The management of the male urethra in radical cystectomy remains a dilemma.[72] According to the literature the risk of a recurrent tumour in the urethra after cystectomy is between 6% and 12%.[17,50,73–79]

Stöckle *et al.*[79] recommended single-stage urethrectomy for all patients with multifocal carcinomas of the bladder. According to Skinner[72] and Zingg and coworkers,[80] the indications for simultaneous urethrectomy are the presence of tumour tissue in the distal prostatic or membranous urethra, stromal involvement of the prostate by the transitional bladder carcinoma, or in preoperatively diagnosed urethral tumours. A routine prophylatic, synchronous urethrectomy increases operative time, blood loss and postoperative mortality and prevents the construction of an intestinal low-pressure bladder substitute. A partial urethrectomy is inadequate, since a recurrent tumour may still occur later in the remaining distal part of the urethra.[77,81,82]

Urinary diversion and bladder reconstruction

Ablative surgery obviously requires some form of urinary diversion or the reconstruction of an orthotopic bladder reservoir.

The urological surgeon who intends to carry out a radical cystectomy should be skilled in the techniques of the different methods of urinary diversion and bladder reconstruction. The type of urinary drainage appropriate to the individual patient should be selected on the basis of the extent of the tumour in the bladder, lymph node status, involvement of the prostatic urethra, morphological and functional situation of the upper urinary tract, performance status, operability, sex, mental status and general state of the patient.

Whenever it is possible we use a form of internal urinary diversion: in selected female patients the ureterosigmoidostomy, and in men the ileal low-pressure bladder substitute (which was developed by Studer[83] in our hospital)thus enabling the patient to void per vias naturales. If these forms of urinary diversion are not possible, we prefer the ileal conduit as the method of choice. In exceptional situations permanent nephrostomy or cutaneous ureterostomies are performed.

In a five-year period from 1985 to 1989, 129 radical cystectomies were carried out at our hospital: 56 bladder replacements, 8 ureterosigmoidostomies, 54 ileal conduits and 3 continent pouches. In the remaining patients cutaneous ureterostomies or permanent nephrostomies were used.

Provided the patients are carefully selected for each form of urinary diversion mentioned, it is our experience that the type of urinary drainage employed does not have any effect on the patients' survival rate in the first five-year period after cystectomy. However, when looking at the outcome of 269 patients who underwent a radical cystectomy at our institution between 1971 and 1988, a significant deterioration of the survival rates at 5–10 years after surgery was noted for patients who had a ureterosigmoidostomy. Five of the patients who were lost to follow-up died from uraemia or metabolic acidosis. This reflects the importance of the continuous follow-up of every patient with any form of urinary diversion and is certainly also true for those with an intestinal bladder substitute.

Operative mortality

There has been a continuous fall in operative mortality over the past few years, from 14.0% to less than 1% today.[7,27,84–89]

Among the 83 patients operated on at the Department of Urology, Berne, between 1971 and 1976 the perioperative mortality was 2.4%, but in 79 cases between 1977 and 1982 it fell to 1.2%. In 155 patients who underwent a radical cystectomy between 1983 and 1989 it was 0.8%.

Postoperative complications

The major non-specific early complications are cardiovascular, pulmonary and septic disorders.[7,64,84,85,87,90,91]

The major specific complications are urinary or intestinal fistulas. In 1982, Thomas and Riddle[92] reported an incidence of 10% ureteroenteric leakages, 7% enteroenteric leakages and 3% complex fistulas. Clark[35] reported in 1978 a 20% incidence of ureteroileal leakages caused at least in part by full-dose preoperative radiation therapy. Today intestinal and urinary fistulas probably occur in less than 1% of cases.[93]

Operative mortality and postoperative complications have been markedly reduced in the last 10 years. Better patient selection, adequate preoperative preparation, non-traumatic operative technique, sophisticated suture material, meticulous technique for restoring bowel continuity and the ureteroenteric anastomoses, intensive postoperative care (high caloric nutrition, physiotherapy, peridural anaesthesia), and optimal postoperative urinary drainage are basic principles for early good results after radical cystectomy.

Survey of results

Five-year survival following radical surgery is summarized in Table 14.4 and local recurrence rates in Table 14.5. Overall, the five-year actuarial survival rate after radical cystectomy and lymphadenectomy in localized tumours invading muscle is between 40% and 60%. Between 60% and 80% die within the first five postoperative years, and the majority die of their tumour, virtually all because of distant metastases. In this context systemic recurrences occur within the first two years.[27,101] It is interesting to note that there are no appreciable differences in the actuarial survival curves with regard to depth of muscular invasion when only those patients without lymph node involvement and no evidence of distant metastases are compared. The analysis of the survival data shows that the prognosis of bladder cancer worsens with increasing depth of tumour invasion. This might be explained by the fact that the more advanced the invasive growth of the cancer, the higher the probabilities of metastatic spread to the lymph nodes and of distant metastases.

Reviewing the literature, it can be observed that the initially poor results of cystectomy alone were substantially improved between 1960 and 1970 when preoperative radiotherapy was also used. Today equivalent results of combination radiotherapy/surgery can be obtained with radical surgical alone.[24,27,39,99,102–104] This obviously misleading comparison with historical controls was probably caused by several circumstances. Firstly, improved preoperative staging techniques (bone scan, axial computer tomography, etc.) excluded poor-risk patients with metastatic diseases which were previously not detectable. Secondly, improved pre- and postoperative care has reduced operative mortality and early morbidity.

This retrospective comparison has been substantiated by the results of a randomized trial by the Southwest Oncology Group. Patients who had their pelvis

Table 14.4   Five-year survival after radical cystectomy with and without preoperative radiotherapy (T and pT categories are not always distinguished)

Authors	Preoperative radiotherapy (Gy)	Five-year survival (%)		
		pT2	*pT3*	*pT4*
van der Werf-Messing (1975)[57]	40	–	50	–
Prout (1976)[94]	45	65	38	6
Wallace and Bloom (1980)[95]	40	–	33	–
Miller (1977)[96]	50	–	53	–
Smith and Whitmore (1982)[36]	40	44	38	22
	20 (true pelvis)	50	58	25
	20 (whole pelvis)	67	43	33
Prout (1976)[94]	–	47	31	20
Pearse *et al.* (1978)[97]	–	64	33	18
Bredael *et al.* (1980)[98]	–	53	30	25
Mathur *et al.* (1981)[91]	–	86	50	40
Skinner (1984)[27]	–	64	69	36
Jacobi *et al.* (1983)[99]	–	57	46	32
Studer *et al.* (1983)[24]	–	44	47	45

Source: Jacobi *et al.*[99]

Table 14.5   Local recurrence rate after cystectomy

Authors	Preoperative radiotherapy	Local recurrence
Chan and Johnson (1978)[100]	5000 cGy	8%
Skinner (1984)[27]	1600 cGy	9%
Skinner (1984)[88]	None	7%
Jacobi *et al.* (1983)[99]	None	6.4%
Montie *et al.* (1984)[39]	None	9%

irradiated with 40 Gy before radical cystectomy did no better than those with radical cystectomy alone.[105] Today, however, the same effect is apparently achieved by radical cystectomy in combination with a bilateral radical pelvic lymphadenectomy.

A local tumour recurrence can be seen as a consequence of inadequate radical tumour extirpation in a patient with an extensive, invasive carcinoma, or because of small presacral lymph node metastases remaining after lymphadenectomy. Local spillage of tumour cells during cystectomy can result in local recurrent tumour.[106] Therefore, inadvertent opening of the bladder wall during cystectomy must be avoided. The incidence of pelvic recurrence is between 6% and 9% (see Table 14.5).

Cystectomy and urinary diversion in elderly patients

Total cystectomy with pelvic lymph node dissection and urinary diversion can be done in elderly patients with acceptable mortality and morbidity. According to the published results, the mortality rate lies between 0 and 6% and is slightly higher than the 1% rate for patients less than 70 years old. In our own series the perioperative mortality in patients older than 70 years was not significantly different from the mortality in younger patients (1.8% versus 1.2%). For evident reasons, these favourable results reflect the careful patient selection at our institution. On the other hand, they show that age by itself is not necessarily a contraindication to radical surgery which is often better tolerated than other treatments such as full-dose radiation therapy or systemic chemotherapy.[88,107–111]

The complication rate does not differ significantly from our experience with younger patients (see Table 14.6).

Table 14.6   Radical cystectomy in elderly patients

Authors	Number of patients	Age (years)	Perioperative mortality	Hospital stay (days)	Compli-cation rate
Zincke (1982)[108]	19	>80	5.3%	22	–
Drago and Rohner (1983)[109]	28	>70	0%	21	–
Skinner (1984)[88]	77	>65	3.9%		31%
Wood *et al.* (1987)[110]	38	>70	5.3%	14	34%
Berne series (1989)[7]	65	>70	1.8%	26	32%

Radical cystectomy for patients with bladder tumours not invading the musculature

It is evident that the prognosis is excellent for those patients with a superficial tumour who have a cystectomy if the tumours are truly superficial. However, for many patients radical cystectomy could be considered as over-treatment. Therefore, the large majority of patients with superficial bladder tumours of stage Ta or T1, even with concomitant carcinoma-in-situ, deserve first a trial of transurethral resection and intravesical therapy.[112] The TUR should consist of an extended resection of the tumour, and the material for histological examination must include muscle fragments of the bladder wall in order to evaluate the depth of tumour invasion, with multiple mucosal biopsies and resection biopsies of the prostate. In cases of tumours of stage pT1, grade 3, the TUR should be repeated to ensure a critical evaluation of the tumour invasion. In our view, postoperative intravesical treatment is mandatory, and we prefer intravesical application of Bacillus Calmette-Guérin (6 weeks course, 120 mg BCG Pasteur, 1 instillation/week).

Patients with persistent positive cytology or biopsy after BCG belong to a high-risk group at risk from early progression within a few months.[112] Cystectomy as a therapeutic option is clearly indicated.

If transurethral resection plus BCG fails, a radical operation is the treatment of choice.

Conclusions

Local control of advanced bladder cancer is possible today through the use of surgery alone. This form of curative treatment is possible only in those patients in whom extensive dissemination into regional lymph nodes or into other organ systems has not yet taken place. Since, at the time of diagnosis, dissemination has already taken place in about 40–60% of locally advanced bladder cancers, a five-year survival rate of 35–60% is the most that can be achieved in these patients by means of surgery alone.

Because invasive bladder carcinoma is often already a systemic disease at the time of diagnosis, it should also be treated systemically. Trials with preoperative or postoperative systemic treatments are not yet conclusive.[113–116] However, more effective and less toxic systemic chemotherapy is required if the survival and quality of life of patients with advanced bladder tumours is to be improved substantially.

We feel that until we have a potent form of systemic treatment, radical cystectomy, which today still offers the best chance of local control of disease, should not be abandoned until prospective randomized trials prove that there is a better form of treatment for patients with non-metastatic, invasive bladder cancer.

References

1. Silverberg E, Lubera JA. Cancer statistics 1988. *CA* 1988; **38**: 5–22.
2. Prout GR, Kopp J. Evaluation and management of patients with primary bladder cancer: protocols of the National Bladder Cancer Collaborative Group A. In: Denis L, Murphy GP, Prout GR, Schröder F (eds), *Controlled Clinical Trials in Urologic Oncology*, vol. 13. New York: Raven Press, 1984: 221–40.
3. Newman LH, Tannenbaum M, Droller MJ. Muscle-invasive bladder cancer: does it arise *de novo* or from pre-existing superficial disease? *Urology* 1988; **32**: 58–62.
4. Brawn PN. The origin of invasive carcinoma of the bladder. *Cancer* 1982; **50**: 515–19.
5. Kaye KW, Lange PH. Mode of presentation of invasive bladder cancer: reassessment of the problem. *J Urol* 1982; **128**: 31–3.
6. Hopkins St C, Ford KS, Soloway MS. Invasive bladder cancer: support for screening. *J Urol* 1983; **130**: 61–3.
7. Danielson DA. *Resultate nach radikaler Zystektomie wegen eines Blasenkarzinomes.* Thesis, University of Berne, 1990.
8. Skinner D. Editorial comment on SC Hopkins *et al.*, 'Invasive bladder cancer: support for screening' (reference 6).
9. Heney NM, Ahmed S, Flanaghan MJ, *et al.* Superficial bladder cancer: progression and recurrence. *J Urol* 1983; **130**: 1083–6.
10. Anderström C, Johansson S, Nilsson S. The significance of lamina propria invasion on the prognosis of patients with bladder tumours. *J Urol* 1980; **124**: 23–6.
11. Jakse G, Loidl W, Seeber G, *et al.* Stage T_1 grade G_3 transitional cell carcinoma of the bladder: an unfavorable tumor? *J Urol* 1987; **137**: 39–43.
12. Abel PD, Hall RR, Williams G. Should pT_1 transitional cell cancers of the bladder still be classified as superficial? *Br J Urol* 1988; **62**: 235–9.

13. Pocock RD, Ponder BA, O'Sullivan JP, *et al.* Prognostic factors in non-infiltrating carcinoma of the bladder: a preliminary report. *Br J Urol* 1982; **54**: 711–15.

14. Lutzeyer W, Rübben H, Dahm H. Prognostic parameters in superficial bladder cancer: an analysis of 315 cases. *J Urol* 1982; **127**: 250–2.

15. Althausen AF, Prout GR, Daly JJ. Non-invasive papillary carcinoma of the bladder associated with carcinoma-in-situ. *J Urol* 1976; **116**: 575–80.

16. England HR, Paris AMI, Blandy JP. The correlation of T_1 bladder tumour history with prognosis and follow-up requirements. *Br J Urol* 1981; **53**: 593–7.

17. Gowing NFC. Urethral carcinoma associated with cancer of the bladder. *Br J Urol* 1960; **32**: 428–38.

18. Seemayer TA, Knaack J, Thelmo WL, Wang NS, Ahmed MN. Further observations on carcinoma-in-situ of the urinary bladder: silent but extensive intraprostatic involvement. *Cancer* 1975; **36**: 514–20.

19. Culp OS, Utz DC, Harrison EG. Experience with ureteral carcinoma-in-situ detected during operations for vesical problems. *J Urol* 1967; **97**: 679–82.

20. Skinner DC, Richie JP, Cooper PH, Walsman J, Kaufman JJ. The clinical significance of carcinoma-in-situ of the bladder and its association with overt carcinoma. *J Urol* 1974; **112**: 68–71.

21. Jewett HJ, Strong GH. Infiltrating carcinoma of bladder: relation of depth of penetration of bladder wall to incidence of local extension and metastases. *J Urol* 1946; **55**: 366–72.

22. Skinner DG. Management of invasive bladder cancer: a meticulous pelvic node dissection can make a difference. *J Urol* 1982; **128**: 34–6.

23. Whitmore WF. Management of invasive bladder neoplasms. *Sem Urol* 1983; **1**: 4–10.

24. Studer UE, Ruchti E, Greiner RM, Zingg EJ. Faktoren, welche die Ueberlebensrate nach totaler Zystektomie wegen Harnblasencarcinom beeinflussen. *Akt Urol* 1983; **14**: 70–7.

25. Camey M. Lymphadénectomie associetée à la cystectomie totale. *J d'Urol* 1985; **91**: 695–6.

26. Bloom HJG, Hendry WF, Wallace DM, Skeet RG. Treatment of T_3 bladder cancer: controlled trial of preoperative radiotherapy and radical cystectomy versus radical radiotherapy: second report and review. *Br J Urol* 1982; **54**: 136–51.

27. Skinner DG, Lieskowski G. Contemporary cystectomy with pelvic node dissection compared to preoperative radiation therapy plus cystectomy in management of invasive bladder cancer. *J Urol* 1984; **131**: 1069–72.

28. Zincke, H, Patterson DE, Utz DC, Benson RC. Pelvic lymphadenectomy and radical cystectomy for transitional cell carcinoma of the bladder with pelvic nodal disease. *Br J Urol* 1985; **57**: 156–9.

29. Skinner DG. Editorial comment on KI Whishnow *et al.* 'Incidence, extent and location of unsuspected pelvic lymph node metastases in patients undergoing radical cystectomy for bladder cancer' (reference 66).

30. Studer UE, Wallace DMA, Ruchti E, Zingg EJ. The role of pelvic lymph node metastases in bladder cancer. *World J Urol* 1985; **3**: 98–103.

31. Leadbetter WE, Cooper JF. Regional gland dissection for carcinoma of the bladder: a technique for one-stage cystectomy, gland dissection, and bilateral uretero-enterostomy. *J Urol* 1950; **63**: 242–9.

32. Laplante M, Brice M. The upper limits of hopeful application of radical cystectomy for vesical carcinoma: does nodal metastasis always indicate incurability? *J Urol* 1973; **109**: 261–4.

33. Dretler SP, Ragsdale BD, Leadbetter WE. The value of pelvic lymphadenectomy in the surgical treatment of bladder cancer. *J Urol* 1973; **109**: 414–16.
34. Reid EC, Oliver JA, Fishman IJ. Preoperative irradiation and cystectomy in 135 cases of bladder cancer. *Urology* 1976; **8**: 247–50.
35. Clark PB. Radical cystectomy for carcinoma of the bladder. *Br J Urol* 1978; **50**: 492–5.
36. Smith JA, Whitmore WF. Regional lymph node metastasis from bladder cancer. *J Urol* 1981; **126**: 591–3.
37. Splinter TAW, Scher HI (eds), *Chemotherapy for Invasive Bladder Tumors: Proceedings of an International Workshop, San Francisco.* New York: Alan Liss, 1989.
38. Yagoda A. Progress in treatment of advanced urothelial tract tumors. *J Clin Onc* 1985; **3**: 1448–50.
39. Montie JE, Straffon RA, Stewart BH. Radical cystectomy without radiation therapy for carcinoma of the bladder. *J Urol* 1984; **131**: 477–82.
40. Gervasi LA, Mata J, Easley JD, *et al.* Prognostic significance of lymph nodal metastases in prostate cancer. *J Urol* 1989; **142**: 332–6.
41. Marshall VF. Current clinical problems regarding bladder tumors. In: *Bladder Tumors: A Symposium.* Philadelphia: Lippincott, 1956: 1–9.
42. Murphy GP. Development in pre-operative staging of bladder tumors. *Urology* 1978; **11**: 109–15.
43. Richie JP, Skinner DG, Kaufman JJ. Radical cystectomy for carcinoma of the bladder: 16 years of experience. *J Urol* 1975; **113**: 186–9.
44. Voges GE, Tauschke E, Stöckle M, Alken P, Hohenfellner R. Computerized tomography: an unreliable method for accurate staging of bladder tumors in patients who are candidates for radical cystectomy. *J Urol* 1989; **142**: 972–4.
45. Sawczuk IS, de Vere White R, Palmer Gold R, Olsson C. Sensitivity of computed tomography in evaluation of pelvic lymph node metastases from carcinoma of bladder and prostate. *Urology* 1983; **21**: 81–4.
46. Salo JO, Kivisaari L, Rannikko S, Lehtonen T. The value of CT in detecting pelvic lymph node metastases in cases of bladder and prostate carcinoma. *Scand J Urol Nephrol* 1986; **20**: 261–5.
47. Greiner E, Skaleric C, Veraguth P. The prognostic significance of ureteral obstruction in carcinoma of the bladder. *Rad Onc Biol Phys* 1977; **2**: 1095–100.
48. Wood DP, Montie JE, Pontes JE, Levin HS. Identification of transitional cell carcinoma of the prostate in bladder cancer patients: a prospective study. *J Urol* 1989; **142**: 83–5.
49. Prout GR, Griffin PP, Daly JJ, Heney NM. Carcinoma-in-situ of the urinary bladder with and without associated vesical neoplasms. *Cancer* 1983; **52**: 524–32.
50. Schellhammer, PF, Bean MA, Whitmore WF. Prostatic involvement by transitional cell carcinoma: pathogenesis, patterns and prognosis. *J Urol* 1977; **118**: 399–403.
51. Coutts AG, Grigor KM, Fowler JW. Urethral dysplasia and bladder cancer in cystectomy specimens. *Br J Urol* 1985; **57**: 535–41.
52. Wood DP, Montie JE, Pontes JE, Van der Brug Medendorp S, Levin HS. Transitional cell carcinoma of the prostate in cystoprostatectomy specimens removed for bladder cancer. *J Urol* 1989; **141**: 346–9.
53. Johnson DE, Hogan JM, Ayala AG. Transitional cell carcinoma of the prostate: a clinical and morphological study. *Cancer* 1972; **29**: 287–93.
54. Chibber PJ, McIntyre MA, Hindmarsh JR, Hargreave TB, Newsam JE, Chisholm GD. Transitional cell carcinoma involving the prostate. *Br J Urol* 1981; **53**: 605–9.

55. Hall RR. TUR and chemotherapy or radiotherapy for invasive bladder cancer. In: Denis L (ed.), *Management of Advanced Cancer of Prostate and Bladder*. New York: Alan Liss, 1986: 605–12.

56. Hall RR. Transurethral resection and systemic chemotherapy as primary treatment for T_3 bladder cancer: a new chance of function preservation. In: Yagoda, A (ed.), *Bladder Cancer: Future Directions for Treatment*. New York: John Wiley, 1988: 117–22.

57. van der Werf-Messing B. Carcinoma of the bladder treated by preoperative irradiation followed by cystectomy: third report of Rotterdam Radiotherapy Institute. *Cancer* 1975; **36**: 718–22.

58. Magri J. Partial cystectomy: a review of 104 cases. *Br J Urol* 1962; **34**: 74–87.

59. Resnick MI, O'Conor VJ. Segmental resection for carcinoma of the bladder: review of 102 patients. *J Urol* 1973; **109**: 1007–10.

60. Utz DC, Schmitz SE, Fugelso PD, *et al.* A clinicopathologic evaluation of partial cystectomy for carcinoma of the urinary bladder. *Cancer* 1973; **32**: 1075–7.

61. Novick AC, Stewart BH. Partial cystectomy in the treatment of primary and secondary carcinoma of the bladder. *J Urol* 1976; **16**: 570–4.

62. Brannan W, Ochsner MG, Fuselier HA, *et al.* Partial cystectomy in the treatment of transitional cell carcinoma of the bladder. *J Urol* 1978; **119**: 213–15.

63. Skinner DG. Technique of radical cystectomy. *Urol Clin N Am* 1981; **8**: 353–66.

64. Skinner DG, Crawford ED, Kaufman JJ. Complications of radical cystectomy for carcinoma of the bladder. *J Urol* 1980; **123**: 640–3.

65. Skinner DG, Tift JP, Kaufman JJ. High dose, short course preoperative radiation therapy and immediate single stage radical cystectomy with pelvic node dissection in the management of bladder cancer. *J Urol* 1982; **127**: 671–4.

66. Whishnow, KI, Johnson DE, Ro JY, Swanson DA, Babaian RJ, von Eschenbach AC. Incidence, extent and location of unsuspected pelvic lymph node metastases in patients undergoing radical cystectomy for bladder cancer. *J Urol* 1987; **137**: 408–10.

67. Linker DG, Whitmore WF. Ureteral carcinoma-in-situ. *J Urol* 1975; **113**: 777–80.

68. Johnson DE, Whishnow KI, Tenney D. Are frozen-section examinations of ureteral margins required for all patients undergoing radical cystectomy for bladder cancer? *Urology* 1989; **33**: 451–4.

69. Shipley WU, Prout GR, Kaufman DS. Bladder cancer: advances in laboratory innovations and clinical management, with emphasis on innovations allowing bladder-sparing approaches for patients with invasive tumours. *Cancer* 1990; **65**: 675–83.

70. Kabalin JN, McNeal JE, Price HM, Freiha FS, Stamey TA. Unsuspected adenocarcinoma of the prostate in patients undergoing cystoprostatectomy for other causes: incidence, histology and morphometric observations. *J Urol* 1989; **141**: 90–4.

71. de Boccard GA, Chatelanat F, Graber P. Association de l'adénocarcinome de la prostate au carcinome transitionnel de la vessie. *Helv Chir Acta* 1985; **52**: 533–4.

72. Skinner DG. Editorial comment on Stöckle M *et al.*, 'Urethral tumor recurrences after radical cystoprostatectomy: the case for primary cystoprostatourethrectomy?' (reference 79).

73. Poole-Wilson DS, Barnard RJ. Total cystectomy for bladder tumours. *Br J Urol* 1971; **43**: 16–24.

74. Raz S, McLorie G, Johnson S, Skinner DG. Management of the urethra in men undergoing cystectomy for bladder carcinoma. *J Urol* 1978; **120**: 298–300.

75. Faysal MH. Urethrectomy in men with transitional cell carcinoma of the bladder. *Urology* 1980; **16**: 23–6.
76. Beahrs JR, Fleming TR, Zincke H. Risk of local urethral recurrence after radical cystectomy for bladder cancer. *J Urol* 1984; **113**: 264–6.
77. Zabbo A, Montie JE. Management of the urethra in men undergoing radical cystectomy for bladder cancer. *J Urol* 1984; **131**: 267–8.
78. Hickey DP, Soloway MS, Murphy WM. Selective urethrectomy following cystoprostatectomy for bladder cancer. *J Urol* 1986; **136**: 828–30.
79. Stöckle M, Gokcebay E, Riedmiller H, Hohenfellner R. Urethral tumour recurrences after radical cystoprostatectomy: the case for primary cystoprostatourethrectomy? *J Urol* 1990; **143**: 41–3.
80. Zingg EJ, Plowman PN, Wallace DMA, Peters PC, Blandy JP. The treatment of muscle invasive bladder cancer. In: Zingg EJ, Wallace DMA (eds), *Bladder Cancer*. New York: Springer, 1985: 189–234.
81. Schellhammer PF, Whitmore WF. Urethral meatal carcinoma following cystourethrectomy for bladder carcinoma. *J Urol* 1976; **115**: 61–4.
82. Shinka T, Uekado Y, Aoshi H, Komura T, Ohkawa T. Urethral remnant tumors following simultaneous partial urethrectomy and cystectomy for bladder carcinoma. *J Urol* 1989; **142**: 983–7.
83. Studer UE, Ackerman D, Casanova GA, Zingg EJ. Three years' experience with an ileal low-pressure bladder substitute. *Br J Urol* 1989; **63**: 43–52.
84. Whitmore WF, Marshall VF. Radical total cystectomy for cancer of the urinary bladder. *J Urol* 1962; **87**: 853–68.
85. Wajsman Z, Merrin C, Moore R, Murphy GP. Current results from treatment of bladder tumors with total cystectomy at Roswell Park Memorial Institute. *J Urol* 1975; **113**: 806–10.
86. Johnson DE, Lamey SM. Complications of single stage radical cystectomy and ileal conduit diversion: review of 214 cases. *J Urol* 1977; **117**: 171–3.
87. Brannan W, Fuselier HA, Ochsner M, Randrup ER. Critical evaluation of 1-stage cystectomy: reducing morbidity and mortality. *J Urol* 1981; **125**: 640–2.
88. Skinner EC, Lieskowsky G, Skinner DG. Radical cystectomy in the elderly patient. *J Urol* 1984; **131**: 1065–8.
89. Stöckle M, Riedmiller H, Jacobi GH, Hohenfellner R. Radikale Zystektomie beim älteren Patienten. *Br J Urol* 1988; **19**: 310–14.
90. Shoenberg HW, Gregory JG, Murphy JJ. Low-mortality cystectomy in bladder cancer. *J Urol* 1973; **110**: 671–4.
91. Mathur VK, Krahn HP, Ramsey EW. Total cystectomy for bladder cancer. *J Urol* 1981; **125**: 784–6.
92. Thomas DM, Riddle PR. Morbidity and mortality in 100 consecutive radical cystectomies. *Br J Urol* 1982; **54**: 716–19.
93. Ackermann R, Ebert T. Komplikationen und Spätfolgen nach radikaler Zystektomie. *Urologe* 1985; **24**: 150–5.
94. Prout JP. The surgical management of bladder carcinoma. *Urol Clin N Am* 1976; **3**: 1.149–75.
95. Wallace DM, Bloom HJG. The management of deeply infiltrating (T3) bladder carcinoma: controlled trial of radical radiotherapy versus preoperative radiotherapy and cystectomy. *Br J Urol* 1976; **48**: 587–94.
96. Miller LS. Bladder cancer: superiority of preoperative irradiation and cystectomy in clinical stage B2 and C cancer. *Cancer* 1977; **39**: 973–80.

97. Pearse HD, Reed RR, Hodges CV. Radical cystectomy for bladder cancer. *J Urol* 1978; **119**: 216–18.
98. Bredael JJ, Croker BP, Glenn JF. The curability of invasive bladder cancer treated by radical cystectomy. *Eur Urol* 1980; **6**: 206–10.
99. Jacobi GH, Klippel FF, Hohenfellner R. 15 Jahre Erfahrung mit der radikalen Zystektomie ohne präoperative Radiotherapie beim Harnblasenkarzinom. *Akt Urol* 1983; **14**: 63–9.
100. Chan RC, Johnson DE. Integrated therapy for invasive bladder carcinoma: experience with 108 patients. *Urology* 1978; **12**: 549–52.
101. Timmer PR, Hartlief HA, Hooijkaas JA. Bladder cancer: pattern of recurrence in 142 patients. *Int J Radio Onc Biol Phys* 1985; **II**: 899–905.
102. Fossa S, Ous S, Tveter K, *et al.* Treatment of T2/T3 bladder carcinoma: total cystectomy with and without preoperative irradiation. *Eur Urol* 1986; **12**: 158–63.
103. Radwin HM. Radiotherapy and bladder cancer: a critical review. *J Urol* 1980; **124**: 43–6.
104. Wijkström H, Edsmyr F, Nilsson B. Treatment of invasive grade 3 transitional cell bladder cancer. *Eur Urol* 1987; **13**: 300–4.
105. Crawford ED, Das S, Smith JA. Preoperative radiation therapy in the treatment of bladder cancer. *Urol Clin N Am* 1987; **14**: 4.781–7.
106. Whitmore WF. Integrated irradiation and cystectomy for bladder cancer. *Br J Urol* 1980; **52**: 1–9.
107. Zingg EJ, Bornet B, Bishop MC. Urinary diversion in the elderly patient. *Eur Urol* 1980; **6**: 347–51.
108. Zincke H. Cystectomy and urinary diversion in patients eighty years or older. *Urology* 1982; **19**: 139–42.
109. Drago JR, Rohner TJ. Cystectomy and urinary diversion: a safe procedure for elderly patients. *Urology* 1983; **21**: 17–19.
110. Wood DP, Montie JE, Maatman TJ, Beck GJ. Radical cystectomy for carcinoma of the bladder in the elderly patient. *J Urol* 1987; **138**: 46–8.
111. Stöckle M, Alken P, Engelmann U, Jacobi GH, Riedmiller H, Hohenfellner R. Radical cystectomy—often too late? *Eur Urol* 1987; **13**: 361–7.
112. Herr HW, Badalament RA, Amato DA, Laudone VP, Fair WR, Whitmore WF. Superficial bladder cancer treated with bacillus Calmette-Guérin: a multivariate analysis of factors affecting tumor progression. *J Urol* 1989; **141**: 22–9.
113. Logothetis CJ, Johnson DE, Chong C, *et al.* Adjuvant cyclophosphamide, doxorubicin, and cisplatin chemotherapy for bladder cancer: an update. *J Clin Onc* 1988; **6**: 1950–6.
114. Logothetis CJ, Dexeus F, Sella A, *et al.* A prospective randomized trial comparing ASCA to MVAC chemotherapy in advanced metastatic urothelial tumors. *J Urol* 1989; **141**: 216A.
115. Scher H, Herr H, Sternberg C, *et al.* Neo-adjuvant chemotherapy for invasive bladder cancer: experience with the M-VAC regimen. *Br J Urol* 1989; **64**: 250–6.
116. Sternberg CN, Yagoda A, Scher HI, *et al.* Methotrexate, vinblastine, doxorubicin, and cisplatin for advanced transitional cell carcinoma of the urothelium. *Cancer* 1989; **64**: 2448–58.

15 Cytotoxic chemotherapy for locally advanced and metastatic bladder cancer

Wadih Arap and Howard I Scher

Bladder tumours encompass a broad clinical spectrum of disease that includes superficial tumours that have little impact on survival, invasive tumours with an increasing metastatic risk, and *de novo* metastatic disease. The latter two categories are responsible for an estimated 12 000 deaths annually in the United States.[1] In the past decade, significant advances have been made in the chemotherapy of urothelial tract malignancies, and a proportion of patients are enjoying long-term disease-free survival. However, the majority of patients with metastatic tumours still succumb to disease. The toxicities of treatment can be considerable, and these may be unacceptable in a population of patients who are mainly elderly. The selection of patients who require chemotherapy in locally advanced disease is critical, and there is considerable controversy as to whether chemotherapy is best applied in the preoperative or postoperative setting.[2] This chapter will focus on the advances in chemotherapy, review what has been learned from adjuvant and neo-adjuvant approaches, and discuss some of the ongoing studies designed to investigate combined modality approaches to improve the prospects for survival.

Single-agent studies in metastatic disease

Patients with metastatic disease include those who present *de novo*, and those who progress after primary treatment for localized disease. The ability to deliver chemotherapy will vary within these groups. For example, prior radiation therapy predisposes to greater myelosuppression following treatment.[3] Patients with ureteric obstruction or long ileal conduits have variable methotrexate kinetics and are predisposed to mucositis at seemingly non-toxic doses of the drug.[4] These factors must be considered when selecting treatment for an individual patient.

A variety of single agents have demonstrated activity as outlined in Table 15.1.

Table 15.1   Single agents for urothelial tract tumours

	CR + PR	% CR + PR	95% Confidence
Cisplatin			
Single institution	70/206	34	20–40%
Randomized trials	55/315	17	37–55%
Carboplatin	21/186	15	11–19%
CHIP	7/39	18	6–30%
Methotrexate			
'Low' dose	68/236	29	23–35%
'High' dose	16/57	45	37–50%
Adriamycin	47/274	17	13–22%
Vinblastine	6/38	16	4–28%
Cyclophosphamide	30/98	31*	22–40%
5-fluorouracil	22/141	17*	11–25%
Mitomycin-C	5/42	13*	2–22%
Gallium nitrate	7/26	27	11–48%

Adapted from Sternberg C, Scher H. Advances in the treatment of urothelial tract tumors. *Urol Clin – Am* 1987; **14**: 373–87.
*Reflects early trials using varied doses, schedules and response criteria.

The optimal dose and schedule of these agents is not well defined. In general, responses to single agents are partial and of short duration, while there are only anecdotal reports of complete responses and long-term survival.

Methotrexate is most frequently administered on a weekly or twice-weekly basis in a dose range of 30–40 mg/m^2 with an overall response rate of 30% (95% confidence limits 25–35%). Administration of higher doses, greater than 100 mg with or without leucovorin rescue, has not been shown conclusively to improve outcome. Although cumulative data suggest a slight improvement (45%, 95% confidence 32–58%) using 'high' dose regimens, this has not been tested in a randomized trial.[5] Methotrexate analogue development has been slow. Activity was shown for 10-deaza-aminopterin in patients who progressed on methotrexate.[6] Trimetrexate (TMQ) showed a 16% (95% confidence interval 1–25%) response rate in 31 patients, including 28 who had progressive disease on M-VAC (methotrexate, vinblastine, Adriamycin and cisplatin).[7] Dichloromethotrexate, cleared via the hepatic route, has also shown activity in combination with cisplatin. This may be beneficial for patients with pleural effusions, ascites or compromised renal function where the toxicity of the parent compound may be excessive.[8] Recently, pirotexim has shown activity in refractory tumours.[9] To date, however, no investigational antifolate has replaced the parent compound in combination chemotherapy programmes.

Cisplatin is felt to be the most active single agent in urothelial tract tumours. Response, when it occurs, is usually rapid, and the drug can probably be discontinued if no response is seen in 1–2 cycles. The usual dose is 70 mg/m^2, and it is unclear whether higher doses of 100–120 mg/m^2 improve outcome. Response rates vary depending on case selection. For example, considering only single institution studies reporting similar dose schedules, an overall response rate of 34% (95% confidence interval 28–40%) is observed. However, reviewing results in the cooperative group setting, one observes a more modest 17% response rate (95% confidence interval 13–22%). In one series of pretreated patients, no responses were observed.[10] The primary limitation of this compound is the inability to utilize adequate doses in patients with compromised renal function. In some cases, divided doses are used,[3] but it is unclear whether this strategy results in equivalent therapeutic efficacy.

Reviewing single-agent studies is increasingly difficult in the era of combination chemotherapy. Care must be taken to evaluate selection criteria, with attention to whether or not patients had received prior chemotherapy and, if so, with which agents. The doses administered and sites of disease can also affect outcome. For example, durable responses are rarely seen in bone or in liver.[11] This is apparent when considering trials with the cisplatin analogue carboplatin. Interest in this compound is based on improved patient tolerance, lack of nephrotoxicity, and the close correlation between the degree of myelosuppression and the area under the concentration/time curve (AUC).[12] The latter correlates directly with the level of renal function.[13] Considering trials in patients with prior chemotherapy, no re-sponses are observed. Reviewing only trials of patients who were chemotherapy-naive, and who received myelosuppressive doses, an overall response rate of 15% (21/186, 95% confidence limits 11–19%) was observed. Yet, even in patients with no prior chemotherapy, response rates vary from 0 to 26%.[14–17] In some cases this may be the result of inadequate dosing. One study suggested a schedule depen-dency with response in 21% (4/19) of cases treated with a continuous infusion regimen.[18] Another platinum analogue, *cis*-dichloro-*trans*-dihydroxy-*bis*-isopropylamine platinum IV (CHIP) was reported to show responses in 4 out of 25 cases (16%, 95% confidence interval 5–35%)[17] and 3 out of 14 cases (21%, 95% confidence interval 7–35%)[14] respectively. The results seem to suggest a slightly lower response rate when compared with cisplatin.

Other single agents that have shown activity include doxorubicin (Adriamycin, ADR), which produced an overall response rate of 17% (95% confidence interval 12–21%) in a dose range of 30–70 mg/m^2 every 3–4 weeks.[5] A dose response curve has been suggested.[18] In contrast, vinblastine (VLB) has shown a response rate of 16% (95% confidence interval 4–28%) in 38 patients treated with 0.1–0.15 mg/kg or 4–6 mg/m^2 intravenously every week.[5] However, the trials as reported do not allow a definite dose-response evaluation.

The literature on 5-fluorouracil is heterogeneous with respect to case selection criteria, dose, and schedule. Cumulatively, responses have been observed in 17% (95% confidence limits 11–25%) of cases. The toxicity profile, in particular its lack of myelosuppression and nephrotoxicity, and potential lack of cross-resistance with contemporary combination programmes, has sparked renewed interest in this agent. Activity has been shown recently when combined with cisplatin,[20] leucovorin (Scher *et al.*, unpublished) and interferon.[21]

Interest in gallium nitrate stemmed from the observation of responses in 7 of 26 patients (95% confidence limits 11–48%) who had progressed on cisplatin-based regimens.[22] Nephrotoxicity was dose-limiting in this trial and this may be in part related to the weekly bolus schedule of administration. More recently, activity of this compound was confirmed with the demonstration of partial remissions in 4 of 23 patients (17.4%, 95% confidence limits 2–33%) treated with doses greater than 350 mg/m^2 for 5 days by continuous infusion. All had progressed on combination chemotherapy with M-VAC (methotrexate/vinblastine/Adriamycin/cisplatin).[23,24] Further studies are warranted.

Combination chemotherapy in metastatic disease

A number of combination programmes have undergone evaluation in urothelial tract tumours. Most contain cisplatin with or without methotrexate. These include cisplatin with methotrexate (DDP/MTX), cisplatin with Adriamycin and cyclophosphamide (CISCA/CAP), cisplatin with methotrexate and vinblastine (CMV), and M-VAC. Using these combinations, responses have been reported in up to 70% of cases.[25–28] While controversy exists over whether combinations are superior to single agents[29] and which regimen should be considered 'front-line' therapy, the results of two randomized trials support the use of M-VAC, developed at Memorial Hospital in 1983, as 'standard therapy' for this disease.

The first compared M-VAC with single-agent cisplatin and showed an advantage for the combination with respect to complete response rate (13% versus 3%), overall response rate (34% versus 9%, $p = 0.01$), and of greater importance, overall survival (12.6 versus 8.7 months, $p = 0.02$).[30] It is noteworthy that the median survival for M-VAC in the randomized trial was similar to that observed in the Memorial Hospital series.[3] While it is too early to compare the proportions of long-term survivors, one would expect a lower rate in the randomized trial based on the lower proportion of complete responders (26% versus 13%). The second randomized trial compared M-VAC with CISCA and also showed a survival advantage; 18.4 versus 9.3 months ($p = 0.0003$) for the M-VAC regimen.[31]

Controversy exists over the relative superiority, if any, of M-VAC versus CMV,[27] which differ in respect of the inclusion of Adriamycin in the former, and a higher dose (100 mg/m^2 versus 70 mg/m^2) of cisplatin in the latter. While a formal randomized comparison has not been undertaken, it is noteworthy that the median survival for completely responding patients treated with M-VAC exceeds 38 months, compared with 14 months for patients treated with the CMV regimen.[32] At present, when considering chemotherapy for urothelial tract tumours, combination chemotherapy should be considered standard.

Other investigators have reported lower response rates and shorter response duration with M-VAC.[33–35] Case selection may explain part of the differences observed. The toxicities of this regimen can be considerable and include myelosuppression, sepsis, mucositis, nephrotoxicity and peripheral neuropathy.[3,28] Toxic deaths have also been reported. Others have attempted to modify the regimen by deletion of the day 14 or 21 doses of methotrexate and vinblastine.[36] Compromising dose, however, may compromise outcome. Still others have substituted epi-adriamycin for Adriamycin in the hopes of developing a less myelosuppressive and less cardiotoxic regimen. Preliminary data are encouraging, although longer follow-up of these programmes is required.[37,38]

The combination of carboplatin and methotrexate has also been investigated. In two studies, overall response rates of 50% and 53% were observed, although complete responses were documented in only 6% and 12% respectively.[39,40] Harland and Fenwick applied these agents using a modified regimen. Flexible doses designed to give an area under the concentration/time curve (AUC) of 6 mg/ml per minute for carboplatin and a steady-state plasma level of 2–5 μM of methotrexate were administered. Of 32 evaluable patients, complete and overall responses were observed in 6 cases (15%; 95% confidence limits 5–32%) and 15 cases (47%; 95% confidence limits 30–64%) respectively.[41] Further studies of pharmacodynamically based regimens are important.

More recently a combination programme designed specifically to be less nephrotoxic and less myelosuppressive than the parent M-VAC regimen has been reported by Waxman and coworkers.[42,43] The regimen substitutes carboplatin for cisplatin, and mitozantrone for Adriamycin. The results in 21 patients with meta-static disease showed complete responses in 5 cases (23%) and an overall response in 11 cases (52%; 95% confidence limits 27–68%). While a formal comparison with M-VAC has not been undertaken, this regimen may be particularly useful for elderly patients with intercurrent diseases who cannot tolerate full doses of M-VAC.

Clearly, however, to improve survival requires an increase in the proportion of patients who achieve complete remission status. In the case of urothelial tract tumours, new agents and combinations must be developed. One of the most important treatment variables related to the use of chemotherapy involves dose and dose intensity.[44] This is rarely controlled in clinical trials. In many cases, combination programmes significantly compromise the ability to deliver adequate doses of each of the active agents. Such is the case for urothelial tract tumours.

The recent availability of haematopoietic growth factors represents a novel approach with the potential to affect outcome significantly, both with respect to patient tolerance of chemotherapy and response. At the Memorial Hospital, treatment cycles with M-VAC plus granulocyte colony stimulating factor (G-CSF) were compared with treatment cycles with M-VAC alone in the same patient. The results showed that a higher percentage of patients were eligible to receive full doses of chemotherapy on day 14 and 21 as planned (100% versus 29%, $p = 0.0015$), significantly fewer days (3 versus 32) with an absolute neutrophil count below 1000 cells/mm^3 ($p = 0.0039$), and less mucositis (11% versus 44%, $p = 0.041$) during cycles that included the growth factor. Patient tolerance was therefore improved.[45]

Trials designed to escalate components of the M-VAC regimen without growth factor support have met with limited success. In one study at the Memorial Hospital, high-dose methotrexate (1000 mg/m^2 with leucovorin rescue) was given and the cycle interval shortened from 28 to 21 days in the hope of increasing the proportion of complete responders. The trial was unsuccessful as toxicities were increased, resulting in a net reduction in the delivered dose with no increase in the complete response rate.[46] Increasing the dose of Adriamycin to 45 mg/m^2 also produced excessive toxicity. Thus, the maximal dose of Adriamycin in this regimen without growth factor support is 30 mg/m^2 (Seidman and Scher, unpublished). This is a modest dose relative to that used in most single-agent studies. A second study evaluated granulocyte macrophage colony-stimulating factor (GM-CSF) plus escalated doses of M-VAC in patients who had progressed on M-VAC with or without CISCA. This group is generally refractory to therapy.[47] The relative dose intensity of the growth-factor-supported regimen compared with conventional M-VAC was 1.43. The results showed a complete and overall response rate of 23% and 40% respectively. Taken together these studies show not only that growth factor can support improved tolerance, but also that clinically significant increases in response rate, a prerequisite to increasing the cure fraction, may be possible with the agents presently available.

One additional study suggests a steep dose-response relationship for Adriamycin in urothelial tract tumours. In this programme, Adriamycin 60 mg/m^2 was followed 12 hours later by cisplatin 60 mg/m^2, in a circadian fashion on a monthly basis. In 35 evaluable patients, complete responses were observed in 8 (23%) and an overall response of 58% observed.[48] Whether the outcome was related to the higher Adriamycin dosage, or the timing of the chemotherapy is unclear. Nevertheless, the data do suggest that the use of haematopoietic growth factors may lead to a clarification of the role of Adriamycin in urothelial tract tumours. Attempts to derive similar data for cisplatin are inconclusive. Nevertheless, extrapolating from other diseases, such as testicular cancer, suggests that an increase in dose from 70 to 100 mg/m^2 can be clinically significant.[49]

Chemotherapy for invasive disease

The results obtained using combination chemotherapy programmes in metastatic disease led to incorporation of chemotherapy in the treatment of patients with invasive (T2–4 N0 M0) disease.[2] The aim is to treat micrometastases, the cause of systemic failure, and to exploit the inverse relationship between tumour burden and curability[50] and the higher sensitivity of small-volume high-growth-fraction tumours.[51] The observed increase in the likelihood of response for patients with advanced nodal versus metastatic disease provides an additional rationale for this approach.[3,29]

The adjuvant and neo-adjuvant approaches are contrasted in Table 15.2. Classically, adjuvant therapy includes treatment after a radical cystectomy and pelvic lymph node dissection. It also includes treatment after a visibly complete endoscopic resection.[52] The major problem with this approach is the inability to document response. Thus, treatments are selected and continued empirically. Patient acceptance and tolerance of toxicities can compromise the outcome. The major advantage, at least following radical surgery, is that the need for treatment is

Table 15.2   Comparison of adjuvant and neo-adjuvant therapies

	Neo-adjuvant	Adjuvant
Rationale		
1. Early treatment of micrometastases		
A. Inverse relationship of tumour burden and cure	+	+
B. Small tumours may be more chemosensitive due to higher growth fraction	+	+
C. Decreased chance of spontaneous resistance	+	+
Factors favouring neo-adjuvant therapy		
1. Chemosensitivity determined case by case *in vivo*		
A. Response assessment *in vivo*	+	−
B. Prognostic information of response versus non-response	+	−
C. Organ preservation possible	+	−
2. 'Downstaging' of the primary tumour can		
A. Decrease the extent and need for additional therapy	+	−
B. Convert an 'unresectable' to a 'resectable' lesion	+	−
C. Drug delivery not compromised by previous surgery or radiation therapy	+	−
3. Endpoint of treatment more precise	+	−
4. Potential for accelerated growth after surgery	+	−
5. Better patient tolerance	+	+/−
Factors favouring adjuvant therapy		
1. Case selection		
A. Clinical *v* pathological staging error	−	+
B. Need for therapy based on pathological as opposed to clinical criteria	−	+
C. Exposure of more patients 'cured' by local therapies to cytotoxic agents	−	+
2. Timing of definitive local therapy		
A. Jeopardize curative therapy by prolonged treatment with ineffective agents	−	+
B. Refusal of potentially curative therapy	−	+

Adapted from Scher H. Chemotherapy of invasive bladder cancer: neo-adjuvant versus adjuvant. *Sem Onc* 1990; **17**: 555–64.

based on pathological criteria, resulting in a smaller number of patients treated with chemotherapy who are not at risk for development of metastatic disease. Further, removal of the bladder eliminates the problem of new tumour formation, and eliminates concerns that delaying definitive treatment may compromise outcome by allowing a 'resectable' tumour to become 'unresectable'. With the more widespread availability of internal urinary reservoirs, this approach is favoured by many physicians.[53]

The major advantage of the neo-adjuvant approach is that, with a marker lesion in the bladder, an *in vivo* assessment of chemosensitivity is possible. This allows individualization of treatment to the point of maximal response. In some cases the extent of the local therapy required can be reduced, permitting organ preservation. Examples include the use of concurrent radiation and chemotherapy following induction,[54] or use of a partial as opposed to a radical cystectomy to achieve local control. Response in the primary tumour also provides prognostic information, although a cause and effect relationship cannot be inferred.[55] Drug delivery is not compromised in the preoperative setting, which improves dose intensity.

The drawback with the neo-adjuvant approach relates to the difficulty in accurately assessing response. Despite clinical 'understaging' in a significant proportion of patients, to base the need for treatment on clinical criteria probably results in more patients being 'ovcrtrcatcd' with systcmic chemotherapy who do not require it.[2,56] This is particularly relevant for studies that include patients with T2 lesions with a low metastatic risk.

The problem with both strategies is an inability to predict accurately which patients ultimately require treatment because of a high risk of metastases and those who are destined to be cured by local strategies alone using currently available clinical, biological and pathological parameters. The choice of chemotherapy is not based on a predetermined sensitivity, but rather is chosen empirically. Of greater importance is that few randomized trials with adequate numbers of patients and with adequate follow-up have been reported.[57,58] Further, some randomized trials have a large beta error, reporting no difference between two treatment policies when one does exist. This is due to the enrolment of small numbers of patients relative to the expected differences outcome. The general applicability of an approach is difficult to ascertain, as few studies report the number of eligible versus treated patients. In addition, few of the ongoing randomized trials are studying combinations based on cisplatin and methotrexate, considered to be 'state of the art' in the 1990s.

Adjuvant therapy

Assessing the role of chemotherapy in the postoperative adjuvant setting highlights some of the difficulties. Most early studies were limited by inclusion of small numbers of patients and utilizing chemotherapy that produced low complete response rates.[3] Recently, two trials were reported that have the potential to affect clinical practice significantly. At MD Anderson, the survival distributions of 339 patients treated by radical cystectomy with or without CISCA were compared.[59] Treatment was advised in patients with a high risk of recurrence, defined by the presence of vascular or lymphatic invasion (37 cases), extravesical tumour (50 cases), node positive disease (24 cases) or extension into the pelvic viscera (22 cases). The criteria used to select which high-risk patients received (71 cases) or did not receive (62 cases) chemotherapy were not stated. The survival distributions of these two groups were compared with low-risk patients (206 cases) who did not show adverse pathological features. The results showed a shift in the survival distributions for high-risk patients treated with chemotherapy to one which was similar to that of the low-risk untreated group. Five-year survival rates of 76%, 70% and 37% were reported for low-risk, and treated and untreated high-risk patients, respectively. In a subset analysis, treatment benefit was only observed in patients with locally extensive, extravesical or microscopic node positive disease. No benefit was observed for patients with vascular/lymphatic invasion in the primary tumour.

In a second trial, patients with P3, P4 ± N+ disease after radical cystectomy and pelvic node dissection were randomized either to adjuvant chemotherapy with CAP or observation. The investigators reported the number of patients referred, the number randomized and the number who received therapy. During the study period, 453 cystectomies were performed; 241 showed pathological features that met protocol criteria for therapy. Of these 241 patients, 43 were medically excluded, and 101 (52%) of the remaining 198 patients agreed to participate in the study. Ten patients with non-transitional cell histologies were excluded from the analysis. Administration of adequate doses was a major problem; 11 of 44 (25%) of the patients randomized to chemotherapy did not receive any, and only 21 (48%) patients completed all four cycles. Nevertheless, the percentage of chemotherapy-treated patients who were free of disease at three years was 70% compared with 46% for the observation group ($p = 0.001$); the median survivals were 4.25 and 2.41 years respectively.[60] In a subset analysis, benefit was again restricted to patients with none or a single microscopically involved lymph node.

While strongly suggestive, these studies cannot be considered definitive. In the former study the factors used to select patients for therapy were unclear, and the second study was limited by small numbers. In addition, the second study was terminated early, before the planned 75 patients per arm were accrued. Thus, confirmatory trials using the best available combinations will be required before adjuvant therapy can be routinely recommended.

Neo-adjuvant therapy

The difficulties and limitations of neo-adjuvant chemotherapy have been well summarized and include differences in selection, staging, restaging, and criteria of response.[52] While definitive conclusions on the role of neo-adjuvant therapy await completion of ongoing randomized trials, several preliminary conclusions can be drawn based on reported results.

These trials have shown that chemotherapy alone can produce tumour regression in the bladder. Response assessments based on clinical (cystoscopic) criteria as opposed to pathological (laparotomy) criteria, result in the higher 'response' rates. As an example, using M-VAC at the Memorial Hospital for patients with invasive (T2–4 N0 M0) disease, the proportion of patients free of tumour assessed cystoscopically was 50% (42/84; 95% confidence limits 39–61%) as opposed to 23% (14/60; 95% confidence limits 13–34%) based on a pathological examination of the bladder removed by surgery. Further, the proportion of complete pathological responses, the most important consideration if one is considering a bladder-sparing approach, decreases with increasing depth of tumour. In our M-VAC experience, 43% of T2 versus only 8% of T4 tumours were pathologically free of disease.[61] The pathology of the primary tumour is also important, as non-transitional cell or mixed-histology tumours are less chemosensitive. Finally, carcinoma-in-situ tends to be less responsive to systemic chemotherapy; an *in situ* component may be the only remaining disease in the bladder after treatment.

A variety of regimens have been evaluated in the neo-adjuvant setting with essentially similar results with respect to the primary tumour. As shown in Table 15.3, the complete pathological response at the time of surgery ranged from 22% to 43%. This clearly shows that chemotherapy alone does not eliminate the need for some form of definitive local treatment for the majority of patients. While some controversy exists on the type of local therapy that should be advised after chemotherapy, in general, most groups advise radical surgery, although other cases have shown that attempts at bladder preservation can be safely tried with the combination of radiation and chemotherapy.[54]

Table 15.3   'Complete' pathological response in the bladder using combination chemotherapy

Agent(s)	No trials	Evaluable	Complete response at cystectomy	95% confidence interval
DDP/5FU	1	16	7 (43%)	19–68%
DDP/MTX	2	75	26 (35%)	24–45%
CMV	3	71	22 (31%)	20–42%
CAP	4	83	18 (22%)	13–31%
M-VAC	7	138	42 (30%)	23–38%

DDP = cisplatin; 5-FU = 5-fluorouracil; MTX = methotrexate; CAP = cyclophosphamide, Adriamycin, cisplatin; CMV = cisplatin, methotrexate, vinblastine; M-VAC = methotrexate, vinblastine, Adriamycin, cisplatin.

Reprinted from Scher H. Chemotherapy for invasive bladder cancer: neo-adjuvant versus adjuvant. *Sem Onc* 1990; **17**: 555–64.

Future perspectives

While significant progress has been made in the treatment of urothelial tract tumours, long-term survival is limited to a select few. The use of haematopoietic growth factors has the potential to improve the outcome for an additional proportion of patients, but ultimately, new agents and strategies will be required. The problem of drug resistance remains a major obstacle, and as more is understood of the mechanisms involved, more selective therapies can be designed. For example, resistance to two of the agents in M-VAC (namely, Adriamycin and vinblastine) are mediated in part by the mdr1 gene.[62] Attempts are ongoing to identify prospectively those tumours with high levels of expression which may be more amenable to treatment with drugs that do not act through this mechanism.

Considering the relatively low proportion of complete responses that result with presently available chemotherapy, and that only an increase in complete response rate can affect cure fraction, improved survival for patients treated in the adjuvant or neo-adjuvant setting should be demonstrated in prospective trials with long follow-up.[58,63] These trials are important, but few consider the reluctance of patients and physicians to participate in these studies.[64] Such considerations are important when designing protocols if they are to answer the question and be completed on a timely basis.

Most important for patients with invasive disease will be the ability to predict which tumours are destined to metastasize and which will ultimately remain localized and be cured by strategies directed exclusively to the primary tumour. For example, high NM23 RNA levels have been shown to correlate with low metastatic potential,[64] while 63% of patients with aneuploid tumours with high levels of the surface antigen T138 were dead in two years.[65] These or other markers may allow more rational treatment recommendations.

Clearly to improve the outcome of patients with urothelial tract tumours will require a combined modality approach. The uniform recommendation of one strategy over another is becoming antiquated. With an improved understanding of tumour biology, drug resistance, advances in chemotherapy and in surgery, an improvement in the care and outcome of these patients is possible in the 1990s.

Acknowledgements

The work reported here was supported by National Institutes of Health grant CA-05826 from the National Cancer Institute, National Institutes of Health, Department of Health and Human Services, Bethesda, MA, and the Frederick R Adler Education Fund (W Arap).

References

1. Silverberg E, Boring CC, Squires TS. Cancer statistics, 1990. *CA* 1990; **40**: 9–26.
2. Scher HI. Chemotherapy for invasive bladder cancer: neo-adjuvant *vs* adjuvant. *Sem Onc* 1990; **17**: 555–64.
3. Sternberg CN, Yagoda A, Scher HI, *et al.* M-VAC for advanced transitional cell carcinoma of the urothelium: efficacy, and patterns of response and relapse. *Cancer* 1989; **64**: 2448–58.
4. Fossa SD, Heilo A, Bormer O. Unexpectedly high serum methotrexate levels in cystectomized bladder cancer patients with an ileal conduit treated with intermediate doses of the drug. *J Urol* 1990; **143**: 498–500.
5. Yagoda A. Chemotherapy of urothelial tract tumours. *Cancer* 1987; **60**: 574–85.
6. Ahmed T, Yagoda A, Scher H, *et al.* 10-deaza-aminopterin: a new antifolate for bladder cancer. *Invest New Drugs* 1986; **4**: 171–4.
7. Witte R, Elson P, Khandekar J, Trump D. Trimetrexate (TMQ) in advanced urothelial carcinoma (AUC): a phase-II evaluation by the Eastern Cooperative Oncology Group (ECOG). *Proc Am Soc Clin Onc* 1990; **9**: 148.

8. Natale RB, Grossman HB, Crawford ED, *et al.* Combination cisplatin and dichloromethotrexate in advanced bladder cancer: a Southwest Oncology Group (SWOG) study. *Proc Am Soc Clin Onc* 1986; **5**: 104.

9. Clendeninn NJ, Savaraj N, Benedetto P, *et al.* Compassionate use of oral pirtrexim in bladder cancer: an effective drug after progression on MVAC chemotherapy? *Proc Am Assoc Cancer Res* 1991; **32**: 186.

10. Tannock I, Gospodarowicz M, Evans WF. Chemotherapy for metastatic transitional cell carcinoma of the urinary tract: a prospective trial of methotrexate, adriamycin and cyclophosphamide (MAC) with *cis*-platin for failure. *Cancer* 1983; **51**: 216–19.

11. Geller NL, Sternberg CN, Penenberg D, *et al.* Prognostic factors for survival of patients with advanced urothelial tumors treated with M-VAC chemotherapy. *Cancer* 1991; **67**: 1525–31.

12. Canctta R, Goodlow J, Smaldonc L, *et al.* Pharmacologic characteristics of carboplatin: clinical experience. In: Bunn P, Canetta R, Ozols RF, Rozencweig M (eds), *Carboplatin (JM-8): Current Perspectives and Future Directions.* Philadelphia: WB Saunders, 1990: 19–38.

13. Van Echo DA, Egorin MJ, Aisner J. The pharmacology of carboplatin. *Sem Onc* 1989; **16** (suppl 5): 1–6.

14. Seynaeve C, Rodenburg C, Kok TC, *et al.* First line chemotherapy with carboplatin (CBDCA) or iproplatin (CHIP) in metastatic transitional cell carcinoma of the urinary tract. *Proc Am Soc Clin Onc* 1990; **9**: 592.

15. Harstrick S, Schultz H, Keizer J, *et al.* Single-agent carboplatin in genitourinary malignancies. European Association of Urologists IXth Congress, Amsterdam, June 1990.

16. Akaza H, Hagiwara M, Deguchi N, *et al.* Phase-II trial of carboplatin in patients with advanced germ-cell testicular tumors and transitional cell carcinomas of the urinary tract. *Cancer Chemother Pharmacol* 1989; **23**: 181–5.

17. Micetich KC, Creekmore SP, Vogelzang N, Fisher RI. A phase-II study of a 24-hour infusion of carboplatin in patients with urinary tract malignancy. In: Bunn P, Canetta R, Ozols RF, Rozencweig M (eds), *Carboplatin (JM-8): Current Perspectives and Future Directions.* Philadelphia: WB Saunders, 1990: 83–92.

18. Trump DL, Elson P, Madajewicz S, *et al.* Randomized phase-II evaluation of carboplatin and CHIP in advanced transitional cell carcinoma of the urothelium. *J Urol* 1990; **144**: 1119–22.

19. O'Bryan RM, Baker LH, Gottlieb JE, *et al.* Dose-response evaluation of adriamycin in human neoplasms. *Cancer* 1977; **39**: 279–85.

20. Quintens H, Chevallier D, Benizri E, *et al.* Neo-adjuvant chemotherapy and transurethral resection in T2–4 Nx M0 bladder cancer. European School of Oncology Conference on Bladder Cancer, Venice, Italy, April 1990.

21. Logothetis C, Dexeus F, Amato R, *et al.* 5-fluorouracil and alpha interferon in the treatment of refractory urothelial tract tumours. *J Natl Cancer Inst* 1991; **83**: 286–8.

22. Crawford ED, Saiers JH, Baker LH. Treatment of metastatic bladder cancer with gallium nitrate. *Proceedings of the 13th International Congress of Chemotherapy* 1983; 240:12.1.7/A4,84.

23. Seidman A, Scher HI, Sternberg CN, *et al.* Gallium nitrate: an active agent in advanced refractory transitional cell carcinoma. *Cancer* (in press).

24 Seligman PA, Crawford ED. Treatment of advanced transitional cell carcinoma (TCC) of the bladder with constant infusion of gallium nitrate. *Proc Am Soc Clin Onc* 1991; **10**: 168 (534).

25. Stoter G, Splinter TAW, Child JA, *et al.* Combination chemotherapy with cisplatin and methotrexate in advanced transitional cell cancer of the bladder. *J Urol* 1987; **137**: 663–7.
26. Logothetis CJ, Samuels ML, Ogden S, *et al.* Cyclophosphamide, doxorubicin and cisplatin chemotherapy for patients with locally advanced urothelial tumors with or without nodal metastases. *J Urol* 1985; **134**: 460.
27. Harker WG, Meyers FJ, Freiha FS, *et al.* Cisplatin, methotrexate, and vinblastine (CMV): an effective chemotherapy regimen for metastatic transitional cell carcinoma of the urinary tract (a Northern California Oncology Group Study). *J Clin Onc* 1985; **3**: 1463–70.
28. Sternberg C, Yagoda A, Scher H, *et al.* Preliminary results of methotrexate, vinblastine, adriamycin and cisplatin (M-VAC) in advanced urothelial tumors. *J Urol* 1985; **133**: 403–7.
29. Scher H. Should single agents be standard therapy for urothelial tract tumors? *J Clin Onc* 1989; **10**: 694–7.
30. Loehrer PJ, Elson P, Kuebler JP, *et al.* Advanced bladder cancer: a prospective intergroup trial comparing single-agent cisplatin (CDDP) versus M-VAC combination therapy (INT 0078) (abstract). *Proc Soc Clin Onc* 1990; **9**: 132.
31. Logothetis C, Dexeus F, Sella A, *et al.* A prospective randomized trial comparing CISCA to MVAC chemotherapy in advanced metastatic urothelial tumors. *J Clin Onc* 1990; **8**: 1050–5.
32. Lo R, Freiha FS, Torti FM. CMV for metastatic urothelial tumors. In: Johnson DE, Logothetis CJ, von Eschenbach AC (eds), *Systemic Therapy for Genitourinary Cancers*. Chicago: Year Book Medical Publishers, 1989: 59–63.
33. Connor JP, Olsson CA, Benson MC, Rapoport F, Sawczuk H. Long-term follow-up in patients treated with methotrexate, vinblastine, doxorubicin and cisplatin (M-VAC) for transitional cell carcinoma of urinary bladder: cause for concern. *Urology* 1989; **34**: 353–6.
34. Tannock I, Gospodarowicz M, Connolly J, *et al.* M-VAC (methotrexate, vinblastine, doxorubicin, and cisplatin) chemotherapy for transitional cell carcinoma: the Princess Margaret Hospital experience. *J Urol* 1989; **142**: 289.
35. Igawa M, Ohkucki T, Ueki T, *et al.* Usefulness and limitations of methotrexate, vinblastine, doxorubicin and cisplatin for the treatment of advanced urothelial cancer. *J Urol* 1990; **144**: 662–5.
36. Pizzocaro G, Milani A, Piva L, Faustini M. Methotrexate, vinblastine, adriamycin and cisplatin versus methotrexate and cisplatin in advanced urothelial cancer: a randomized study. *Ann Onc* (submitted).
37. Frassoldati A, Federico M, Berri G, *et al.* M-VEC and C-M regimens as neoadjuvant chemotherapy in T2–4 N0 M0 bladder carcinoma. *J Cancer Res Clin Onc* 1990; **116** (suppl): 542, B4.209.24.
38. Rupp W, Ruther U, Bauerle K, *et al.* Phase-II study trial of M-VEC for metastatic urothelial tract tumors. *J Cancer Res Clin Onc* 1990; **116** (suppl): 542, B4.209.25.
39. Dogliotti L, Bertetto O, Berruti A, *et al.* Carboplatin (CBDCA) and methotrexate (MTX) combination chemotherapy in advanced urothelial cancer (UC): a phase-II study. Abstract 1990.
40. Stalder M, Leyvraz S, Bauer J, *et al.* An outpatient treatment for advanced urothelial tract cancer including patients with impaired renal function. *Proc Am Soc Clin Onc* 1990; **9**: A576.

41. Harland SJ, Fenwick E. Carboplatin and methotrexate (MTX) in advanced bladder cancer. *Proc Am Soc Clin Onc* 1989; **8**: A571.
42. Waxman J, Abel P, James N, *et al*. New combination chemotherapy programme for bladder cancer. *Br J Urol* 1989; **63**: 68–71.
43. Waxman J, Barton C, Biruls R, *et al*. Bladder cancer: interrelationships between chemotherapy and radiotherapy. *Br J Urol* (in press).
44. Hryniuk W, Bush H. The importance of dose intensity in chemotherapy of metastatic breast cancer. *J Clin Onc* 1984; **2**: 1281–8.
45. Gabrilove JL, Jakubowski A, Scher H, *et al*. A study of recombinant human granulocyte colony stimulating factor in cancer patients at risk for chemotherapy-induced neutropenia. *New Engl J Med* 1988; **318**: 1414–22.
46. Arap W, Scher H, Sternberg C, *et al*. High-dose methotrexate, vinblastine, adriamycin and cisplatin (HD-MVAC) for urothelial tract tumors (abstract). *Proc Am Ass Cancer Res* 1990; **31**: 187.
47. Logothetis C, Dexeus F, Sella A, *et al*. Escalated (ESC) MVAC (MTX 30 mg/m², adriamycin 60 mg/m², vinblastine 4 mg/m², cisplatin 100 mg/m²) with recombinant human granulocyte macrophage stimulating factor [(rhGM-CSF) Schering Corp] for patients (PTS) with advanced and chemotherapy (CHT) refractory urothelium tumors: a phase-I study. *J Clin Onc* 1990; **8**: 1050–5.
48. Hrushesky WJM, Roemeling RV, Wood PA, *et al*. High-dose intensity, circadian-timed doxorubicin and cisplatin adjuvant chemotherapy for bladder cancer. *Cancer Treat Rep* 1987; **71**: 915–19.
49. Ozols RF. Cisplatin dose intensity. *Sem Onc* 1989; **16** (suppl 6): 22–9.
50. Skipper HE, Schabel FM, Wilcox WS. Experimental evaluation of potential anticancer agents. XII: On the criteria and kinetics associated with curability of experimental leukemia. *Cancer Chemother Rep* 1964; **35**: 1–9.
51. Shackney SE, McCormack GW, Cuchural GJ. Growth rate patterns of solid tumors and their relationship to responsiveness to therapy. *Ann Intern Med* 1978; **89**: 107–21.
52. Scher H. Neo-adjuvant treatment of invasive bladder cancer. In: Williams R, Carroll P (eds), *Advances in Urologic Oncology: Treatment Perspectives*. New York: Pergamon Press, 1990: 201–32.
53. Broderick GA, Stone AR, deVere White R. Neo-bladders: clinical management and considerations for patients receiving chemotherapy. *Sem Onc* 1990; **17**: 598–605.
54. Shipley WU, Kaufman DS, Heney NM. Radiation therapy in bladder cancer: can its integration with chemotherapy and transurethral surgery make cystectomy unnecessary? *Oncology* 1990; **4**: 25–32.
55. Splinter TAW, Scher HI, EORTC-GU group, *et al*. The prognostic value of the pT-category after combination chemotherapy for patients with invasive bladder cancer who underwent cystectomy. In: Splinter T, Scher HI (eds), *Neo-Adjuvant Chemotherapy of Invasive Bladder Cancer*. New York: Alan R Liss, 1990: 219–24.
56. Scher H, Herr H, Yagoda A, *et al*. Neoadjuvant M-VAC (methotrexate, vinblastine, adriamycin and cisplatin): the effect on primary bladder tumors. *J Urol* 1988; **139**: 470–4.
57. Geller NL, Scher H, Parmar M, *et al*. Trial design and statistics: can we combine available data to evaluate the effects of neoadjuvant chemotherapy for invasive bladder cancer? *Sem Onc* 1990; **17**: 628–34.
58. Tannock IF. Endpoints of clinical trials in invasive bladder cancer. *Sem Onc* 1990; **17**: 619–27.

59. Logothetis CJ, Johnson DE, Chong C, *et al*. Adjuvant cyclophosphamide, doxorubicin, and cisplatin chemotherapy for bladder cancer: an update. *J Clin Onc* 1988; **6**: 1590–6.
60 Skinner DG, Daniels JR, Russell CA, *et al*. The role of adjuvant chemotherapy following cystectomy for invasive bladder cancer: a prospective comparative trial. *J Urol* 1991; **141**: 459–64.
61. Scher H, Herr H, Sternberg C, *et al*. M-VAC (methotrexate, vinblastine, adriamycin and cisplatin) and bladder preservation. In: Splinter T, Scher HI (eds), *Neo-Adjuvant Chemotherapy of Invasive Bladder Cancer*. New York: Alan R Liss, 1990: 179–86.
62. Dalesio O. Trial design and statistics. In: Splinter T, Scher HI (eds), *Neo-Adjuvant Chemotherapy of Invasive Bladder Cancer*. New York: Alan R Liss, 1990: 57–64.
63. Ling V. P-glycoprotein and multidrug resistance. *Sem Onc* 1989; **16**: 156–65.
64. Steeg PS, Bevilacqua G, Kopper L, *et al*. Evidence for a novel gene associated with low tumor metastatic potential. *J Natl Cancer Inst* 1988; **80**: 200–3.
65. Fradet Y, Tardif M, Bourget L, *et al*. Clinical cancer progression in urinary bladder tumors evaluated by multiparameter flow cystometry with monoclonal antibodies. *Cancer Res* 1990; **50**: 432–7.

Section V

Renal Cell Carcinoma

16 Immunoregulatory therapies in urological cancer

Angus Dalgleish and Paul Sondel

One of the most publicised therapeutic advances in clinical oncology over the last decade has been the clinical testing of defined recombinant human immunoregulatory proteins as a fourth modality, designated 'biological therapy' in the treatment of human cancers. Both recombinant interferons and interleukin-2 have now been tested in some detail. Unfortunately, the more common cancers such as lung and breast have not yet shown encouraging responses. Renal cell carcinoma (RCC), however, is one of the cancers which has responded to these therapeutic approaches.

In 1987 in the USA there were approximately 22000 new cases of RCC and 9500 deaths. In the UK there were 2300 deaths. Prior to the development of biological therapies the principal hope for cure was surgical resection. However, over 50% of patients with RCC present with metastatic disease and many with local disease are too far advanced to be resected. The prognosis is therefore bleak, with a 74% mortality at one year and 96% mortality at three years. For those with advanced disease, late recurrences post-resection can occur in approximately 10% of patients. Moreover, paraneoplastic syndromes can contribute to morbidity.

Radiotherapy, chemotherapy and hormonal therapy rarely affect RCC and new therapies have been actively explored. A well-documented, but exceedingly rare (<1%), feature of RCC is the phenomenon of spontaneous remission of metastatic disease, a process that is believed to be due to the host's antitumour immune response.[1]

A number of approaches to manipulate the immune system in RCC have met with some suggestion of clinical antitumour response, including testing with the BCG bacillus, immune RNA, transfer factor and infusion of autologous tumour cells. The early 'responses' claimed for some of these therapies, reviewed in detail by Quesada,[2] were probably due to clinically 'minor responses' (less than 50% shrinkage of all measurable tumour mass) rather than bona fide 'complete' or partial (>50% shrinkage) responses. Since then, well-documented partial and occasional complete responses have been noted using well-controlled and reproducible regimens using human recombinant interferons or interleukin-2.

This chapter does not attempt to provide a detailed and comprehensive review of the literature of the interferons and interleukins. Instead we overview the major landmarks and developments with regard to how biological response modifiers (BRMs) might be used in protocols either singly or in combination with other treatments, which it is hoped will lead to enhanced response rates in urological cancers.

Interferons

The interferons (INFs) are a family of secreted proteins that were originally characterized by their ability to interfere with virus infection.[3] Subsequently, cytostatic activities were reported. The INFs can exert a wide range of regulatory actions both on normal tissues (mainly those cells of the immune system) and tumour cells (Table 16.1). Potentially useful effects in cancer therapy include a direct antiproliferative effect and augmentation of expression of tumour cell membrane antigens. This latter effect is particularly important as some tumours are thought to escape immunoregulatory controls by down-regulation of their MHC class I antigens. Endogenously produced interferons need to be induced or activated and are readily released in response to virus infection. The antiviral activity of INFs is exerted on the host cell (rendering it resistant to virus replication) and not on the virus itself. In order to express biological activity, interferon needs to bind to specific saturable high-affinity receptors on the plasma membrane.

Table 16.1   Biological effects of interferon

Antiproliferative	Non-toxic slowing of all the phases of the cell cycle
Effects on oncogene expression	Inhibition of tumour proliferation correlates with reduced oncogene expression
Phenotypic reversion and loss of tumourigenic potential	Tumour cells revert to more normal morphology
Immunomodulatory effects	Modulates the cytotoxic activity of monocytes and natural killer cells and augments tumour cell membrane expression of MHC antigen increases
Differentiation	May effect tumour stem cell differentiation and maturation

INFs can be divided into two distinct groups. Type 1 INFs, which include alpha and beta INFs, are released by many cell types following viral infection and by certain INF 'inducers' such as soluble oligonucleotides. Type 2 (gamma) or 'immune' INF is released by activated T lymphocytes. In addition to augmented MHC class I expression on cell membranes induced by type 1 INF treatment, type 2 INF also induces increased expression of class II MHC molecules.

INFs are now produced biotechnically as cloned recombinant products, although

some preparations in clinical use have been produced by activated human leuko-
cytes or fibroblasts, and include a variety of different molecular types. There are at
least 14 homologous species of alpha-interferon, and a number of reviews document the *in vitro* activities of the INFs in detail.[4–6]. Prior to evaluating INFs in the
clinical setting, activity can be assessed in a variety of assays, some of which are
particularly useful for comparing new INFs, and combinations of INF and chemotherapy. Two of these assays have been particularly important.[4] The human
tumour clonogenic assay tests detect cytostatic effects on tumour cells *in vitro*, and
human tumour xenograft models can be used to measure the influence of the test
agent on the growth of human tumour implants transplanted into immuno-
compromised mice.

A summary of studies in these models of INFs leads us to conclude that an INF is
a biological response modifier (BMR) in that it modifies the host immune response
to malignant cells, and that in addition INFs have the capacity to directly inhibit cell
proliferation. These activities vary in magnitude against different tumours.

Clinical studies of interferons

Alpha-interferon has been extensively tested in phase I, II and III trials. Toxicity is
dose-related and includes fever, chills, fatigue, anorexia, nausea, myalgia and
myelosuppression. The high response rates of up to 80% in hairy cell leukaemias,
and 30% in certain other leukaemias and lymphomas, are well known. In contrast,
gamma-interferon does not appear to be effective in these conditions.

In RCC a number of studies reviewed by Muss[7] suggest no clear dose-response
relationship, although doses under 5×10^6 units a day tend to be associated with
lower response rates. Gamma-interferon does not appear to be as active, with only
four responses in 54 patients. There appears to be no relationship between
response and age, sex or disease-free interval. Asymptomatic patients respond
better than symptomatic patients, and the continued presence of a primary tumour
does not preclude a response. Patients with small pulmonary metastases are most
likely to respond and those with bone metastases are least likely to do so.

Antibodies may develop against INFs and may be more of a problem in some
preparations than others. Although the viral effects of interferon may be neutralized
by some antibodies and these are more likely to be associated with failure of clinical
response, a relationship between antibody production and clinical response or lack
of it has yet to be conclusively demonstrated.[8] A change of preparation is
recommended when neutralizing antibodies are suspected of inhibiting clinical
response. There is *in vitro* synergy between INFs and various chemotherapeutic
agents, but there is no synergy demonstrable in clinical studies combining INF with
chemotherapy in renal cell cancer.[9,10]

Interleukins

The role of interleukins (ILs) in acquired disease has been reviewed elsewhere.[11]
Only one, interleukin-2, has been tested to any degree for RCC at the present time.

IL-2 is an immunoregulatory molecule produced by activated T cells and previously known as T cell growth factor.[12,13] IL-2 binds specific cell surface receptors which results in functional signalling in a variety of cell types including T, B, NK, monocytes and oligodendritic cells. It is worth noting that IL-2 was developed as a result of the search for human retroviruses. It was considered that as putative retroviruses may only be present in a few lymphocytes, and then only at low copy number, attempts to isolate them would be fruitless unless the target populations— and hence the integrated retroviruses—could be expanded. Work in this field led to the discovery of the T-cell growth factor now known as IL-2, the use of which eventually led to the isolation of both the human leukaemic viruses (HTLV-I, HTLV-II) as well as the cytopathic viruses (HIV-1, HIV-2) which are the causative agents of AIDS.[13,14]

The identification and cloning of the IL-2 gene has led to the production of large quantities of IL-2 by using recombinant technology, allowing extensive characterization including preclinical and clinical studies.

There are two components of the IL-2 receptor, the alpha and beta chains. The alpha chain is a 55 kD protein recognized by the TAC monoclonal antibody. The beta chain is a 75 kD protein which is found constitutively on resting T and NK cells. IL-2 is secreted *in vivo* following recognition of antigen by antigen-specific T lymphocytes. Contact with antigen induces surface expression of the beta chain of the IL-2 receptor (IL-2R). Those cells which express both alpha and beta receptors can proliferate rapidly in response to low levels of IL-2, and some of these cells can mediate destruction of antigen-bearing cells. As IL-2 concentrations increase, cells expressing only the beta receptor are also activated as they associate with newly synthesized TAC chains to form a high-affinity receptor complex. After IL-2 treatment some IL-2 responsive cells mediate direct destruction of transformed cells; others release lymphokines and cytokines which can themselves activate a cascade of immune responses, which may result in toxic effects on tumour cells.

Mechanisms of anti-tumour action

Murine models have demonstrated that IL-2 is active against non-immunogenic as well as immunogenic tumours and may exert its antitumour effects by a variety of mechanisms.[15,16] Immunogenic tumours can be induced by oncogenic viruses, chemical carcinogens or physical agents such as ultraviolet radiation.

These tumours can be prevented by immunizing with non-viable tumour or tumour fragments. Immunogenic tumours express tumour-specific antigens on their surface allowing them to be recognized by specific cytotoxic T cells bearing appropriately rearranged T cell receptor molecules (the α,β/CD3 complex). This requires the co-recognition of autologous MHC class 1 major histocompatibility complex antigens which are also present on the surface of the tumour cells. The MHC antigens serve to present the tumour-specific antigens to autologous cytotoxic T cells. Protection is antigen-specific in that only the immunizing tumour is recognized. Immune spleen cells transferred to naive animals can protect them against subsequent tumour challenges. This is the role model for adoptive immunotherapy.[17,18] However, spontaneously arising murine neoplasms differ from 'immunogenic' tumours in that they are often functionally non-immunogenic and do not appear to express tumour-specific antigens that can be recognized by autologous or syngeneic cytotoxic T lymphocytes. These tumours are more representative of clinical tumours seen in humans, very few of which can be classified as immunogenic using current *in vitro* techniques.

Non-MHC-restricted cytotoxicity was first described in a small population of human lymphocytes that have neither B nor T cell markers. These cells, initially designated null cells for their lack of known B or T cell surface markers and absence of characterizable function, can mediate destruction *in vitro* of certain cultured tumour cell lines. Killing by these 'natural killer' (NK) cells does not appear to involve MHC-restricted recognition of target cells, and no role for the T cell receptor complex has been identified for NK cells. Unfortunately, most tumour cell lines and fresh tumour preparations have been resistant to 'resting' NK cells.

Upon exposure to high doses of IL-2 they become activated along with other T and B cells and are able to destroy most tumour cell lines and tumour tissue preparations *in vitro*. This reaction has been designated the 'lymphokine activated killer' (LAK) phenomenon, and these heterogeneous cells referred to as LAK cells, the majority of which are activated NK cells.[19-25]

In mouse models, IL-2 has been used to treat immunogenic and non-immunogenic tumours. It is considered that the murine non-immunogenic tumour is a more realistic model for human tumours than is the immunogenic variety. Early murine studies suggested that IL-2 responses in humans would likely result in highly variable tumour responses and depend upon many factors including tumour mass, dissemination, susceptibility of tumour cells, growth rate and host/tumour immune interactions. Clinical protocols using IL-2 were based upon pre-clinical testing in animals, particularly murine studies. These murine studies are reviewed in detail elsewhere.[26,27] However, the following are the main points which affected the design of early human trials. Firstly, IL-2 has a short half-life and needs to remain in contact with IL-2 receptors for many hours in order to induce non-MHC-restricted antitumour activity. In these studies toxicity was closely related to antitumour efficacy and dependent on an active immune system. Secondly, infusions of splenocytes cultured in the presence of IL-2 *in vitro* did not enhance the toxicity of high-dose IL-2 treatments *in vivo* but appeared to enhance antitumour activity against certain murine tumours. Thirdly, prolonged administration of lower doses of IL-2 was more effective than high-dose intravenous boluses. Finally, efficacy was greatest when the tumour burden was small. From these observations clinical trials proceeded.

Clinical aspects

Initial studies with recombinant IL-2 in mice showed that, in addition to inducing tumour responses, high-dose IL-2 regimens had severe (at times, life-threatening) transient systemic toxicities. Human studies have confirmed the toxicity profile seen in mice with regard to fever, chills, capillary leakage, pulmonary oedema, dermatitis, hepatocellular injury and renal dysfunction. As described below, significant responses were seen in RCC and melanoma in approximately 20% of patients.[28-30] Most clinical responses were partial, lasting only a few months although occasional prolonged complete responses have been seen. Some patients with colorectal cancer and lymphomas also showed responses to IL-2, and these tumours are under further investigation at a variety of centres. Much of this early work was performed by Dr Steven Rosenberg and his colleagues at the National Cancer Institute. They had been impressed with observations that some murine tumours respond better to IL-2 when combined with infusions of syngeneic LAK cells activated with IL-2 *in vitro*.

The initial report on LAK and IL-2 treatment by Rosenberg and colleagues included three patients with renal cell carcinoma who showed a partial response of their pulmonary metastases.[28]

Subsequent reports from the National Cancer Institute and other centres using the same regimen have shown that approximately 20% of patients with RCC and melanoma have measurable (>50%) shrinkage of all tumour.[29-35] A few patients have experienced complete responses and occasional patients have had sustained remissions for over a year. The toxicity reported with bolus IL-2 and LAK treatments is severe and many patients require intensive care. A number of patients responded to IL-2 (bolus) alone without LAK therapy. Trials evaluating IL-2 alone, given either as a bolus or continuous infusion, versus IL-2 together with LAK cell infusions have since been reported,[29,30] and results are similar with both approaches, although the complete response rate may be higher when LAK cells are included.

Sondel and others[35-40] have looked at continuous as opposed to bolus IL-2 administration. Initial studies showed that toxicity to the same daily dose given as a bolus was qualitatively similar when given continuously for seven consecutive days, but was not as severe. These patients showed marked immunological changes such as transient lymphopenia during the IL-2 infusion (probably representing redistribution out of the blood vessels), rebound lymphocytosis and enhanced LAK activity measured *in vitro* after cessation of IL-2.[36] Despite the striking immunological results none of these initial 25 patients showed any measurable antitumour response.

A modified protocol whereby continuous IL-2 is given for four days a week with three days off for a total of a month was associated with transient partial responses in 3 of 12 patients with RCC.[38] Other investigators have used similar protocols and confirmed the lower toxicity profile of continuous IL-2 as compared with bolus IL-2, as well as the more striking immune activation and *in vivo* induction of LAK activity.

Clearly the use of IL-2 as therapy for RCC (and melanoma) is hopeful but far from satisfactory. Many questions remain unanswered with regard to dose and scheduling of IL-2. In addition, the importance of *in vitro* expanded LAK cells has yet to be resolved. The considerable time, facilities required and total cost of preparing LAK cells dictate that any advantage of LAK and IL-2 over IL-2 alone will have to be considerable to justify continued development. In the meantime, studies using IL-2 alone or with other biologicals, in doses that can be tolerated for longer time periods, are encouraging, although much further evaluation is necessary.

Immune-cell/tumour-cell target interactions

Specific cytotoxic T lymphocyte responses as well as non-specific responses (LAK) may occur against tumour cells. The ligands involved in these interactions are shown in Fig. 16.1. The activation of cytotoxic T cells is dependent on an antigen-specific interaction whereby the T cell receptor complex sees antigen in association with self MHC antigens. These MHC molecules are also bound by CD4 and CD8 molecules on the T cell for class II and class I antigens respectively.

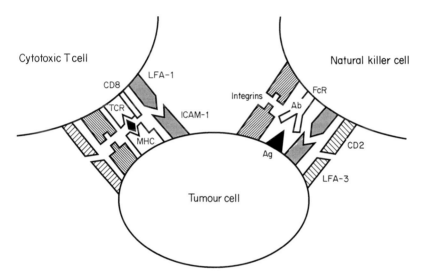

Fig. 16.1   Target interactions.

LAK cells may interact with their targets via the Fc IgG receptor (CD16), CD2, or a variety of other cellular adhesion molecules such as LFA-1, ICAM, LFA-3 and possibly the integrins, which are a set of adhesion-related molecules that bind target molecules. Enhancement of immune responses may be achieved by binding an appropriate antibody to the FcR of the effector cell simultaneously with the tumour target which would lead to antibody-directed cell-mediated cytotoxicity (ADCC) and lysis of the tumour. Alternatively, antibodies to CD2 or CD3 could activate LAK cells or T cells directly and ultimately induce antitumour effects via this activation. Additionally, INF could enhance expression of MHC molecules or tumour antigens themselves. Based on this understanding, a number of combination therapies are worthy of consideration, such as IL-2 and other biological response modifiers (e.g. INF and tumour necrosis factor), as well as combinations using monoclonal antibodies (MAbs) in addition to standard chemotherapy and radiotherapy regimens.

Specific strategies

IL-2 in combination with MAbs should represent a means of selectively enhancing the antitumour effects of IL-2, and this is under investigation. A potential problem is that humans will mount an anti-mouse response which could permit the antibody to bind to normal cells and increase toxicity. To circumvent these anti-mouse responses, chimeric antibodies with murine-derived binding sites and human-antibody constant regions have been developed, and these should avoid significant anti-mouse responses as well as improving FcR binding and, it is hoped, the ADCC potential.

Low-dose IL-2 will greatly enhance ADCC when used with antibodies directed against a number of tumour-associated antigens.[41,42] *In vitro* and murine data suggest that non-specific antibodies such as those against CD3 will also enhance IL-2 induced antitumour activity.

Molecularly engineered antibodies, designated 'heteroconjugates' or 'bifunctional antibodies', which have antigen binding sites with two different specificities, such as one for a tumour antigen and another for an effector cell surface molecule, such as CD2 or CD3, may have an important role in enhancing IL-2 induced lysis. With the advent of single-chain monoclonal antibody production in bacteria such as *E. coli* (which avoids laborious hybridoma production) in conjunction with the polymerase chain reaction which allows the rapid expansion of specific sequences, it should be possible to manufacture large quantities of MAb chimeras and hetero-conjugates to order. The clinical evaluation of these products together with IL-2 should prove rewarding.

IL-2 and INF and other BRMs

Antitumour synergy between INF and IL-2 has been reported in murine tumour models.[43,44] A number of clinical trials are now under way combining IL-2 with alpha, beta and gamma INFs. Other BRMs in combination with IL-2 are also under trial at a number of centres; these include IL-4 and tumour necrosis factor (TNF). TNF-α enhances antitumour responses in a number of animal models.[45]

IL-2 and chemotherapy

It has been suggested that cyclophosphamide has a selective antisuppressor cell effect which enhances the efficacy of IL-2 in murine models. Mitchell and colleagues have reported that pretreatment with cyclophosphamide allows outpatient administration of IL-2 in patients with melanoma with results as good as those of IL-2 and LAK, with considerably less toxicity.[46] It will also be interesting to look at the effect of standard chemotherapy regimens combined with IL-2 where chemotherapy is given initially to reduce tumour volume and then IL-2 to reduce residual disease. Such an approach is being tried in patients with leukaemia where there is a high chance of relapse.

Tumour infiltrating lymphocyte therapy (TIL)

Further refinements of IL-2 therapy include identifying those T cells which appear to be specific for tumour antigens and selectively expanding them *in vitro*. For some melanoma patients such tumour-specific lymphocytes have been found following IL-2 stimulated growth of lymphocytes found within the tumour. These tumour infiltrating lymphocytes are cultured and expanded *in vitro* and administered intravenously in the same way as LAK cells with IL-2. In their initial report, Rosenberg and colleagues reported exciting responses using this approach in patients with melanoma.[47] However, calculation of a true response rate is difficult as nearly 50% of patients who were eligible to be enrolled in this treatment and had a tumour biopsy performed to grow TIL cells were not able to subsequently receive the TIL therapy owing to poor cell harvest or tumour progression during *in vitro* expansion.

Although murine data suggest that TIL cells are up to 100 times more potent on a cell-to-cell basis than LAK cells at eliciting antitumour effects *in vivo*, this will need further detailed evaluation against experimental tumours, as there are currently no data suggesting analogous efficacy for TIL from renal cell cancers. In fact, the TIL obtained from renal cancers resemble peripheral blood derived LAK cells rather than tumour-specific T cells.

Antigen-specific tumour reactive T lymphocytes, unlike NK-derived LAK cells, theoretically have an advantage in that they should be specific for the tumour and bind to the tumour and not affect normal tissues. There is some evidence that this may be the case for melanomas. Experiments now being conducted at the NIH, Bethesda, USA, have labelled lymphocytes by gene transfer in order to assess the number or percentage of labelled cells that home to tumour tissue.

Local treatment

If tumour-specific lymphocytes mediate most of the antitumour activity, then exposing them alone to IL-2 could theoretically reduce the amount of IL-2 required. Local administration of IL-2 injected directly into the tumour has therefore been tried. Few tumours lend themselves to this approach. Using locally injected IL-2, Pizza and colleagues reported that 3 out of 6 patients with superficial bladder cancer underwent complete responses.[48] Further confirmation of this initial report is still required. Forni and colleagues have injected IL-2 into tumours of the head and neck and noted partial responses, particularly in those patients who had associated lymphadenopathy into which IL-2 was also injected.[49]

At Northwick Park Hospital (NPH) we are currently treating patients with advanced breast cancer with local injections of IL-2 into the tumour and their draining lymph nodes where accessible. Clearly this approach does not readily lend itself to RCC! Anecdotal observations suggest that IL-2 administered locally as well as systemically may have a role in sensitizing tumours to radiotherapy or chemotherapy, and it will be important to demonstrate or refute these observations before designing new protocols.

Local treatments using interferon injected into the base of warts or superficial carcinomas of the urogenital tract, such as cervical dysplasia, have also been tested experimentally. Great care must be taken in the case of cancer especially when more radical treatment is known to be curative in some of these conditions. Nevertheless, local administration may yet play an important role in treating accessible tumours especially if they sensitize the tumour to other therapies. Continuation of local therapy may also be tried, apart from IL-2 and interferon. Tumour necrosis factor (TNF) may be more useful locally than systemically, especially in combination with IL-2. As its name suggests, TNF causes central tumour necrosis whereas IL-2 induces antitumour activity mainly at the periphery. If significant advances do occur in local therapy it will still be necessary to improve systemic treatments in the majority of the tumours for which BRMs are being used at the present time, because of metastatic spread.

Conclusions

The most important questions to answer at the moment are how the modest benefit currently obtained using IL-2 can be augmented by combined approaches, and whether or not LAK activity is the primary mechanism for the antitumour effect of IL-2. It is of interest that responses may occur after IL-2 administration has ceased, which is reminiscent of the fact that most interferon responses may take at least 2–3 months using low-dose regimens. The totally unpredictable way one patient will undergo a complete response and another with the same tumour will maintain disease progression, in spite of treatment, argues strongly for other selective factors which govern responses to BRMs. It would be extremely useful if some assay could differentiate between patients likely and unlikely to respond to a certain therapy. Combination therapies using low-dose IL-2 and TNF are now under trial in a variety of tumours at a number of centres throughout the world. The results will be awaited with interest. The results of other combinations with chemotherapy, radiotherapy and monoclonal antibodies will also be known over the next few years, and it can only be hoped that these will lead to a significant benefit in tumour response. In the meantime, a persistent problem in the use of high-dose IL-2 is the toxicity with its concomitant need for hospitalization. Our experience suggests lower doses ($3 \times 10^6 U/m^2/d$) can be given in the hospital without requiring intensive care support. Even lower doses ($1-2 \times 10^6 U/m^2/d$) can be well tolerated on an outpatient basis. IL-2 dose titrations, either up or down, should be based on individual patient tolerance.[40]

If IL-2 combined with other approaches has a place in the treatment of urological cancer it may not necessarily be due solely to maximizing 'LAK' activity by high-dose IL-2, but may include more subtle effects on the immune system that might allow less toxic IL-2 regimens to be combined with other treatments as effective therapy.

References

1. Freed SZ, Halperin JP, Gordon M. Idiopathic regression of metastases from renal cell carcinoma. *J Virol* 1977; **118**: 538–42.
2. Quesada JR. Biologic response modifiers in the therapy of metastatic renal cell carcinoma. *Sem Onc* 1988; **15**, 396–407.
3. Isaacs A, Hindemann J. Virus interference. 1: The interferon. *Proc R Soc Lond (Biol)* 1957; **147**: 258–67.
4. Trotta PP. Preclinical biology of alpha interferons. *Sem Onc* 1986; **13** (suppl 2): 3–12.
5. Taylor-Papadimitriou J. Effects of interferons on cell growth and function. In: Billiau A (ed.), *Interferon: General and Applied Aspects*. Amsterdam: Elsevier, 1984: 139–66.
6. Vikek J, DeMacyer E (eds). *Interferons and the Immune System*, vol. 2. New York: Elsevier, 1984.
7. Muss H. The role of biological response modifiers in metastatic renal cell carcinoma. *Sem Onc* 1988; **15**: 30–4.
8. Steis RG, Smith JW, Urba WJ. Resistance to recombinant interferon alpha-2a in hairy cell leukaemia associated with neutralising anti-interferon antibodies. *N Engl J Med* 1988; **318**: 1409–13.
9. Figlin RA, deKernion JB, Maldazys J, Sarna G. Treatment of renal cell carcinoma with α (human leukocyte) interferon and vinblastine in combination: a phase I–II trial. *Cancer Treat Rep* 1985; **69**: 263–7.
10. Bergerat JP, Herbrecht R, Dufour P, *et al.* Combination of recombinant interferon alpha-2A and vinblastine in advanced renal cell cancer. *Cancer* 1988; **62**: 2320–4.
11. Malkovsky M, Sondel PM, Strober W, Dalgleish AG. The interleukins in acquired disease. *Clin Exp Immunol* 1988; **74**: 151–61.
12. Morgan DA, Ruscetti FW, Grallow R. Selective *in vitro* growth of T-lymphocytes from normal human bone marrows. *Science* 1978; **193**: 1007–8.
13. Smith KA. Interleukin-2: inception, impact and implications. *Science* 1988; **240**: 1169–76.
14. Dalgleish AG, Malkovsky M. Advances in human retroviruses. In: Klein G, Weinhouse P (eds), *Advances in Cancer Research*, vol. 51. New York: Raven Press, 1988: 307–60.
15. Shu S, Clion T, Rosenberg SA. Generation from tumour bearing mice lymphocytes with *in vivo* therapeutic efficacy. *J Immunol* 1987; **139**: 295–304.
16. Cheever MA, Greenberg PD, Fefer A, Gillis S. Augmentation of the antitumour therapeutic efficacy of long-term cultured T-lymphocytes by *in vivo* administration of purified interleukin-2. *J Exp Med* 1982; **155**: 968–80.
17. Borden EC, Sondel PM. Lymphokines and cytokines as cancer treatment: immunotherapy realised (in press).
18. Voss SD, Weil Hillman G, Hank J, Sosman J, Sondel PM. The clinical immunobiology of IL-2: potential modified uses for improved cancer treatment (in press).
19. Grimm EA, Mazumder A, Zhang HZ, *et al.* The lymphokine-activated killer cell phenomenon: lysis of NK-resistant fresh solid tumour cells by IL-2 activated autologous human peripheral blood lymphocytes. *J Exp Med* 1982; **155**: 1823–41.
20. Phillips JH, Lanier LL. Dissection of the lymphokine-activated killer phenomenon: relative contribution of peripheral blood natural killer cells and T lymphocytes to cytolysis. *J Exp Med* 1986; **164**: 814–25.
21. Mule JJ, Shu S, Schwartz SL, *et al.* Adoptive immunotherapy of established metastases with LAK cells and recombinant interleukin-2. *Science* 1984; **225**: 1487–9.

22. Rosenberg SA, Mule JJ, Spiess PJ, *et al.* Regression of established pulmonary metastases and subcutaneous tumour mediated by the systemic administration of high dose recombinant interleukin-2. *J Exp Med* 1985; **161**: 1169–88.

23. Thompson JA, Peace DJ, Klarnet JP, *et al.* Eradication of disseminated murine leukaemia by treatment with high-dose interleukin-2. *J Immunol* 1986; **137**: 3675–80.

24. Peace DJ, Cheever MA. Toxicity and therapeutic efficacy of high dose interleukin-2: *in vivo* infusion of antibody to NK attenuates toxicity without compromising efficacy against murine leukaemia. *J Exp Med* 1989; **169**: 161–73.

25. Bubenik J, Indrova M. The anti-tumour efficacy of human recombinant interleukin-2: correlation between sensitivity of tumours to the cytolytic effect of LAK cells *in vitro* and their susceptibility to interleukin-2 immunotherapy *in vivo*. *Cancer Immunol Immunother* 1987; **24**: 269–71.

26. Talmadge JE, Phillips H, Schindler J, Tribble H. Systemic preclinical study on the therapeutic properties of recombinant IL-2 for the treatment of metastatic disease. *Cancer Res* 1987; **47**: 5725–32.

27. Ettinghausen SE, Rosenberg SA. Immunotherapy of murine sarcomas using lymphokine activated killer cells: optimization of the schedule and route of administration of recombinant IL-2. *Cancer Res* 1986; **46**: 2784–92.

28. Rosenberg SA, Lotze MT, Muul LM, *et al.* Observations on the systemic administration of autologous lymphokine activated killer cells and recombinant IL-2 to patients with metastatic cancer. *N Engl J Med* 1985; **313**: 1485–92.

29. Rosenberg SA, Lotze MT, Muul LM, *et al.* A progress report on the treatment of 157 patients with advanced cancer using lymphokine-activated killer cells and interleukin-2 or high dose interleukin-2 alone. *N Engl J Med* 1987; **316**: 889–97.

30. West WH, Tauer KW, Yannelli JR, *et al.* Constant infusion recombinant interleukin-2 in adoptive immunotherapy of advanced cancer. *N Engl J Med* 1987; **316**: 898–905.

31. Schoof DD, Gramolini BA, Davidson DL, *et al.* Adoptive immunotherapy of human cancer using low-dose recombinant interleukin-2 and lymphokine activated killer cells. *Cancer Res* 1988; **48**: 5007–10.

32. Fisher RI, Coltman CA, Doroshow JH, *et al.* Metastatic renal cancer treated with interleukin-2 and lymphokine-activated killer cells: a phase II clinical trial. *Ann Int Med* 1988; **108**: 518–23.

33. Dutcher JP, Creekmore S, Weiss GR, *et al.* A phase II study of interleukin-2 and lymphokine-activated killer cells in patients with metastatic malignant melanoma. *J Clin Oncol* 1989; **7**: 477–85.

34. Phillips JH, Gemlo BT, Myers WW, *et al. In vivo* and *in vitro* activation of natural killer cells in advanced cancer patients undergoing recombinant interleukin-2 and LAK cell therapy. *J Clin Oncol* 1987; **5**: 1933–41.

35. Sondel PM, Kohler PC, Hank JA, *et al.* II: Clinical and immunologic effects of Recombinant IL-2 given by repetitive weekly cycles in patients with cancer. *Can Res* 1988; **48** (9): 2561–7.

36. Sosman JA, Kohler PC, Hank JA, *et al.* Repetitive weekly cycles of interleukin-2. II: Clinical and immunologic effects of dose, schedule, and addition of indomethacin. *J Natl Cancer Inst* 1988; **80**: 1451–61.

37. Albertini MR, Sosman JA, Hank JA, *et al.* The influence of autologous LAK cell infusions on the toxicity and antitumour effect of repetitive cycles of IL-2. *Cancer* 1990; **66**: 2457–64.

38. Sosman JA, Kohler PC, Hank JA, *et al.* Repetitive weekly cycles of recombinant human

interleukin-2: responses of renal carcinoma with acceptable toxicity. *J Natl Cancer Inst* 1988; **80**: 60–4.

39.   Hank JA, Kohler PC, Hillman GW, *et al. In vivo* induction of the lymphokine-activated killer (LAK) cells generated *in vivo* during administration of human recombinant IL-2. *Cancer Res* 1988; **48**: 1965–72.

40.   Goldstein D, Sosman JA, Hank JA, *et al.* Repetitive weekly cycles of interleukin-2 (IL-2): the effect of outpatient treatment with a lower dose of IL-2 on non-MHC restricted killer activity. *Cancer Res* 1989; **49**: 6832–9.

41.   Kawase I, Komuta K, Hara H, *et al.* Combined therapy of mice bearing a lymphokine-activated killer-resistant tumour with recombinant interleukin-2 and an anti-tumour monoclonal antibody capable of inducing antibody-dependent cellular cytotoxicity. *Cancer Res* 1988; **48**: 1173–9.

42.   Hank JA, Robinson RR, Surfus J, Mueller BM, Reisfeld RA, Kong-Cheung N, Sondel P. Augmentation of antibody dependent cell mediated cytotoxicity following *in vivo* therapy with recombinant interleukin-2. *Can Res* 1990; **50** (17): 5234–9.

43.   Agah R, Malloy B, Sherrod A, *et al.* Successful therapy of natural killer-resistant pulmonary metastases by the synergism of γ-interferon with tumour necrosis factor and interleukin-2. *Cancer Res* 1988; **48**: 2245–8.

44.   Zimmerman RJ, Gavny S, Chan A, *et al.* Sequence dependence of administration of human recombinant tumor necrosis factor and IL-2 in murine tumor therapy. *J Natl Cancer Inst (USA)* 1989; **81**: 227–31.

45.   McIntosh JK, Mule JJ, Merino MJ, *et al.* Synergistic anti-tumour effects of immunotherapy with recombinant interleukin-2 and recombinant tumour necrosis factor-α. *Cancer Res* 1988; **48**: 4011–17.

46.   Mitchell MS, Kempf RA, Harel W, *et al.* Effectiveness and tolerability of low-dose cyclophosphamide and low-dose intravenous interleukin-2 in disseminated melanoma. *J Clin Oncol* 1988; **6**: 409–25.

47.   Rosenberg SA, Packard BS, Aebersold PM, *et al.* Use of tumour-infiltrating lympho-cytes and interleukin-2 in the immunotherapy of patients with metastatic melanoma: a preliminary report. *N Engl J Med* 1988; **319**: 1676–80.

48.   Pizza G, Severini G, Menmiti D, De Vinci C, Corrado. Tumour progression after intralesional infection of IL-2 in bladder cancer: preliminary report. *Int J Cancer* 1984; **34**: 359–67.

49.   Cortesina G, Stefani A, Grovarelli M, *et al.* Treatment of recurrent squamous cell carcinoma of the head and neck with low doses of IL-2 injected perilymphatically. *Cancer* 1988; **62**: 2482–5.

17 Embolization of the kidney

Tetsuro Kato

Arterial embolization of renal cell cancer has been practised since the early 1970s. The anatomical features of the kidney allow a ready access to the renal artery by percutaneous catheterization under radiographic monitoring. Since renal cell carcinoma is relatively resistant to chemotherapy as well as to radiotherapy, and most tumours have a hypervascular structure which might be well controlled by an ischaemic manoeuvre, many urologists have employed this technique of vascular occlusion as a means of tumour control.[1]

Embolization has been used preoperatively to facilitate nephrectomy, by decreasing operative time and blood loss, and as a palliative measure to control symptoms such as pain and haemorrhage. It has also been used to enhance other therapies such as hyperthermia, chemotherapy or immunotherapy, to stimulate the host–immune response, and as an adjunct to intravascular targeting of anticancer drugs.

A variety of embolic materials and techniques have been investigated to improve treatment and these include mechanical embolization, chemoembolization and radioembolization. Mechanical embolization as introduced by Almgard and associates[2] simply involves devascularization with embolic or sclerosing materials. Chemoembolization utilizes a drug-carrier complex, which is designed to act as both an embolic material and a controlled drug-release device.[3-6] Radioembolization is an approach to interstitial irradiation by radioactive seeds which are intra-arterially infused and lodged in the tumour vascular beds.[7]

Despite early enthusiasm, the place of embolization remains controversial and its use often regarded sceptically.[8] This may be attributed in part to a lack of systematic studies. Despite the controversies and scepticism, this treatment modality remains in current practice. In this chapter the author reviews the other investigators' and his own experiences, describing the present and future role of embolization.

Methods

Embolization is currently practised by percutaneous arterial catheterization under fluoroscopic monitoring. It is essential to identify all of the tumour feeding arteries by aortography, in order to achieve a substantial therapeutic response. A localized, small tumour is usually fed by an intrarenal branch of the renal artery, while an invasive, large tumour often has well-developed parasitic arteries. All of these feeding arteries should be individually treated.

The aim of mechanical embolization is complete and permanent devascularization. Muscle chips, blood clots and other autologous tissues of patients were first used as embolic material, but were inconvenient. Subsequently, various synthetic materials were introduced. Among them, Gelfoam (solidified gelatin), a haemostatic material in surgery, has been most commonly used. Though this biodegradable material is convenient to use, recanalization usually occurs within a few weeks. Accordingly, non-absorbable materials were investigated. These included isobutyl-2-cyanoacrylate,[9] polyvinyl alcohol[10] and steel coils.[11] However, these solid materials do not achieve peripheral devascularization. Finally, liquid materials such as ethanol[12] and an oily contrast medium[13] were employed. Ethanol acts as a sclerosing agent. The oily contrast medium remains preferentially in tumour vascular beds and can be used as a visual marker of the embolized area. It should be recognized that complete occlusion of main feeding arteries often promotes the development of a collateral circulation (Fig. 17.1).

Chemoembolization is achieved by using a drug-carrier complex which acts as both an embolic material and a drug-release device. The early experience of the author revealed that the simple combination of embolization and intra-arterial chemotherapy failed to provide a substantial enhancement of therapeutic effect due to rapid efflux of the drug.[4,5] The author and associates developed ethylcellulose microencapsulated mitomycin C (MMC microcapsules) with a mean diameter of approximately 200μm, which can be infused through an arterial catheter. The ethylcellulose membrane is a semipermeable structure, releasing the encased drug at a prescribed rate when in contact with body fluids. The intra-arterially infused microcapsules are entrapped by the arteriolar beds and slowly release the drug into the surrounding parenchyma. Both the arteriolar haemostasis and the sustained-release properties of the microcapsules will enhance the preferential distribution of the drug within the target sites, and the destruction of the vascular as well as perivascular structure will promote the intra-parenchymal drug migration. In addition, the preferential activation of mitomycin C in hypoxic conditions[14] will make MMC microcapsules the best candidate for chemoembolization. These possible advantages were demonstrated by animal and clinical studies, being reflected by an enhancement of antitumour effects and a decrease in systemic drug toxicity.[3–6,15]

Where selective catheterization is possible, chemoembolization can be applied to various tumour lesions. But, for tumours which have arteriovenous fistulae, the fistulae should be occluded by mechanical embolization prior to micro-capsule infusion to prevent efflux of microcapsules. Thus in the majority of cases

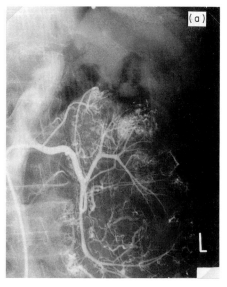

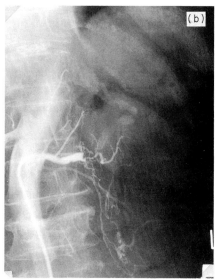

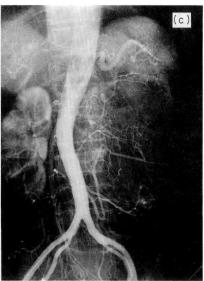

Fig. 17.1 Angiograms of left renal cell carcinoma (*a*) before, (*b*) immediately after, and (*c*) three weeks after Gelfoam embolization. The tumour vascular beds completely disappeared by occlusion of the renal artery (*b*), but the aortogram three weeks after embolization showed development of collateral circulations which resulted in regrowth of the tumour.

of renal cell carcinoma, microcapsule chemoembolization should be preceded by Gelfoam embolization. The occlusion of fistulae should be kept at a minimum, so as to leave the peripheral vascular beds for the microcapsules and prevent the development of collateral circulations. Chemoembolization can also be performed with other drug-carrier complexes which have the same function as that of microcapsules.[16]

Radioembolization is carried out by transcatheter arterial infusion of radioactive particles. Lang used ^{125}I seeds with a size of 0.8 × 4.3 mm and applied a fractionated infusion to obtain homogeneous radiation.[7] Unfortunately, this technique has not been repeated by other institutions.

With all of these methods, outflow of the embolic materials should be avoided by careful radiographic monitoring. The arteriovenous fistulae should be closed by a large volume of embolic material such as Gelfoam pieces or steel coils. Movement of embolic material can be prevented by using a balloon catheter together with contrast medium. Despite such precautions, distant embolization has been experienced which, fortunately, in the majority of the cases has not been symptomatic or fatal. Large embolic materials which embolize a proximal portion of the affected area will allow the development of collateral circulations. On the other hand, ethanol or tiny materials such as Gelfoam particulates with a particle size less than 10 μm cause peripheral embolization, and may result in serious and fatal infarction in the affected normal tissues such as the intestine.[17]

Antitumour effect

There were initial hopes of achieving complete responses of tumours by devascularization. In fact, many urologists felt that the reduction in tumour mass after embolization was more significant than that obtained by chemotherapy or external irradiation. Unfortunately, it was soon recognized that the prompt tumour response mainly comes from the reduction of vascular beds of the hypervascular tumours.

Mebust and associates[18] reported the results of treatment of 27 patients who were subjected to mechanical embolization with Gelfoam pieces and steel coils. Twenty (75%) of these patients had a tumour reduction of about 30%, but the others had no tumour reduction. Kaisary and associates[19] employed the same method in the treatment of 49 patients. Surgical specimens revealed that there remained histologically viable tumour cells in 34 cases (70%). In general, the necrotic changes caused by embolization are proportional to the degree of devascularization,[20] but tumour tissues seem to be more resistant to embolization than the normal renal tissues. The tumour resistance to devascularization was suggested by a histological study[21] as well as an *in vitro* culture system.[22]

Ethanol embolization was expected to produce infarction of the whole kidney including tumours. However, Klimberg and associates[23] found that tumour infarction was not complete in 25 cases treated by ethanol embolization, despite the fact that renal blood flow was completely blocked in all of the cases.

A preliminary study on MMC microcapsule chemoembolization combined with Gelfoam embolization showed that a substantial tumour reduction of greater than 50% in area was found in 68% of 22 tumours thus treated, while Gelfoam embolization combined with conventional MMC infusion failed to provide such a substantial response in 10 tumours examined.[5] This result indicated the superiority of MMC microcapsule chemoembolization over conventional embolization, though the evaluation was based on the combined findings of radiograms, echograms and surgical specimens. Subsequent analysis based on CT scans[24] showed that MMC microcapsule chemoembolization exerted an objective tumour remission of greater than 50% in 8 (26%) of 31 tumours (Fig. 17.2) and a tumour remission of less than 50% but greater than 25% in 10 (32%).

Review of the available data will show the limitations of achieving tumour eradication by devascularization alone. This is attributable either to incomplete

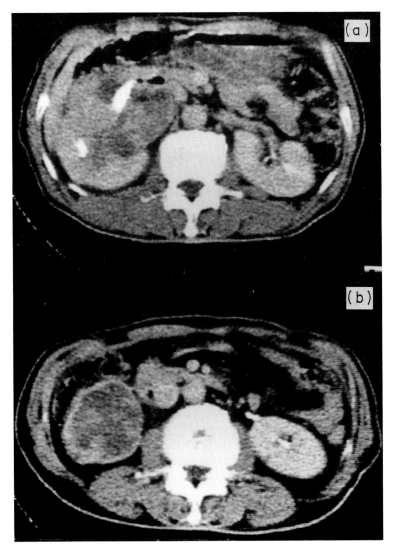

Fig. 17.2   CT scans of right renal cell carcinoma (*a*) before and (*b*) four weeks after MMC microcapsule chemoembolization. A marked tumour reduction in association with visualization of the inferior vena cava was achieved.

peripheral embolization, recanalization of the occluded vessels, difficulty in embolizing the collateral vessels, development of a collateral circulation due to neoplastic angiogenesis, a high resistance of tumour cells to ischaemia, or a combination of all factors.[2] These problems could possibly be overcome by combining embolization with other therapeutic manoeuvres, so that a better response might be obtained.

Palliative measures

Renal cell carcinoma typically tends to metastasize to bone, causing intractable pain. Although radiotherapy is the common treatment for osseous metastases, embolization is also of value. Devascularization of the feeding arteries of osseous lesions has been reported to provide a remarkable improvement in symptoms such as pain and neurological disorders in the majority of patients treated, although the number of patients treated were small.[25–27]

Lang[28] treated 77 patients by radioembolization utilizing ^{125}I seeds. He stated that 40 patients with osseous metastases fared better than 37 patients with metastases to other sites. Remission of tumour activity was experienced in 55% of the patients with osseous metastases for two years and 38% for five years. The best results were encountered in 11 patients with solitary osseous metastases; remission of tumour activity was 60% for two years and 40% for five years.

Courtheoux and associates[29] applied MMC microcapsule chemoembolization to thoracic and lumbar spine metastases in nine patients, the primary tumour in two patients being renal cell carcinoma. The treatment was fractionated two or three times. All patients obtained remarkable improvement of symptoms. In eight patients, pain completely resolved in seven and decreased in one. Furthermore, motor-sensory disorders were improved in five patients. Extensive biopsy specimens in two patients showed no tumour cells in one and only a few tumour cells in the other. The author treated two patients who had radio-resistant osseous metastases of the femur (Fig. 17.3) or the pelvis. In both cases, the severe pain at the metastatic site subsided within a few days of chemoembolization and the effect persisted for more than four months. None of the eleven patients in both series experienced any complications or side-effects.

Arterial catheterization for metastatic lesions often requires a skilful technique, but is successful in most cases especially for solitary osseous metastases. Considering the high response rate, embolization is a worthwhile practice in the treatment of osseous metastases. The degree and duration of therapeutic effects by chemoembolization and radioembolization are likely to be superior to mechanical embolization.

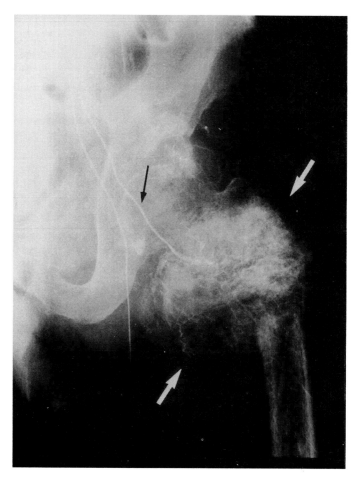

Fig. 17.3   Selective arteriogram of a metastasis from right renal cell carcinoma to the left femoral head. Infusion of MMC microcapsules reduced the severe pain which was resistant to radiotherapy.

Chemoembolization as an aid to surgery

Many urologists have the impression that preoperative embolization facilitates nephrectomy, especially for a larger tumour, by decreasing the vascularity and creating perinephric oedema.[8,23,30,31] Reduction of operative time and blood loss have been reported,[32,33] while such an advantage was not supported by others.[18,30] The reports disregard such factors as the stage and vascularity of individual tumours, the degree of devascularization, the interval to nephrectomy and/or the surgical skill of individual urologists. Some urologists seem to be prejudiced against embolization because of its morbidity and the delay in nephrectomy.

The author's experience of MMC microcapsule chemoembolization is as follows.

The mean intraoperative blood loss was 364 ± 112 (SD) millilitres in cases with the preoperative adjuvant embolization and 659 ± 509 ml in the cases without.[24] The mean weight of the surgical specimens was 493 g for the former group and 408 g for the latter, and all of the surgery was done by the same surgeon. These data support the benefit of preoperative chemoembolization with respect to decrease of tumour bulk.

This preoperative manipulation is useful for highly invasive tumours which may be initially considered as inoperable. The author treated four patients with huge tumours of the right kidney which were directly invading the caval wall. Chemo-embolization repeated two to five times at monthly intervals led to a marked reduction of the primary lesion, so that radical surgery was considered to be possible. At surgery, access to the vessels was relatively easy because of shrinkage of the tumour. The renal vessels were first identified. The intracaval tumour was removed with the associated caval wall, the defects of the cava were patched with an artificial vascular graft, and finally a nephrectomy was performed. Ligation or transection of the interior vena cava was not needed. Of the four patients, three are alive without tumour at 1, 4, and 10 years after surgery, and one died of cancer at 18 months.

Metastatic lesions, especially osseous metastases, are also a candidate for preoperative embolization. Roscoe and associates[34] applied this technique to eight patients with spinal metastases. Effective devascularization was achieved in six patients, resulting in a significant reduction of intraoperative blood loss. The average blood loss in the eight patients was 940 ml, compared with 1975 ml in 20 non-embolized patients. They claimed that preoperative embolization of spinal metastases, though it demands technical skills, is effective in devascularizing these lesions without serious neurological complications.

The experiences of these other investigators and this author support the efficacy and safety of preoperative embolization and/or chemoembolization for primary as well as metastatic lesions. This technique is a most effective preoperative measure for highly invasive and haemorrhagic lesions.

Immunological response

Since the suggestion by Almgard and associates,[2] stimulation of the immune system by embolization or subsequent tumour necrosis has attracted the attention of many investigators. If the immune system were enhanced, embolization could play an important role in the treatment of this disease. Wallace and associates[35] described an enhancement of delayed cutaneous reaction, but this was not confirmed by others.[19] Bakke and associates[36] found increased natural killer (NK) cell activity for 96 hours after embolization, and speculated that it might be related to the production of interferon resulting from macrophage activation due to tumour necrosis. Johnson and Kalland[37] also found elevated NK cell activity following devascularization of experimental renal tumours. Wright and associates[38] showed that the reticuloendothelial system was stimulated when embolization was combined with intra-arterial injection of BCG, and suggested that this method might be valuable for advanced renal cell carcinomas. In addition, increase of T cell population,[39] lymphocyte transformation[40] and monocyte to macrophage maturation[18] were found in some cases where embolization was followed by nephrectomy either alone or in combination with chemotherapy.

Sato and associates[41] showed that NK cell activity and OKT4/8 ratios in the peripheral blood were continuously augmented in 67% and 83% of the patients, respectively, for up to four weeks after microcapsule chemoembolization. In the patients with enhancement of these immunological parameters, the mature NK cell population (Leu7$^-$OKT16$^+$) also showed a continuous increase for four weeks after chemoembolization. These findings indicate that chemoembolization increases NK cell activity in association with OKT$^+$T cell activation and, at the same time, enhances maturation of NK cells in approximately two-thirds of the patients.

Swanson and associates[42] subjected 100 patients with stage IV disease to embolization in combination with delayed nephrectomy and progesterone administration. They found beneficial responses to the metastatic lesions in 28 of these patients; complete remission in 7 patients; partial remission in 8; and stable disease for more than one year in 13. It should be noted that all of the lesions in the responders were pulmonary metastases. The survival of 28 responders was significantly higher than that of the remaining 72 non-responders. Dreikorn and associates[43] also reported a case of complete remission of lung metastases after similar therapy. Kaisary and associates[19] found no response in metastatic lesions, but suggested a prolonged survival by embolization and delayed nephrectomy. These reports, which suggested an augmentation of the immune system by embolization, stimulated the interest of other investigators. They failed to confirm any therapeutic responses to this kind of therapy.[18,30,44–46] Unfortunately, no controlled study has been performed.

The author has not seen any response of metastatic lesions to chemoembolization. However, retrospective analysis of 66 patients with stage IV disease, who were subject to chemoembolization, appeared to provide some suggestion of an effect.[2,24] Of these, 23 patients received some biological response modifiers (BRM) such as an inactivated streptococcus preparation (OK-432) or interferon, while the other 43 received no BRM. Nephrectomy was performed in 7 patients (30%) of the BRM group and 17 (39%) of the non-BRM group. The survival of the BRM group (median survival, 12 months) was significantly better ($p = 0.02$) than that of the non-BRM group (median survival, 5 months). It may be that the combination of BRM administration with chemoembolization of the primary lesions promoted an immunologic response which resulted in the prolongation of survival.

The available data indicate that tumour necrosis by devascularization may in some cases affect the immune system. The immune response may be determined by the degree of infarction in the tumour tissue in relation to normal renal tissues and individual responsiveness. Generally the immune response is ineffective in producing significant remission of visible tumours or improved patient survival, but it may control micrometastases and so delay the progression of disease.

Effect on survival

Embolization has been widely employed as a preoperative measure for stages I to III tumours with a hope that this treatment might improve the prognosis after nephrectomy. But there have been very few systematic studies which analysed the outcome of patients.

Guiliani and associates[46] reported 104 patients who underwent nephrectomy with or without preoperative embolization. They found no significant difference in the relative mortality, of 1.10 in 73 patients with embolization and 0.87 in 31 without embolization, and concluded that embolization did not affect the postoperative survival. Kaisary and associates[19] found postnephrectomy metastases in one of 18 patients with stage I disease, 3 of 9 with stage II and 3 of 5 with stage III, and doubted the adjuvant effect of preoperative embolization. Klimberg and associates[23] seemed to support the effect of embolization, but they did not present data to be discussed.

The results of MMC microcapsule chemoembolization were as follows. Abe and associates[47] reported the results of 43 patients who had stages I to III disease and underwent nephrectomy after chemoembolization during the period from 1978 to 1983, comparing them with a control group of 52 patients who underwent nephrectomy without chemoembolization during the period 1971 to 1983. The survival rate of stage I patients did not differ significantly between the two groups, while the survival rates of the stage II and III chemoembolization group were significantly better than those of the corresponding control group. Subsequently, the author analysed the survival of 102 patients who had stages I to III disease and underwent nephrectomy during the period 1978 to 1986. Sixty-eight of these patients received preoperative chemoembolization, while 34 did not. A single chemoembolization was performed in 80% of the 68 patients and repeated 2–5 times in the others. The median total dose of the microcapsules expressed as mitomycyn C activity was 20 mg with a range of 5–120 mg, and the median interval to nephrectomy was 19 days with a range of 1–183 days. Again, there was no difference in survival rate between the two groups of stage I patients, but the survival rate of the stage II and III chemoembolized group was significantly improved as compared with that of the controls (Fig. 17.4). These retrospective studies may indicate the adjuvant advantage of preoperative chemoembolization in terms of survival.

The trend for an improved prognosis for invasive tumours by chemoembolization may be due to the increased ease of curative surgery due to tumour reduction, sterilization of intraoperative tumour dissemination, cytostatic or cytocidal effects on micrometastases due to drug release into the systemic circulation,[4] or the augmented immune response,[41] or combinations of all these effects. However, as shown in the survival curves, an adjuvant effect of chemoembolization decreased as time passed (Fig. 17.4), implying only an early advantage to this technique.

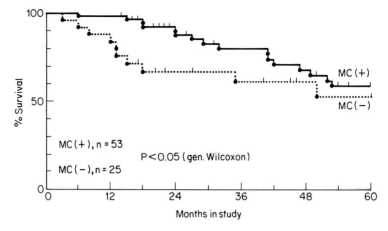

Fig. 17.4 Survival curves of stages II and III renal cell carcinomas after nephrectomy. The survival of the group with preoperative MMC microcapsule chemoembolization (MC+) was significantly better than that of the group without the adjuvant (MC−). Both groups were treated during 1978 to 1986.

Side-effects and complications

The postembolization syndrome, which includes local pain, fever and abdominal symptoms such as nausea and vomiting, is a common occurrence. The syndrome is proportional to the completeness of devascularization, especially in the normal renal tissue. When the tumour is selectively embolized, the syndrome is mild and usually lasts for approximately one week. Since the pain is often severe it may need to be controlled by epidural anaesthesia. The patient and the family should be informed of these expected side-effects.

Laboratory tests show a leukocytosis, elevations of serum enzymes such as glutamic-pyruvic transaminase, glutamicoxaloacetic transaminase and lactic dehydrogenase and an increase of erythrocyte sedimentation rate. Mebust and associates[18] reported that in 72% of the patients, serum creatinine levels rose transiently by 0.6 mg on average after embolization. Renal failure, which relates to the dose of contrast medium and contralateral renal function,[8,24] is uncommon. However, hydration should be performed to encourage excretion of the contrast medium.

Distant embolization by the inadvertent outflow of embolic materials is the most serious complication. Fortunately, in most cases where relatively larger embolic materials were used, distant embolization was asymptomatic, and manageable.[48–50] On the other hand, smaller or liquid embolic materials are hazardous and may result in irreversible or lethal complication. Tragic cases, where extensive intestinal necrosis occurred by retrograde regurgitation of Gelfoam particulates[51] and ethanol,[18,52] have been reported. Since this kind of complication could not be prevented even with careful manipulation utilizing a balloon catheter, Mebust and associates[18] warned against the use of ethanol.

Of 173 patients who underwent MMC microcapsule chemoembolization in combination with Gelfoam embolization, fever occurred in 65% of the patients, pain in 58%, gastrointestinal discomfort in 35%, abnormal renal and hepatic function in 17%, and myelosuppression in 24%, but all were reversible. The fever, pain and gastrointestinal symptoms were considered attributable mainly to the concomitant Gelfoam embolization. Distant embolization was observed in five patients (3%), but they were asymptomatic. All patients tolerated the treatment well.

The mortality of embolization was reported to be 2–3%,[53,54] and the majority of the lethal complications were encountered in the patients who had other serious underlying diseases or suffered from contralateral necrosis due to the excess dose of contrast medium. This author has experienced no lethal complications in 173 patients subjected to chemoembolization in combination with Gelfoam embolization. Recent advances in techniques have significantly decreased the mortality and made the overall complication rate acceptable.

Conclusions

Both the biological diversity of renal cell carcinoma and the lack of controlled studies make a true analysis of the effects of new treatment modalities difficult to evaluate. This is also true of embolization. A review of the literature and the author's experience imply only a limited antitumour effect of mechanical embolization. It should be recognized that a complete and persistent devascularization can be rarely achieved in invasive tumours, and the tumours are usually resistant to ischaemia. Chemoembolization has been developed to overcome these problems.

However, mechanical embolization often provides definite benefit as a preoperative measure for invasive and haemorrhagic primary and metastatic lesions, reducing the surgical morbidity. In addition some tumours, initially considered inoperable, may become operable. This treatment is also useful for control of painful osseous metastases, even if the tumours are resistant to radiotherapy. These advantages, which seem greater with chemoembolization, require wider acceptance.

The influence of embolization on survival is still uncertain. Preoperative mechanical embolization seems not to improve the prognosis of stage I to III disease. There has been no study of whether embolization will prolong the survival of stage IV disease or not. Although mechanical embolization may stimulate the immune system in a proportion of patients, changes in immune parameters do not reflect tumour response and survival. It may be that the combination of embolization with other therapies such as nephrectomy, hormones or biological response modifiers will affect the survival, and this requires verification in future controlled studies.

MMC microcapsule chemoembolization exerts an enhanced antitumour effect as compared with mechanical embolization and improves survival of patients with stage II and III disease. This effect comes mainly from the drug action on the kidney as the effect of devascularization by the capsular material is relatively small. Over ten years of experience suggest that this kind of cancer therapy may have application to other malignant tumours.

References

1. Kato T, Sato K, Abe R, Moriyama M. The role of embolization/chemoembolization in the treatment of renal cell carcinoma. In: Murphy GP, Khoury S (eds), *Therapeutic Progress in Urological Cancers*. New York; Alan R Liss, 1989: 697–705.
2. Almgard LE, Fernstrom I, Havering M, Ljungquist A. Treatment of renal carcinoma by embolic occlusion of the renal circulation. *Br J Urol* 1973; **45**: 474–9.
3. Kato T, Nemoto R. Microencapsulation of mitomycin C for intra-arterial infusion chemotherapy. *Proc Jpn Acad* 1978; **54**(B): 413–17.
4. Kato T, Nemoto R, Mori H, Kumagai I. Sustained-release properties of microencapsulated mitomycin C with ethyl-cellulose infused into the renal artery of the dog. *Cancer* 1980; **46**: 15–21.
5. Kato T, Nemoto R, Mori II, Takahashi M, Tamakawa Y. Transcathcter artcrial chemoembolization of renal cell carcinoma with microencapsulated mitomycin C. *J Urol* 1981; **125**: 19–24.
6. Kato T, Nemoto R, Takahashi M, Tamakawa Y, Harada M. Arterial chemoembolization with microencapsulated anticancer drug: an approach to selective cancer chemotherapy with sustained effects. *JAMA* 1981; **245**: 1123–7.
7. Lang EK. Superselective arterial catheterization as a vehicle for delivering infarcts. *Radiology* 1971; **98**: 391–9.
8. Williams G. Angioinfarction in renal adenocarcinoma. In: deKernion JB, Pavone-Macalusso (eds), *Tumor of the Kidney*. Baltimore: Williams & Wilkins, 1986.
9. Dotter CT, Goldman ML, Roesch J. Instant selective arterial occlusion with isobutyl-2-cyanoacrylate. *Radiology* 1975; **115**: 227–30.
10. Chuang VP, Soo CS, Wallace S. Ivalon embolization in abdominal neoplasms. *Am J Roentgenol* 1981; **136**: 729—33.
11. Gianturco C, Anderson JH, Wallace S. Mechanical devices for arterial occlusion. *Am J Roentgenol* 1975; **124**: 428–35.
12. Ellman BA, Parkhill BJ, Curry TS, Marcus PB, Peters PC. Ablation of renal tumours with absolute ethanol: a new technique. *Radiology* 1981; **151**: 619–29.
13. Konno T, Maeda H, Iwai K, Tashiro S, Maki S, Morinaga M, Hiraoka T, Yokoyama I. Effect of arterial administration of high molecular weight anticancer agent SMANCS with lipid lymphographic agent on hepatoma. *Eur J Cancer Clin Onc* 1983; **19**: 1052–65.
14. Kennedy KA, Rockwell S, Sartorelli AC. Preferential activation of mitomycin C to cytotoxic metabolite by hypoxic tumor cell. *Cancer Res* 1980; **40**: 2356–60.
15. Kato T. Encapsulated drugs in targeted cancer therapy. In: Bruck SD (ed.), *Controlled Drug Delivery*, vol. 2. Boca Raton, FL: CRC Press, 1983.
16. Fujimoto S, Miyazaki M, Endoh F, Okui K, Sugibayashi K, Morimoto Y. Effects of intra-arterially infused biodegradable microspheres containing mitomycin C. *Cancer* 1985; **55**: 522–6.
17. O'Cornell KJ. Angioinfarction. In: Javadpour N (ed.), *Cancer of the Kidney*. New York: Thieme-Stratton, 1984.
18. Mebust WK, Weigel JW, Less KR, Cox GG, Jewel WR, Krishnan EC. Renal cell carcinoma–angioinfarction. *J Urol* 1984; **131**: 24–7.
19. Kaisary AV, Williams G, Riddle PR. The role of preoperative embolization in renal cell carcinoma. *J Urol* 1984; **131**: 641–5.
20. McIvor J, Kaisary AV, Williams G, Grant RV. Tumor infarction after preoperative embolization of renal carcinoma. *Clin Radiol* 1984; **35**: 59–64.

21. Teasdale C, Kirk D, Jeans WD, Penry JB, Tribe CT, Slace N. Arterial embolization in renal carcinoma. *Br J Urol* 1982; **54**: 616–19.
22. Bailey GA, Bells JA, Kandzar SJ, McClung JE, Horton JA. *In vitro* growth of renal cell carcinoma after preoperative renal infarction. *Urology* 1984; **24**: 456–8.
23. Klimberg I, Hunter P, Hawkins IF, Drylie DM, Wajsman Z. Preoperative angioinfarction of localized renal cell carcinoma using absolute ethanol. *J Urol* 1985; **133**: 21–4.
24. Kato T. Renal cancer. In: Taguchi T, Nakamura M (eds), *Arterial Infusion Chemotherapy*. Tokyo: Gan-to-Kagakuryohosha, 1989.
25. Waneck R, Jantsch HS, Karnel F, Lechner G. Embolization of bone metastases. *Hamostaseologie* 1989; **9**: 37–43.
26. Nagato Y, Nakano Y, Abe M, Takahashi M, Kohno S. Osseous metastases from hepatocellular carcinoma: embolization for pain control. *Cardiovasc Intervent Radiol* 1989; **12**: 159–63.
27. Braedel HU, Zwergel U, Knopp W. Embolization of pelvic metastases from renal cell carcinoma. *Eur Urol* 1984; **10**: 380–4.
28. Lang EK. ^{125}I embolotherapy of renal tumours. In: Loehr E, Leder L-D (eds), *Renal and Adrenal Tumors*. Berlin: Spinger-Verlag, 1987.
29. Courtheoux P, Alachkar F, Casasco A, Adam Y, Derlon JM, Courtheoux F, L'Hirondel JL, Theron J. Chemoembolization of lumbar spine metastases: a preliminary study. *J Neuroradiol* 1985; **12**: 151–62.
30. Christensen K, Dyreborg U, Anderson JF, Nissen HM. The value of transcatheter embolization in the treatment of renal carcinoma. *J Urol* 1985; **133**: 191–3.
31. Ritchie AWS, Chisholm GD. Management of renal carcinoma. *Br J Urol* 1983; **55**: 591–4.
32. Singsaas MW, Chopp RT, Mendez R. Preoperative renal embolization as adjunct to radical nephrectomy. *Urology* 1979; **15**: 1–4.
33. Sparwasser H, Lampante L, Derschum W, Habighorst LV, deLeon F. Nierenarterienverschluss durch Spiralembolisation nach Gianturco. *Akt Urol* 1979; **10**: 155–8.
34. Roscoe MW, McBroom RJ, Louis ES, Grossman H, Perrin R. Preoperative embolization in the treatment of osseous metastases from renal cell carcinoma. *Clin Orthop Relat Res* 1989; **238**: 302–7.
35. Wallace S, Chuang VP, Swanson D, Bracken B, Hersh EM, Ayala A, Johnson D. Embolization of renal carcinoma: experience with 100 patients. *Radiology* 1981; **138**: 563–70.
36. Bakke A, Goethlin JH, Haukaas SA, Kallan T. Augmentation of natural killer cell activity after arterial embolization of renal carcinoma. *Cancer Res* 1982; **42**: 3880–3.
37. Johnson G, Kalland T. Enhancement of mouse natural killer cell activity after dearterialization of experimental renal tumors. *J Urol* 1984; **132**: 1250–3.
38. Wright KC, Soo CS, Wallace S, McDonald MW, Ayala A. Experimental percutaneous renal embolization using BCG-saturated Gelfoam. *Cardiovasc Intervent Radiol* 1982; **5**: 260–3.
39. Carmignani G, Belgrano E, Puppo P, Cornaglia P. T and B lymphocyte levels in renal cancer patients: influence of preoperative transcatheter embolization and radical nephrectomy. *J Urol* 1977; **118**: 941–3.
40. Nakano H, Nihira H, Toge T. Treatment of renal cancer by transcatheter embolization and its effects on lymphocyte proliferative response. *J Urol* 1983; **130**: 24–7.
41. Sato K, Abe R, Moriyama M, Kato T. Immune parameters of peripheral blood in

chemoembolization with microencapsulated anticancer drugs. *Jpn J Cancer Chemother* 1989; **16**: 73–7.

42. Swanson DA, Johnson DE, Essenbach AC, Chuang VP, Wallace S. Angioinfarction plus nephrectomy for metastatic renal cell carcinoma. *J Urol* 1983; **130**: 449–52.

43. Dreikorn K, Terwey B, Drings P, Horsch R, Palmtaf H, Roessler W. Complete regression of multiple pulmonary metastases in a patient with advanced renal cell carcinoma treated by occlusion of the renal artery with subsequent radical nephrectomy and progesterone. *Eur Urol* 1983; **9**: 254–6.

44. Bakke A, Goethlin J, Hoisaeter PA. Renal malignancies: outcome of patients in stage 4 with or without embolization procedure. *Urology* 1985; **26**: 541–3.

45. Gottesman JE, Scardino P, Crawford ED, McCracken JD, Grossman HB. Infarction–nephrectomy for metastatic renal carcinoma. *Urology* 1985; **25**: 248–50.

46. Kurth KH, Clinqualbre J, Oliver RTD, Schulman CC. Embolization and subsequent nephrectomy in metastatic renal cell carcinoma. In: Kurth KH, Debruyne FMJ, Schroeder FH, Spinter TAW, Wagener TDJ (eds), *Progress and Controversies in Oncological Urology*. New York: Alan R Liss, 1984.

47. Abe R, Kato T, Mori H, Sato K, Moriyama M, Tamakawa Y, Unno K, Goto K. Mitomycin C microcapsules in renal cell carcinoma. *J Jpn Soc Cancer Ther* 1985; **20**: 535–41.

48. Klein FQ, Texter JH, Mendez-Picol G. Complications of the Gianturco coil in preoperative infarction of renal cell carcinoma. *J Urol* 1981; **125**: 105–7.

49. Chuang VP, Wallace S, Swanson DA. Technique and complications of renal carcinoma embolization. *Urol Radiol* 1981; **2**: 223–8.

50. Milewski JB, Malewski AS, Malanowska S, Borkowski A, Skowtowdki IA, Tomankowicz Z, Sawkra E. Embolization in patients with renal carcinoma. *Int Urol Nephrol* 1981; **13**: 221–9.

51. Mukamel E, Hader H, Nissen I, Sernadio C. Widespread dissemination of Gelfoam particles complicating the renal circulation. *Urology* 1979; **15**: 194–7.

52. Mulligan BD, Espinosa GA. Bowel infarction: a complication of ethanol ablation of a renal tumor. *Cardiovasc Intervent Radiol* 1983; **6**: 55–7.

53. Marx FJ, Chaussy CH, Moser E. Grenzen und Gefahren der palliativen Embolisation inoperabler Nierentumoren. *Urologe* 1982; **21**: 206–10.

54. Hemingway AP, Allison DJ. Complications of embolization: analysis of 410 procedures. *Radiology* 1988; **166**: 669–72.

18 Endocrine aspects of renal cell carcinoma ——————

Jonathan Waxman

Annually in the UK, 2300 people die from renal cell cancers,[1] and the median survival of patients with metastatic disease is 9 months. The scientific basis for hormonal therapies comes from the empirical observation of the effects of treatment in animals. Renal cell carcinomas in oestrogen-treated or orchiectomized Syrian golden-haired hamsters were shown to regress with testosterone or progestogen therapy, and from this model hormonal therapies developed. Bloom subsequently reported a 30% response rate to progestogens given to patients with metastatic renal cell carcinomas.[2] This initial positive finding was not confirmed in other series. However, responses to endocrine therapies are seen in a minority of patients and their molecular basis is intriguing.

Steroid hormone receptors

In tumours such as breast and prostatic cancer where there is a high order of response to hormonal therapies, receptors for steroid hormones are found and it is these receptors that are thought to mediate response. Renal cell carcinomas also contain steroid hormone receptors. It was initially hypothesized that the receptors were located in the tumour cell cytoplasm. Steroids were thought to enter the cell passively, bind with receptor, and the receptor–steroid complex transported into the cell nucleus, to bind with DNA. This concept is now thought to be incorrect. New histological fixation techniques have shown that the receptor is a membrane-bound glycoprotein. Only small amounts are located in the cytoplasm, and after binding the receptor–steroid complex rapidly translocates to the cell nucleus.

The structure of the steroid hormone receptor has been characterized and the receptor genes cloned, using the techniques of molecular biology. The structure of the oestrogen receptor has been identified and contains a 66 amino acid segment which is the DNA binding domain and a 2551 amino acid component that binds to 17 beta oestradiol. The gene that encodes this receptor has marked homology to the avian erythroblastosis virus genome and is called v-ErbA. Interaction of receptor with DNA leads to modulation of transcription, by recruitment of transcription factors including RNA polymerase. The target genes for steroid receptors contain *cis* elements in 5′ flanking regions. Single base changes within these short *cis* elements abrogate steroid responsiveness. The genes for the steroid hormone receptors are part of a large 'super gene family' of regulatory molecules. These include the receptors for thyroid stimulating hormone, vitamin D_3, retinoic acid, oestrogen, androgen, progesterone and glucocorticoid.[3]

Steroid hormone receptors in renal cell carcinomas

Renal cell carcinomas contain receptors for steroid hormones and these include dihydrotestosterone, 17 beta oestradiol and progesterone. In one series, 11 of 55 renal cancers were oestrogen receptor positive, 4 of 55 were progesterone receptor positive, and 10 of 53 were testosterone receptor positive.[4] Twelve of 62 tumours assayed for steroid hormone binding were found to contain dihydrotestosterone receptors.[5] In another series of 41 renal carcinomas, 30 were androgen receptor positive, 11 were oestrogen receptor positive and 11 were progesterone receptor positive. In these 41 patients, survival directly correlated with receptor positivity and those patients whose tumours expressed more than one receptor survived for longer than those who were receptor negative.[6] In another series, 16 of 19 patients' tumours were testosterone receptor positive, one of 19 was oestrogen receptor positive and 20 were dihydrotestosterone receptor positive. In these patients the level of dihydrotestosterone binding directly correlated with clinical stage and the more advanced tumours had higher levels.[7] There are conflicting data with regard to receptor status in the normal as compared with the tumour-bearing kidney. In one study, progesterone and dihydrotestosterone receptor levels were similar when 20 tumours were compared with 14 autologous kidney biopsies.[7] In a further study, oestrogen and progesterone receptor levels in 19 renal cell tumours were in the same range as levels in eight kidneys from patients with transitional cell carcinoma, renal cyst, or nephrolithiasis.[8]

Parathyroid hormone-related peptide

The mechanisms underlying humoral hypercalcaemia in malignancy have been unravelled and much of this work relates to information garnered from renal cell carcinomas.

A peptide derived from human tumours associated with humoral hypercalcaemia has been sequenced.[9,10] Polyadenylated RNA from a renal carcinoma from a patient with this syndrome was used to construct a cDNA library which was screened with a codon-preference oligonucleotide, synthesized on the basis of a partial N-terminal amino acid sequence from a peptide derived from a human tumour, and a 2.0 kilobase cDNA was identified. The cDNA encoded a 177 amino acid prohormone which contained a 36 amino acid leader sequence which is cleaved to produce a 141 amino acid, mature peptide, parathyroid hormone-related peptide. The first 13 amino acids of the mature peptide have sequence homology with parathyroid hormone, and the N-terminal sequence is thought to be the parathyroid hormone receptor binding region.[11] Parathyroid hormone-related peptide was found to be expressed in most normal human tissue, where its role is undetermined.[12] The gene for parathyroid hormone-related peptide has been mapped to the short arm of chromosome 12, and this is in contrast to the parathyroid hormone gene which has been mapped to the short arm of chromosome 11. The gene for parathyroid hormone-related peptide is complex and contains a six exon, 12 kilobase, single copy sequence, encoding up to five mRNA species. Exons 2, 3 and 4 are similar to the parathyroid hormone gene.[13]

There is some evidence that parathyroid hormone-related peptide might be a growth factor for renal cell carcinomas. This is because the growth of a human renal cell carcinoma cell line which secretes this peptide is inhibited by a polyclonal antiserum raised against parathyroid hormone-related peptide sequences 1–34. There is no growth-promoting effect of added parathyroid hormone-related peptide, but this may not be significant in a saturated system.[14]

Erythropoietin

A small percentage of patients with renal cell carcinomas have polycythaemia at presentation and it is thought that this polycythaemia is secondary to the secretion of erythropoietin by the tumour. The major source of erythropoietin is thought to be renal peritubular cells which are probably capillary endothelial in origin and this has been shown in a mouse hypoxic kidney model. *In situ* hybridization was performed on the tumours from three patients with renal cell carcinomas who had polycythaemia associated with high serum erythropoietin levels. Labelling was associated with tumour cells rather than capillary endothelium. Northern blot analysis after restriction digestion showed no significant erythropoietin gene rearrangement.[15] It is interesting to conjecture why erythropoietin is produced by these tumours, and this may be a normal response to the hypoxia commonly seen in tumours.

Growth factors

The epidermal growth factor is a protein of molecular weight 6000 daltons secreted in large quantities in saliva and throughout the urothelial tract. Its receptor is a four-domain transmembrane protein of molecular weight 175 000 daltons. The binding of epidermal growth factor to its receptor leads to tyrosine kinase activation. There is significant homology between the gene encoding the receptor and the oncogene c-erbB1. Epidermal growth factor receptor content was assayed in 13 renal cell carcinomas and compared with levels in normal surrounding tissue within the nephrectomy specimen. There was a five-fold increase in receptor levels in the tumour as compared with normal surrounding tissue. There was no correlation between receptor levels and tumour grade. An assay was performed of epidermal growth factor levels in tumour as compared with surrounding tissue. Epidermal growth factor receptor levels were five times higher in the 11 tumours studied than in the surrounding normal tissue.[16] This result suggests that epidermal growth factor and its receptor may be involved in an autocrine stimulatory loop in a proportion of renal cell tumours.

In another study, pro-epidermal growth factor, pro-transforming growth factor alpha and epidermal growth factor receptor gene expression were examined in 33 renal cell carcinomas. There was under-expression of the pro-epidermal growth factor gene in 21 tumours analysed and over-expression of the genes for pro-transforming growth factor alpha in 33 tumours and epidermal growth factor receptor in 22 of 23 tumours analysed. Pro-transforming growth factor alpha gene expression correlated with differentiation, being higher in well than in less differentiated tumours.[17] The relevance of these findings is unknown.

Hormonal treatment

A number of different hormonal therapies have been applied to the management of patients with metastatic renal cell cancer. Their attractiveness as a therapy for malignant disease lies in their comparative lack of toxicity as compared with cytotoxic chemotherapy or biological agents.

Progestogens

Medroxyprogesterone acetate was the first progestogen used to treat patients[2] and has been applied in different dosages and schedules to large numbers of patients. At a dosage of 500 mg given intramuscularly daily for six weeks and thereafter twice-weekly, three of 20 patients were seen to have responded. In this study, tumour ploidy was assessed and it was found that those patients who responded had diploid tumours.[18] In a group of 18 patients with advanced disease, medroxyprogesterone acetate was given at a dosage of 800 mg intramuscularly weekly and no responses were reported.[19] Twenty-one patients were treated with 500–1000 mg daily intramuscularly and one partial response was seen.[20] Megestrol acetate was used to treat 85 patients with metastatic renal cell carcinoma at a dosage of 40 mg thrice-daily and four responded.[21] These studies have considered the activity of the progestogens in terms of tumour responsiveness. However, there are additional effects that are important and which are welcomed by patients. These relate to the anabolic qualities of this group of compounds which lead to increased weight and appetite.

Flutamide and tamoxifen

Flutamide is a pure antiandrogen without central effects which competitively binds to the androgen receptor. Twenty-eight patients were treated at a dosage of 250 mg of flutamide thrice-daily orally; 25 patients were assessable and one had a partial response.[5]

Tamoxifen has been used because of the finding of oestrogen receptors within renal cell carcinomas. At a dose of 20 mg twice-daily, responses were reported in 8 of 70 patients.[22]

Conclusion

Conventional hormonal therapies are a relatively ineffective treatment for renal cell carcinomas. The techniques of molecular biology have shown us the extent of the involvement of oncogenes and growth factors in the development of this type of tumour. It is hoped that the next decade will bring new treatments for this condition that are based on the development of peptide antagonists of these growth factors.

References

1. Cancer Statistics: Cause 1987. DH2 no. 14, 1989. HMSO.
2. Bloom HJ. Medroxyprogesterone acetate (Provera) in the treatment of metastatic renal cell cancer. *Br J Cancer* 1971; **25**: 250–65.
3. O'Malley B. The steroid receptor superfamily: more excitement predicted for the future. *Mol Endocrin* 1990; **4** (3): 363–9.
4. Pizzocaro G, Piva L, Salvioni R, Di Fronzo G, Ronchi E, Miodini P, and the Lombardy Group. Adjuvant medroxyprogesterone acetate and steroid hormone receptors in category Mo renal cell carcinoma: an interim report of a prospective randomized study. *J Urol* 1986; **135**: 18–21.
5. Ahmed T, Benedetto P, Yagoda A, *et al.* Estrogen, progesterone, and androgen-binding sites in renal cell carcinoma. *Cancer* 1984; **54**: 477–81.
6. Nakano E, Tada Y, Fujioka H, *et al.* Hormone receptor in renal cell carcinoma and correlation with clinical response to endocrine therapy. *J Urol* 1984; **132**: 240–5.
7. Mukamel E, Bruhis S, Nissenkorn I, Servadio C. Steroid receptors in renal cell carcinoma: relevance to hormonal therapy. *J Urol* 1984; **131**: 227–30.
8. Noronha RFX, Rao BR. Increased dihydrotestosterone receptor levels in high-stage renal adenocarcinoma. *Cancer* 1985; **56**: 134–7.
9. Burtis WJ, Wu T, Bunch C, Wysolmerski JJ, *et al.* Identification of a novel 17,000-dalton parathyroid hormone-like adenylate cyclase-stimulating protein from a tumor associated with humoral hypercalcemia of malignancy. *J Biol Chem* 1987; **262**: 7151–6.
10. Moseley JM, Kubota M, Diefenbach-Jagger H, *et al.* Parathyroid hormone-related protein purified from a human lung cancer cell line. *Proc Natl Acad Sci USA* 1987; **84**: 5048–52.
11. Habener JF, Rosenblatt M, Potts JT. Parathyroid hormone: biochemical aspects of biosynthesis, secretion, action and metabolism. *Physiol Rev* 1984; **64**: 985–1053.
12. Mangin M, Webb AC, Dreyer BE, *et al.* Identification of a cDNA encoding a parathyroid hormone-like peptide from a human tumor associated with humoral hypercalcemia of malignancy. *Proc Natl Acad Sci USA* 1988; **85**: 597–601.
13. Mangin M, Ikeda K, Dreyer BE, Broadus AE. Isolation and characterization of the human parathyroid hormone-like peptide gene. *Proc Natl Acad Sci USA* 1989; **86**: 2408–12.

14. Burton PBJ, Moniz C, Knight DE. Parathyroid hormone-related peptide can function as an autocrine growth factor in human renal cell carcinoma. *Biochem Biophys Res Commun* 1990; **167** (3): 1134–8.
15. Da Silva JL, Lacombe C, Bruneval P, *et al*. Tumor cells are the site of erythropoietin synthesis in human renal cancers associated with polycythemia. *Blood* 1990; **75** (3): 577–82.
16. Ambs KE, Takahashi A, Hering F, Costa S, Huber PR. Epidermal growth factor receptor in adenocarcinoma of the kidney. *Urol Res* 1989; **17**: 251–4.
17. Petrides PE, Bock S, Bovens J, Hofmann R, Jakes G. Modulation of pro-epidermal growth factor, pro-transforming growth factor beta and epidermal growth factor receptor gene expression in human renal carcinomas. *Cancer Res* 1990; **50**: 3934–9.
18. Ljungberg B, Tomic R, Roos G. Deoxyribonucleic acid content and medroxy-progesterone acetate treatment in metastatic renal cell carcinoma. *J Urol* 1989; **141**: 1308–10.
19. Gottesman JE, Crawford ED, Grossman HB, Scardino P, McCracken JD. Infarction-nephrectomy for metastatic renal carcinoma. *Urology* 1985; **25**: 248–50.
20. Kjaer M, Frederikson PL. High-dose medroxyprogesterone acetate in patients with renal adenocarcinoma and measurable lung metastases: a phase-II study. *Cancer Treat Rep* 1986; **70** (3): 431–2.
21. Hahn RG, Bauer M, Wolter J, *et al*. Phase-II study of single agent therapy with megestrol acetate, VP-16-213, cyclophosphamide and dianhydrogalactitol in advanced renal cell cancer. *Cancer Treat Rep* 1979; **63**: 513–5.
22. Al-Sarraf M, Eyre H, Bonnet J, *et al*. Study of tamoxifen in renal cell carcinoma and the influence of certain prognostic factors: a Southwest Oncology Group Study. *Cancer Treat Rep* 1981; **65**: 447–51.

19 Spontaneous regression and responses in renal cell carcinoma _____

Patrick F Keane and Gordon Williams

Spontaneous regression occurs when documented metastatic lesions resolve and no specific therapy has been used to treat them. The first documented case of regression of metastases in humans was recorded by Bumpus[1] in a patient with renal cell carcinoma. In 1966 Everson and Cole[2] documented 176 instances of regression of metastases and 31 (18%) were in patients with metastatic renal carcinoma; this is by far the highest incidence of this phenomenon in humans.

Renal carcinoma is one of the most capricious of human malignancies, both in terms of its presentation and subsequent biological behaviour. The clinical course of this tumour is often unpredictable. Patients with proven metastatic disease at the time of the initial diagnosis may survive for years,[3,4] while patients who have undergone curative radical surgery may survive only to die of metastatic disease 30 years later.[5] Spontaneous regression of metastases in patients with renal carcinoma is well documented and the phenomenon occurs most commonly in those patients with lung secondaries.[3] Spontaneous regression of metastatic renal carcinoma has excited much interest and caused much ink to be spilt in documenting what is a rare occurrence. As always with renal cancer, spontaneous regression is completely unpredictable and the mechanism by which it occurs continues to defy scientific explanation and has been attributed on occasion to divine intervention.[6]

Incidence

Bloom[7] noted two cases of spontaneous regression in 200 cases of renal carcinoma, but on reviewing the literature he estimated that the true incidence was closer to 0.3%. The vast majority of cases of regression occur in patients who have lung metastases alone, which are rarely histologically confirmed. Freed[3] reported 51 cases, 19 of whom had histological confirmation of the secondary lesion.

Thus although there is no doubt that regression of proven metastatic disease occurs, it is probable that the high incidence of regression based on radiological evidence alone may be due to resolution of concomitant inflammatory or infective conditions of the lungs. The majority of cases of regression occur in patients who have had the primary tumour excised, and there are only seven cases reported in the literature in which there has been regression without nephrectomy.[8]

Fairlamb[9] updated Freed's series to a total of 67 cases. The incidence of spontaneous regression was higher in males, with a male to female ratio of 3:1, which is higher than the sex ratio of 1.5–2.0:1 quoted for renal carcinoma. In 60 of the 67 cases (89%) reported, regression was documented in patients with lung metastases. There were four cases of regression of soft tissue metastases, and the remaining three cases occurred in patients with bone secondaries. Fifteen of the 67 patients (22%) were alive at five years, but just under 50% of these patients died of recurrent disease within 15 years.

A solitary case of regression of a brain secondary has been reported,[10] though this patient had been treated with dexamethasone and there was no histological confirmation of the diagnosis. There continue to be sporadic reports of spontaneous regression in the English literature,[11] but no single centre will ever be able to accumulate enough cases to allow a systematic study.

Natural history of advanced renal carcinoma

The natural history of advanced renal carcinoma is important to understand in relation to the results of various treatments.

Holland[12] reported that the crude survival for patients with metastatic renal carcinoma was 4.4% at three years and 1.7% at five years, although in Best's series[13] no patient with stage IV carcinoma was alive after two years. Several adverse prognostic features have been identified,[14] and are listed in Table 19.1. Because of prolonged survival when spontaneous regression is considered, it is essential in interpreting survival figures for the various forms of treatment to have some form of stratification of the patients documented.

As already noted the incidence of spontaneous regression is of the order of 0.3% of cases. Some patients, however, have partial responses or have stable disease for prolonged periods. The precise incidence of spontaneous *response* rates has important implications for assessing treatments used in advanced renal carcinoma.

Table 19.1   Adverse prognostic factors in advanced renal carcinoma

High-grade tumours
Multiple lesions
Liver involvement
Lymphatic involvement
Poor performance status
Malaise
   Weight loss >10%
   Anorexia
   Lethargy

Oliver[4] documented 73 patients with advanced renal carcinoma who underwent a period of surveillance before entering any treatment protocol. Seventy-five per cent of patients had evidence of progression within three months of diagnosis but 10% were progression-free for one year. Within this group three patients had a complete response, two had a partial response and four had stable disease for a period of greater than one year. Oliver estimates that the *spontaneous response rate* for patients with stage IV renal carcinoma is of the order of 7%. It follows that any treatment for such patients must have a response rate significantly better than 7% to be considered useful.

Treatment results in the context of spontaneous regression

Immunotherapy

One popular explanation for spontaneous regression is that it represents a host immune response to the tumour, and this has led clinicians to use immunotherapy, both specific and non-specific, to treat the disease.[15-17]

Almost all patients entered into trials of immunotherapy have excision of the primary tumour as part of their treatment. This may bias results of treatment in that patients entered into immunotherapy protocols are fit for nephrectomy, compared with those patients who may be entered into trials of chemotherapy or hormonal therapy.

Intravenous interferon and infusions of lymphokine activated killer (LAK) cells with interleukin-2 are the most common forms of immunotherapy in use today. The results of clinical trials with biological response modifiers are shown in Table 19.2.

Table 19.2   Regression

Authors	Agent	No.	CR	PR
McCune (1981)[18]	Irradiated tumour cells	14		4
Sahasrahbudhe (1986)[19]	Irradiated tumour cells +cyclophosphamide	20	1	4
Tallberg (1986)[20]	Autologous tumour	127	6	*
Fowler (1986)[21]	Autologous tumour	16	0	0
Morales (1976)[22]	BCG	8	0	5
Ritchie and deKernion (1989)[15]	TNF	10	0	0
Ritchie and deKernion (1989)[15]	Interferons	338	5	34
Schornagel (1988)[23]	Interferon alpha-2A + vinblastine	66	0	4
Ramming (1977)[24]	Immune RNA	20	0	5
Rosenberg (1987)[25]	LAK cells + IL2	36	4	8
Rosenberg (1987)[25]	IL2	21	1	0
Fisher (1988)[26]	LAK cells + IL2	35	2	3

*Five-year survival 24% versus 3.7% in control group.

Responses (CR, PR) with interferon therapy range from 11% to 23%. LAK cells with interleukin-2 therapy has the greatest response rate (33%) of any of the treatment modalities presently available, but the toxicity of the treatment is formidable and intensive care facilities are required to monitor the patient during therapy. This form of treatment has been restricted to specialist centres and seems unlikely to gain widespread acceptance until it becomes available in a less toxic form.

The discovery of tumour infiltrating lymphocytes and their possible isolation and subsequent amplification with lymphokines appears to be the most promising avenue for immunotherapy in the future.[27]

Critical assessment of the results indicates that the responses seen may not reflect a specific antitumour effect but may simply be due to the patients' good general condition. Similarly for interferon therapy, the responses seen are significantly better in patients who have less advanced disease and good performance status.[28] Thus response to treatment may not reflect a specific antitumour effect but rather is simply a predictor of survival. Although response rates to these therapies are encouraging, because of patient selection, it could be argued that treatment may not offer any significant survival advantage as compared with conservative management.

Angio-infarction

Angio-infarction of the primary tumour was used in the hope that infarction of the tumour would not only reduce the blood supply to the tumour but also release a large amount of antigenic material and thus stimulate the hosts' immune response.

Initially it was suggested, based on data from the MD Anderson Hospital, that angio-infarction improved survival in patients with locally invasive or metastatic lung disease. Swanson *et al.*[29] reported on 100 patients from the MD Anderson Hospital treated by angio-infarction with delayed nephrectomy. The majority of the patients in this study also received medroxyprogesterone acetate which complicates the interpretation of results. The overall response rate was 15% (7 complete and 8 partial responses) and if patients who had stabilization of their disease were included as responders the 'response' rate was increased to 28%. However, there was no improvement in these patients' survival following treatment by angio-infarction when compared with an historical control group treated by nephrectomy at the same institution.

Other centres adopted the technique, and Gottesman *et al.*[30] reported only one partial response in 30 patients treated by angio-infarction, suggesting that the treatment was no better than observation alone. Bakke *et al.*[31] found no difference in survival in a group of 44 patients who underwent nephrectomy ($n = 8$), embolization ($n = 18$) or no treatment ($n = 18$). Angio-infarction does not improve survival in patients with secondary disease and does not give reproducible partial responses either.[32]

Surgery

Radical nephrectomy is the treatment of choice for renal cell carcinoma, but the role of surgery in patients with metastatic disease is a matter of some debate. Radical surgery does not induce spontaneous regression of metastatic disease,[32] and therefore the vain hope of inducing spontaneous regression of metastatic deposits is not an indication for surgery. Furthermore the mortality and morbidity of nephrectomy in stage IV disease is considerable and is of the order of 10%.[33] There can be no justification for routine nephrectomy in metastatic renal cell carcinoma. Indications for nephrectomy include symptomatic local disease, troublesome para-neoplastic syndromes or in patients included in experimental treatment protocols. Obviously clinical judgement plays a major role in the selection of patients for surgery.

Patients who have a solitary metastatic lesion at the time of diagnosis represent a specific group of patients and should be considered for surgery with excision of the primary and secondary lesion. Tolia and Whitmore[34] reported that 1–3% of cases of renal cell carcinoma have solitary metastases and survival rates of the order of 30–50% can be achieved. A more recent report[35] of 29 patients with solitary metastases showed that 22 died of metastatic disease with an average disease-free interval of 22 months. Four patients are disease-free and three have died of other causes. From these results it seems that micrometastases are often present at the time of diagnosis of the solitary lesion. Therefore, it would be prudent to observe the patient for some months before proceeding to thoracotomy for an apparently solitary lesion.

References

1. Bumpus HC. The apparent disappearance of pulmonary metastasis in a case of hypernephroma following nephrectomy. *J Urol* 1928; **20**: 185–9.
2. Everson TC, Cole WH. *Spontaneous Regression of Cancer.* Philadelphia: WB Saunders, 1961: 11–87.
3. Freed SZ, Halperin JP, Gordon M. Idiopathic regression of metastases from renal cell carcinoma. *J Urol* 1977; **118**: 538–42.
4. Oliver RTD. Medical management of renal cell carcinoma. In: Oliver RTD (ed.), *Urological and Genital Cancer.* London: Blackwell, 1989: 180–91.
5. Kradjian RM, Bennington JL. Renal carcinoma recurrent 31 years after nephrectomy. *Arch Surg* 1967; **90**: 192–5.
6. Kirk D. Spontaneous regression of metastatic renal carcinoma. *Br J Surg* 1987; **74**: 1–2.
7. Bloom HG. Hormone induced and spontaneous regression of metastatic renal cancer. *Cancer* 1973; **32**: 1066–77.
8. Chapple CR, Gannon MX, Shah VM, Newman J. Spontaneous regression of pulmonary metastases from renal adenocarcinoma before nephrectomy. *Br J Surg* 1987; **74**: 69–70.
9. Fairlamb DJ. Spontaneous regression of metastases of renal carcinoma. *Cancer* 1981; **47**: 2102–6.

10.   Omland H, Fossa Sophie D. Spontaneous regression of cerebral and pulmonary metastases in renal cell carcinoma. *Scand J Urol Neprol* 1989; **23**: 159–60.
11.   Thomas J, Stott M, Royle GT. Spontaneous regression of subcutaneous and pulmonary metastases from renal carcinoma. *Br J Urol* 1989; **63**: 102–3.
12.   Holland JM. Cancer of the kidney: natural history and staging. *Cancer* 1973; **32**: 1030–42.
13.   Best BG. Renal carcinoma: a ten year review 1971–80. *Br J Urol* 1987; **60**: 100–2.
14.   Neves RJ, Zincke H, Taylor WF. Metastatic renal cell carcinoma and radical nephrectomy: identification of prognostic factors and patient survival. *J Urol* 1988; **139**: 1173–6.
15.   Ritchie AWS, deKernion JB. Immunobiology of renal carcinoma. In: Chisholm GD, Fair WR (eds), *Scientific Foundations of Urology*. Oxford: Heinemann, 1990: 540–8.
16.   deKernion JB. Treatment of advanced renal cell carcinoma: traditional methods and innovative approaches. *J Urol* 1983; **130**: 2–7.
17.   Droller MJ. Immunotherapy in genitourinary neoplasia. *J Urol* 1985; **133**: 1–5.
18.   McCune CS, Schapira DV, Henshaw EC. Specific immunotherapy for advanced renal carcinoma: evidence for the polyclonality of metastases. *Cancer* 1981; **47**: 1984–8.
19.   Sahasrahbudhe DM, deKernion JB, Pontes E, *et al.* Specific immunotherapy with suppressor function inhibition for metastatic renal cell carcinoma. *J Biol Response Mod* 1986; **5**: 581–4.
20.   Tallberg R, Tykka H. Specific active immunotherapy in advanced renal cell carcinoma: a clinical longterm follow-up. *W J Urol* 1986; **3**: 234–44.
21.   Fowler JE. Nephrectomy in metastatic renal cell carcinoma. *Urol Clin N Am* 1987; **14**: 749–56.
22.   Morales A, Eidenger D. Bacille Calmette Guerin in the treatment of adenocarcinoma of the kidney. *J Urol* 1976; **115**: 377–80.
23.   Schornagel JH, Verwieii J, Wim W, *et al.* Phase II study of recombinant interferon alpha-2a and vinblastine in advanced renal cell carcinoma. *J Urol* 1987; **138**: 1379–81.
24.   Ramming KP, deKernion JB. Immune RNA therapy for renal cell carcinoma: survival and immunological monitoring. *Ann Surg* 1977; **186**: 459–67.
25.   Rosenberg SA, Lotze MT, Muul LM, *et al.* A progress report on treatment of 157 patients with advanced cancer using lymphokine activated killer cells and interleukin-2 or high-dose interleukin-2 alone. *N Engl J Med* 1987; **316**: 889–97.
26.   Fisher RI, Coltman CA, Doroshaw JH. Metastatic renal carcinoma treatment with interleukin-2 and LAK cells: a phase II clinical trial. *Ann Int Med* 1988; **108**: 518–23.
27.   Holmes EC. Immunology of tumour infiltrating lymphocytes. *Ann Surg* 1985; **201**: 158.
28.   Sarna G, Figlin R, deKernion JB. Interferon in renal cell carcinoma: the UCLA experience. *Cancer* 1987; **59**: 610–13.
29.   Swanson D, Johnson DE, Von Eschenbach AC, *et al.* Angioinfarction plus nephrectomy for metastatic renal cell carcinoma: an update. *J Urol* 1983; **130**: 449–52.
30.   Gottesman JE, Crawford ED, Grossman HB, Scardino P, McCracken JD. Infarction nephrectomy for metastatic renal carcinoma. *Urology* 1985; **25**: 248–50.
31.   Bakke A, Goethlin J, Holsaeter PA. Renal malignancies: outcome of patients in stage 4 with or without embolisation procedure. *Urology* 1988; **32**: 254–8.
32.   Flanigen RC. The failure of infarction and/or nephrectomy in stage IV renal cell cancer to influence survival or metastatic regression. *Urol Clin N Am* 1987; **14**: 757–62.

33. Fowler JE. Failure of immunotherapy for metastatic renal cell carcinoma. *J Urol* 1986; **135**: 22–5.

34. Tolia BM, Whitmore WF. Solitary metastasis from renal cell carcinoma. *J Urol* 1975; **114**: 836–8.

35. Dineen MK, Pastone RD, Emrich LJ, Huben RP. Results of surgical treatment of renal cell carcinoma with solitary metastases. *J Urol* 1988; **140**: 277–9.

Index